Fundamentals of Electrocardiography

Roger W. Jelliffe

Fundamentals of Electrocardiography

With 191 Illustrations

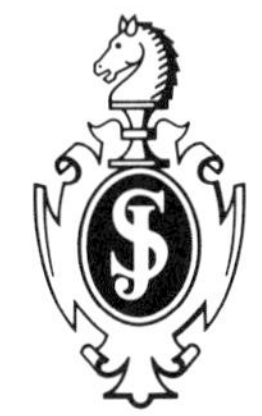

Springer-Verlag
New York Berlin Heidelberg
London Paris Tokyo Hong Kong

Roger W. Jelliffe
Laboratory of Applied Pharmacokinetics
University of Southern California
School of Medicine
Los Angeles, California
USA

Printed on acid-free paper.

© 1990 Springer-Verlag New York, Inc.

Text prepared by author in camera-ready form.

Printed and bound by Edwards Brothers, Inc., Ann Arbor, Michigan, USA.
Printed in the United States of America.

9 8 7 6 5 4 3 2 1

ISBN 0-387-97185-8 Springer-Verlag New York Berlin Heidelberg
ISBN 3-540-97185-8 Springer-Verlag Berlin Heidelberg New York

To my Joyce, Love to Love,
To Ron Selvester and Jack Zinn,
Dick Eckstein and Nick Sperelakis,
and to Bob Richard

Acknowledgements

The full page vectorcardiograph figures are reproduced through the kind permission of Ronald Selvester, M.D., Rancho Los Amigos Hospital, Downey, California. The continuous, 12-lead EKG figures are reproduced through the kind permission of Robert Richard, M.D., Ph.D. Figure 2 and 142 are reproduced from *Electrophysiology of the Heart*, by B.F. Hoffman and P.F. Cranefield, McGraw-Hill Book Company, Inc., New York, 1960, with permission. Figures 186, 187, and 191 are reproduced from *Clinical Electrocardiography* by Robert Grant, copyright 1957, Blakiston Division, McGraw-Hill Book Company, with permission.

The thoughtful and patient secretarial and administrative assistance of Mrs. Georgene Denison, without whom our laboratory would not have run for so many years, and in whose absence this book would not have been completed, the steadfast help of Dr. Julian Rodriguez Larrea, and the more recent assistance of Mrs. Shirley Davenport, are most gratefully acknowledged.

Contents

Chapter Six: The Ectopic Arrhythmias

Chapter Seven: Conduction Disturbances

Chapter Eight: Pulmonary Disease and Pediatric Tracings

Chapter Nine: Drugs, Electrolytes, Pacemakers, and Technical Errors

Normal Things

<u>AN INITIAL VIEW OF THE EKG</u>

The abbreviation "EKG" comes from the German word "elektrokardiogramm", the name given to this record by Dr. Willem Einthoven, the Dutch physician who invented the string galvanometer and this type of electrical record of the heartbeat. It consists of P, Q, R, S, T, and U waves. The <u>P</u> wave is associated with depolarization of the atria, after which they contract. The normal P wave duration is up to 0.12 seconds.

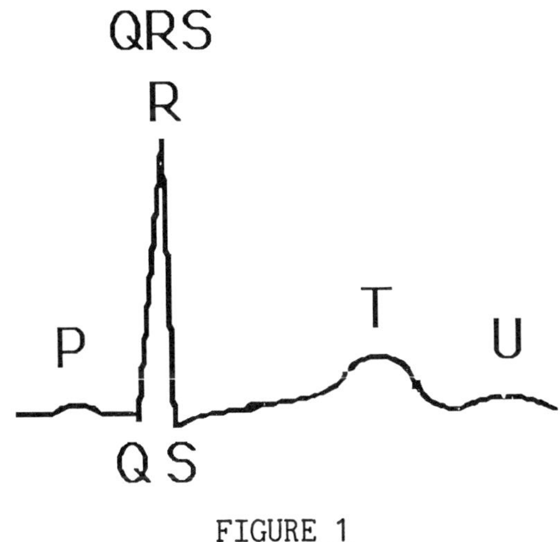

<u>FIGURE 1</u>

The <u>QRS</u> complex reflects the excitation of the ventricles. The Purkinje and ventricular myocardial cells begin their action potentials (phases 0 and 1). The usual QRS duration is up to about 0.10 seconds.

The QRS complex begins from 0.12 to 0.20 seconds after the beginning of the P wave. This interval is known as the normal "P-R" interval. It is somewhat shorter at rapid heart rates and somewhat longer at slow rates.

The QRS complex is followed by the <u>J point</u>, the junctional point between the QRS complex and the <u>ST segment</u>. The ST segment is associated with the plateau (phase 2) of the action potential. The ST segment gradually bends to form the <u>T wave</u>, as shown.

The T wave is associated with the "repolarization" phase of the cells as they pass through phase 3 of their action potentials to regain almost their original resting potential once again. The usual QT duration depends on the heart rate, but is usually not over 0.36 to 0.40 seconds. Finally, the U wave (a normal finding, but often hard to see) may be seen. The U wave is accentuated with hypokalemia and other electrolyte abnormalities, as we will see later.

DEFINITION OF Q, R, S, T, and U WAVES

The following definitions may seem arbitrary. They are. But they are the vocabulary that has developed so that people can describe EKG findings to one another without ambiguity.

A Q wave occurs when the first deflection in the QRS complex is downward in any particular lead. It must occur at the very beginning of the QRS complex, before an R wave (see below). If a downward deflection occurs after a R wave, then it is not a Q wave but an S wave (see below).

An R wave is the first upward deflection of the QRS complex in any particular lead.

An S wave is the first downward deflection after an R wave in any lead.

An R' is the first upward deflection after an S wave.

An S' is the first downward deflection after an R' wave, etc.

The J point is that point where the QRS stops and the ST segment begins, where the spike of the action potential (phases 0 and 1) ends and its plateau (phase 2) begins.

The ST segment is the plateau between the J point and the beginning of the T wave.

The <u>T wave</u> is the slow wave of ventricular "repolarization", when the myocardial cells are in their phase 3, and are regaining their resting potentials once again.

The <u>U wave</u> is a small undulation following a T wave. It is occasionally accentuated in hypokalemia. It is often seen in normal EKG's, and is a normal finding. It may possibly be due to Purkinje fiber "repolarization" (their action potentials last that long!). It is often difficult to tell when a T wave ends and a U wave begins.

<u>CALCULATING THE HEART RATE AND THE OTHER EKG EVENTS</u>

Each small 1 mm. box on the EKG (at the standard recording speed of 25mm/sec) is .04 seconds. Five of them make up 1 large box, which thus represents .20 sec. If an event occurs every large box or every .20 sec, it is occurring 5 times a second, or 300 times per minute.

Let us keep this number of 300, and divide it by the number of large boxes between events. If an event occurs every 2 large boxes, its rate is 300/2, or 150/min. Every 3 large boxes gives a rate of 300/3, or 100/min, and so on, as shown in the table below. Using this table, it is easy to calculate both atrial rates, using the P-P intervals, and ventricular rates, using the R-R intervals.

Number of Large Boxes between Events	Rate (events/minute)
1	300
2	150
3	100
4	75
5	60
6	50
7	43
8	38
9	33
10	30

Careful appraisal of an EKG is just as important as a careful history and physical examination. Look at it.

1. What is the rhythm? What are the atrial and ventricular rates? Are the P waves, QRS complexes, and T waves normal or not?

2. Is there any evidence of improper lead placement?

3. Plot the P, QRS and T axes or vectors in both frontal and horizontal planes, and examine their relationships to each other.

4. Approach the specific abnormalities. Look for hypertrophy, strain, ischemia, conduction abnormalities, electrolyte problems, and infarcts, for example.

5. Write a sentence or two describing the EKG. This is better than a mere listing of the abnormalities that may or may not be present. For example:

This record is within normal limits.

This record is probably within normal limits.

This is a borderline record showing (describe what you see). The presence of (describe what problems come to mind) cannot be excluded.

This is an abnormal record showing (describe features) consistent with (list problems).

Again, when you read an EKG, think of the patient. Is something present which the ward staff should know about now by phone? Sometimes patients on surgical and other services may have unrecognized recent infarcts, for instance. You also may want to end with a suggestion to repeat the EKG, or to repeat it "if clinically indicated". Serial records may be in order to

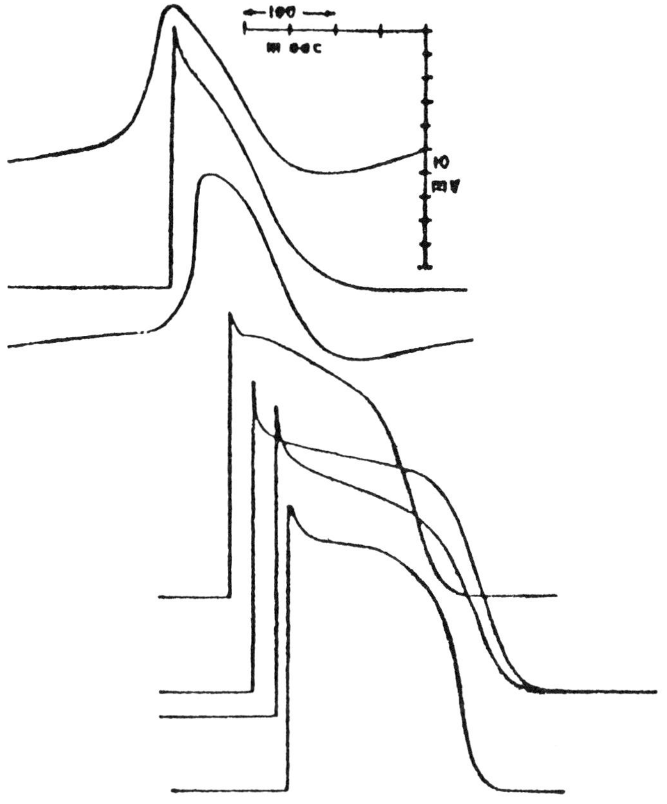

observe the evolutionary changes of an infarct to document it as being of recent origin, or to examine and document <u>any possible recently changing</u> myocardial process.

ELECTRICAL ACTIVITY OF MYOCARDIAL CELLS

The myocardium is not a syncytium, as we used to think. However, many of our customary clinical EKG words and ideas still have reference to those days. They need to be updated. The heart is actually a collection of many individual cells, each electrically isolated from each other except at the intercalated discs. It is likely that some chemical mediator in the inter-calated disc may be responsible for impulse transmission from one myocardial cell to another, in a manner analogous to the role played by acetylcholine in nerve impulse transmission from the motor end plate to striated muscle.

Electrical activity (action potentials) in single myocardial cells can be measured by inserting a microelectrode into them, just as one can insert an electrode into nerve fibers to measure their action potentials. Myocardial action potentials appear different from those of nerve. They are not just a spike, but last longer. Cells of each region of the heart have their own characteristic types of action potential, as shown in Figure 2.

The normal impulse originates in the SA node because it has the most rapid rate of spontaneous firing (about 70/minute). If this activity ceases, the impulse usually originates from the AV node (AV junction), because when left to itself it usually fires spontaneously at about 50-60/minute. If this activity should also cease, the impulse usually then arises from the specia-lized Purkinje fibers of the Bundle of His or its branches. When left to themselves, they usually fire spontaneously at about 30-45/minute.

The cell with the most rapid spontaneous rate of discharge becomes the "pacemaker" for the heart. Generally, the rate of spontaneous discharge of any cell with potential pacemaker capability is governed by the rate of its slow depolarization during diastole (phase 4) from its resting potential to a lesser potential (threshold), at which time the rapid ion movements occur which initiate the spike discharge. This spike is then conducted to the other conducting and myocardial cells. Ischemia, anoxia, drugs, and disease states may impair the cell's ability to make an adequate spike, and thus to initiate and sustain a successfully propagated impulse.

Cells of the atrial conducting system may show spontaneous diastolic (phase 4) depolarization and consequent spontaneous firing (pacemaker activity) under certain conditions (anoxia, ischemia, dilation, sympathomimetic amines, digitalis toxicity, etc.). Most atrial extrasystoles, ectopic atrial rhythms, and atrial tachycardias arise from spontaneous pacemaker activity of the cells of the atrial conducting system. In contrast, the atrial myocardial cells are usually passive, have no depolarization during phase 4, and must be triggered to fire by the activity of some pacemaker cell.

Similarly, cells of the ventricular myocardium are also passive, and must be triggered to fire. Many investigators have tried, basically without success, to initiate spontaneous diastolic depolarization and spontaneous firing in ventricular myocardial cells. Purkinje fibers, though, _are_ capable of such pacemaker activity, and are in fact the source of so-called ventricular extrasystoles and of ventricular arrhythmias.

Usually then, atrial extrasystoles and arrhythmias arise from potential pacemaker cells in the atrial conducting system, _not_ from atrial myocardial cells, just as ventricular extrasystoles and arrhythmias arise from potential pacemaker cells of the His-Purkinje conducting system, _not_ from the ventricular myocardial cells.

HOW SINGLE CELL EVENTS GENERATE THE EKG

Atrial Activity

In general, it is likely that the wave of depolarization may spread from inside the atrium toward the outside, as well as longitudinally over the surface of the atria. Let us now examine the electrical behavior of such a typical slice of atrium, if it were cut away, mounted in a bath, and stimulated at the endocardial end so that the wave of depolarization travelled in a straight line to the other (epicardial) end. This eliminates considerations of axes and vectors at this time.

Consider a strip of atrial muscle as shown in Figure 3. The left (endocardial) end of this strip is stimulated. The wave front travels essentially like a single wave front moving toward the right. When the wave front reaches cell A, that cell is stimulated and gives rise to its individual action potential, as shown by the thicker trace on the upper channel of the scope. Later, when the wave front reaches and stimulates cell B, that cell then similarly gives rise to its action potential, as shown by the thinner trace on the upper channel of the scope.

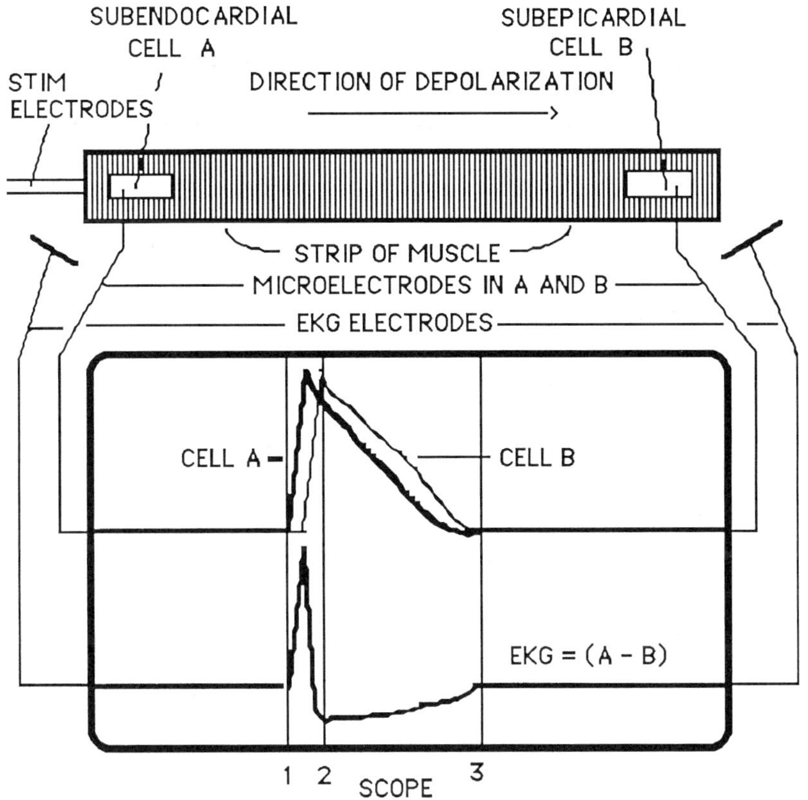

FIGURE 3

However, if external electrodes (an EKG lead, which is, after all, only a type of voltmeter) are used to record the electrical activity of this strip, they will record essentially only the <u>voltage differences</u> occurring between the two leads, (analogous to cell A minus cell B, for example). Let us set this up so that the recording pen writes upward when the voltage difference (Cell A minus Cell B) is positive and Cell A is more positive (less negative) than Cell B, and downward when the difference (Cell A minus Cell B) is negative, and Cell A is then more negative than Cell B.

Thus, when cell A is fired and loses its negativity, an upward deflection will first be seen, as shown on the lower trace on the oscilloscope, just after time line #1. As cell A begins to recover (with no significant plateau phase to its action potential as it is an atrial, not a ventricular, cell) cell B is fired, and there is an instant when the 2 leads are at the same potential and the difference between them is zero. Then cell B reaches the peak of its spike at time line #2, and from then on a slight negative difference exists on the EKG trace, as cell A goes through its phase 3 (repolarizes) slightly ahead of cell B. This difference gradually becomes zero when both cells have fully completed phase 3.

What has been recorded on the EKG trace here is essentially a unidirectional P wave. It comes up at time line #1, then down at time line #2, with no ST segment because the atrial cells have no significant plateau phase to their individual action potentials. A slight negative "T" wave is then inscribed. Clinically, this "atrial T wave" is usually blotted out by the QRS complex and T wave which occur at about this time. However, in atrial tachycardias, the atrial T wave is often seen when the atrial rate is rapid, and in atrial flutter this may become so pronounced as to give an actual sawtooth appearance to the atrial complexes.

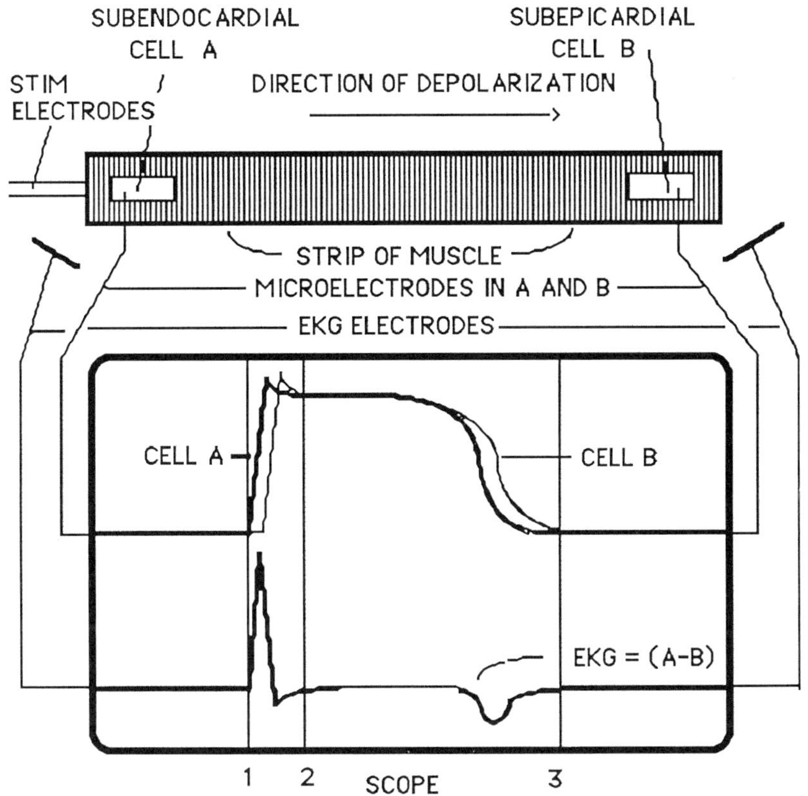

FIGURE 4

Consider now a strip of ventricle mounted and connected in a similar fashion, as shown in Figure 4. As with the atria, a preparation of this type eliminates considerations of axes and vectors for the present, to simplify things. Later on we will consider them again.

The wave of depolarization is rapidly delivered to the endocardial surface of the ventricles by the Purkinje cells, travelling at a speed of 3-4 meters/sec. The wave front then proceeds to the epicardial surface through the myocardium, travelling at a speed of about 1 meter/sec. More on this later. Basically though, the strip in Figure 4 is once again stimulated on the left, at its endocardial end, and the wave front travels to the right, firing first the "typical" subendocardial cell A and then the "typical" subepicardial cell B, as shown on the scope.

Ventricular cells differ from atrial cells in that their action potentials have a very pronounced plateau phase, as shown, probably due to the calcium ion movement and current.

When an EKG lead (analogous to cell A minus cell B) is connected and cell A is fired, a potential difference is created between the two EKG electrodes and an upward deflection is seen on the lower "EKG channel" of the figure (Cell A minus Cell B), as cell A fires its spike on the upper (single fiber) channel of the scope. When the wave front reaches and fires cell B, cell A is now on its plateau. After this, both cells are on their plateaus (time line #2), and no potential difference exists between the two EKG electrodes. The EKG trace thus becomes isoelectric. This isoelectric phase, the ST segment, lasts until cell A begins to repolarize (enters its phase 3), when a _negative_ T wave begins to be inscribed on the EKG channel. This lasts until both cells have repolarized and regained their resting potentials once again. This explanation, though, _fails_ to explain why people usually have _upright_ T waves in most leads.

It is not fully understood why the T wave is upright in normal people. It may be that since the _Purkinje_ fibers fire first, have _very_ _long_ action potentials, and probably repolarize last, as shown in Figure 2, that this is why people have upright T waves. Dogs and horses, however, normally have inverted T waves, and the T wave will be upright or inverted in various other animals.

<u>EVENTS DURING DEPOLARIZATION AND REPOLARIZATION</u>

Based on the above strip or core of myocardium, and on the long action potentials of the Purkinje cells, let us now reconstruct, reexamine and reevaluate what may be happening in this core during depolarization and the cascade of rapid ion movements that follows. The <u>inner third</u> of the strip contains the Purkinje cells with their long-duration action potentials. Because of this, the <u>average</u> duration of the action potential in this region is prolonged ("average" Cell A) so that it regains its resting potential (repolarizes) later than does the outer subepicardial region ("average" Cell B), which contains no Purkinje cells, only ventricular myocardial cells.

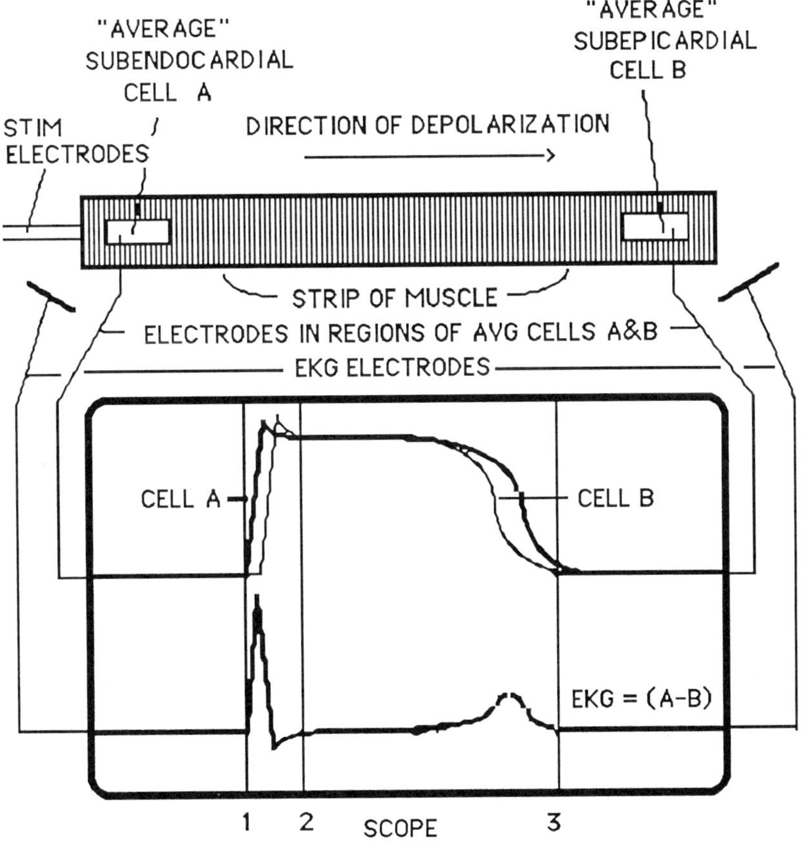

<u>FIGURE 5</u>

As shown in Figure 5, when the "average" Cell A fires, A is less negative (more positive) than "average" Cell B. The pen writes an R wave. Then "average" Cell B also depolarizes. The R wave diminishes, reaches zero for an instant, and then becomes a small S wave as "average" Cell B reaches the peak of its phase zero. Then this is followed by an isoelectric ST segment as all cells are on the plateau (phase 2) of their action potentials. Then, however, the subepicardial "average" Cell B begins to repolarize (phase 3) before "average" Cell A, as B has no Purkinje cells to prolong the average action potential in this subepicardial region. A positive, upright T wave now begins. Finally, the "average" Cell A, with its action potential prolonged by the contribution of the Purkinje cells in this subendocardial region, finally also begins to repolarize, and the positive T wave now diminishes and gradually fades to the isoelectric line. Thus we have a reasonable explanation for the normally upright T wave in people, based on the fact that the Purkinje cells, with their long duration action potentials (also see Figure 2), are localized to the subendocardial region and prolong the average duration of depolarization in that region.

Note that there is no propagated _wave_ of repolarization as there is of depolarization. Instead, each cell regains its own resting potential independently, without any propagated wave or any communication with any other cells.

With the spike (phase 0) of the action potential, the sodium ions run in along their concentration gradient. The Ca ions also begin to be released from storage sites in the vesicles of the longitudinal tubular system, and diffuse to the contractile apparatus. The Ca ions tie up troponin and permit the actomyosin bridges to develop, thus initiating contraction. They also play a significant role in governing the rate of contraction (contractility or power) at any instantaneous resistance (afterload). In college chemistry we saw that the rate at which some chemical reactions proceeded to completion often was a function of the concentration of some of the key reactants. Here the concentration of calcium ions appears to regulate the rate at which the chemical reaction of muscular shortening takes place, thus regulating ventricular contractility (contractile power).

After the Na and Ca ion movements, the Ca is then pumped back by the Na-Ca ATPase from the contractile apparatus back to the vesicles in the longitudinal tubular system (and perhaps to the transverse tubules as well), at the end of the sarcomere, near the Z lines. This permits the muscle to relax. Finally, somewhere during the plateau (phase 2) and mostly during phase 3, K moves out of the cell along its concentration gradient.

All these Na, Ca, and K movements or fluxes cause the action potential, not only because of the transfer of charges, but also in part because some of the <u>potential energy</u> of the <u>resting potential</u> is converted into the <u>kinetic energy</u> of the flowing ions. Since the total energy in the system must remain constant (the conservation of energy), the potential energy also <u>falls</u> during the time of the ion <u>movements</u>. This is similar to pouring yourself a cup of coffee from a large 50 cup coffee urn, and watching the level of the coffee in the pipe at the front. At first, as the coffee was stationary, it had the level appropriate to 50 cups. As the coffee is poured, the level falls markedly as the <u>moving coffee</u> acquires kinetic energy and goes into the cup. When you stop pouring, the level in the pipe rises back up to a level of 49 cups. This is a reasonable hydraulic analogy to some part of the events associated with nerve and muscle action potentials. The regained resting potential, very close to that of the original resting potential, is regained in part because the various rapid ion flows are _over_ and have _ceased,_ and because the intracellular ion _concentrations_ seen by the intramyocardial electrode have _hardly changed_ after this cascade of ions initiated by the spike (phase 0) of depolarization.

During diastole (phase 4), in addition to the various ion leaks that create the slope of phase 4 in pacemaker tissues, the Na-K ATPase pumps Na back out of the cells and K back in again. It is interesting that one can completely shut off the Na-K ATPase and continue to stimulate these myocardial preparations at normal rates for several hours before enough intracellular K is lost so that the resting potential falls low enough to initiate spontaneous firing of Purkinje cells, and ventricular extrasystoles and arrhythmias are generated. All this means that very little Na, Ca, and K actually move across the membrane with each depolarization. Intracellular ion concentrations in the main part of the cell are changed _very little_ with each depolarization cascade.

What are "depolarization" and "repolarization"? They are _not_ opposites, although we used to think so, and many books still suggest this. Depolarization is the _spike_ and the _beginning_ of the whole Na, Ca, and K cascade. Repolarization merely takes place as this cascade is _ended,_ and almost the original resting potential is regained once again. Repolarization is not the same thing as recovery. Repolarization merely indicates that with phase 3, the rapid ion cascade is over. True recovery is achieved only during phase 4, when the ions are more or less all pumped back again during diastole.

Now let us return to consider the heart situated in the body, and the electrical axes and vectors and their various directions in the body.

The magnitude and direction of the recorded EKG voltage depend on the direction of the positive and negative components of the voltage in relation to the recording leads, as shown in Figure 6.

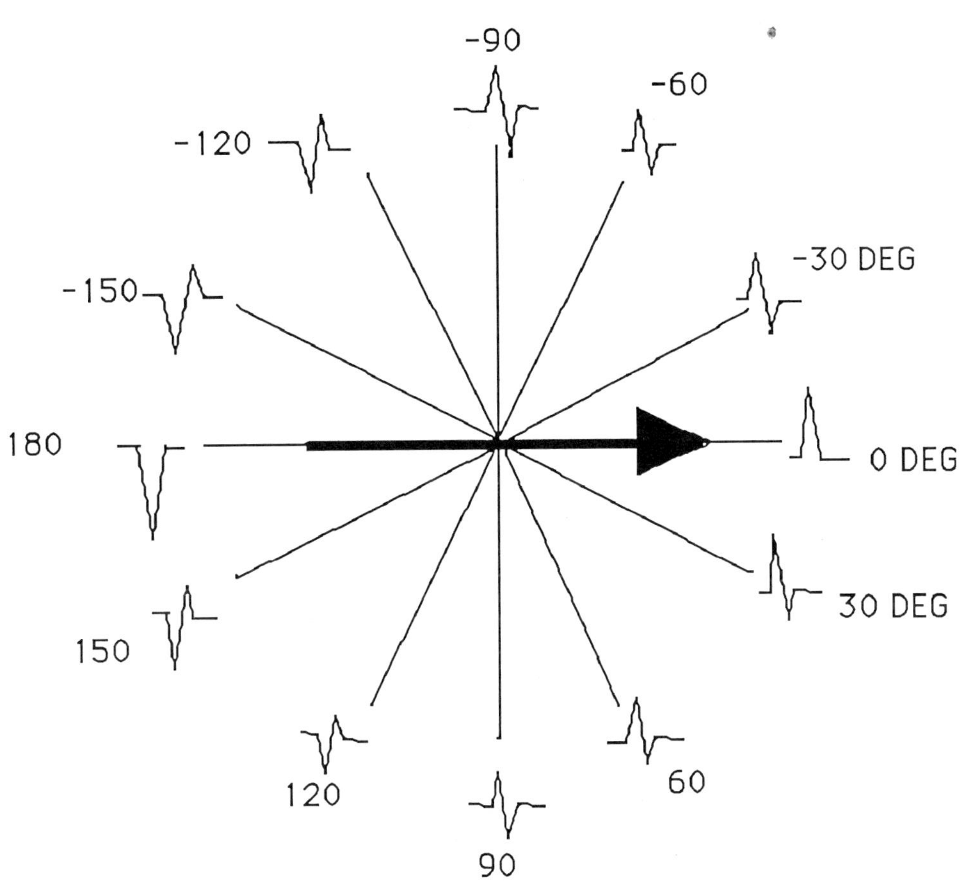

FIGURE 6

17

The angle between the direction of the <u>positivity</u> and the recording bipolar lead determines the appearance of the EKG trace. When the positivity is <u>toward</u> or away from an EKG electrode, an <u>upward</u> or downward deflection is seen respectively. The EKG is simply set up this way. As the direction of positivity becomes perpendicular (90 degrees) to the leads, a biphasic trace is seen with upward and downward deflections of equal amplitude and a net zero deflection. This is analogous to a "null" point in a radio direction finder.

<u>LEAD</u> <u>SYSTEMS</u>: <u>LIMB</u> <u>LEADS</u>

Originally, Einthoven had devised a triangular representation of events within the thorax as seen from the front. This became known as Einthoven's triangle, as shown in Figure 7, with leads 1,2, and 3 shown on it.

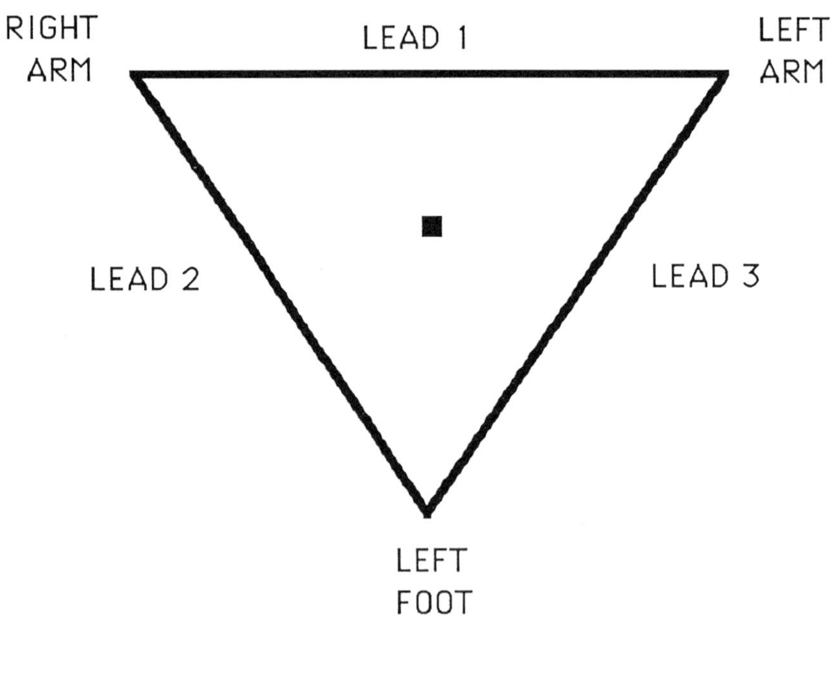

<u>Figure 7</u>

<u>Lead 1</u>. <u>Electrodes</u> <u>on</u> <u>the</u> <u>right</u> <u>arm</u> <u>and</u> <u>Left</u> <u>arm.</u>

1. Deflection is upward when positivity is toward the left arm, and

2. Downward when positivity is toward the right arm.

3. A biphasic deflection or no net deflection is seen when positivity is perpendicular (+90 or -90 degrees) to the line of the lead (zero degrees, straight to the patient's left).

<u>Lead 2</u>. <u>Electrodes</u> <u>on</u> <u>the</u> <u>right</u> <u>arm</u> <u>and</u> <u>left</u> <u>foot.</u>

1. Deflection is upward when positivity is toward the left foot, and

2. Downward when positivity is toward the right arm.

3. A biphasic or no net deflection is seen when positivity is perpendicular (-30 or +150 degrees) to the line of this lead (+60 degrees).

<u>Lead 3</u>. <u>Electrodes</u> <u>on</u> <u>the</u> <u>left</u> <u>arm</u> <u>and</u> <u>left</u> <u>foot.</u>

1. Deflection is upward when positivity is toward the left foot,

2. Downward when positivity is toward the left arm, and

3. Biphasic when positivity is perpendicular (+30 or -150 degrees) to the line of this lead (+120 degrees).

All electrical activity is bipolar in nature. One side of the recording galvanometer is relatively positive and the other relatively negative. During the 1930's, Wilson and others devised lead systems that would "look at" the heart from the right arm, the left arm, and the foot respectively. They wanted to pay attention only to one side of the galvanometer. They therefore devised a "central terminal" by connecting together the other leads except the one in question to the other side of the galvanometer. They were called VR, VL, and VF. The QRS complexes were small, and resistors were added to augment the size of the complexes. These were then called the "augmented unipolar limb leads", and are now known as aVR, aVL, and aVF respectively, as shown in Figure 8.

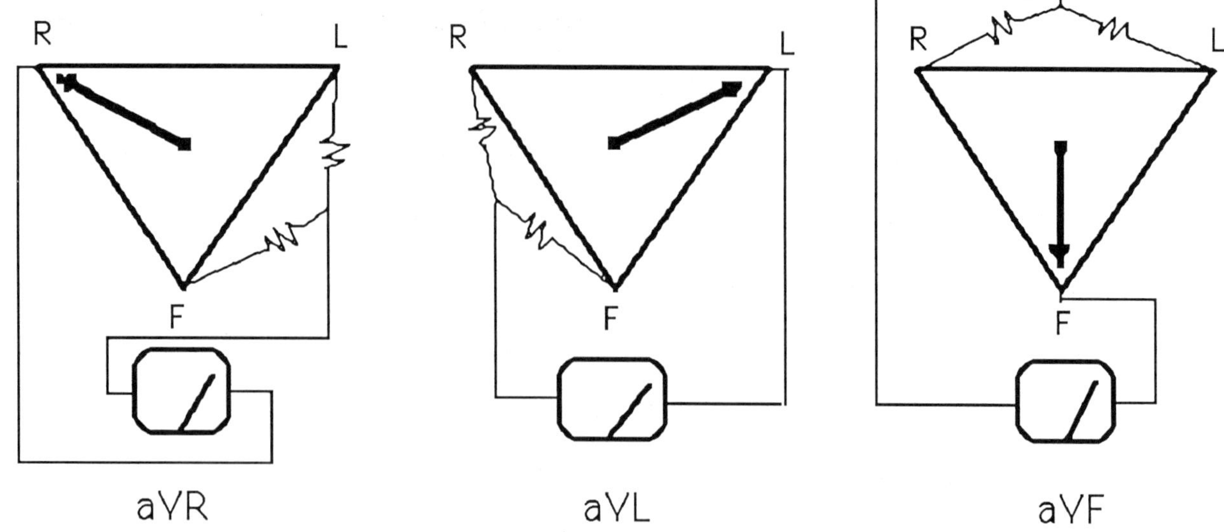

<u>Figure 8</u>

Galvanometer deflection is arranged to be upward when the electrode in question is positive, and positivity is toward that electrode. Deflection is downward when that electrode is negative, and positivity is away from it. There is a biphasic deflection or no net deflection when the positivity is perpendicular to the line of the exploring electrode.

By the use of the central terminal, the real "lead" for the other side of the galvanometer was actually moved to an unknown but central internal point inside the patient somewhere near the heart, as shown by the dots in the center of each triangle of each lead, the origin of each arrow of positivity.

By combining the six limb leads, 1, 2, 3, and aVR, aVL, and aVF, we can now plot the direction of the electrical QRS axis as seen from the front (frontal plane). A six - lead system has become traditional as shown. This has all evolved from Einthoven's triangle, as shown in Figure 9.

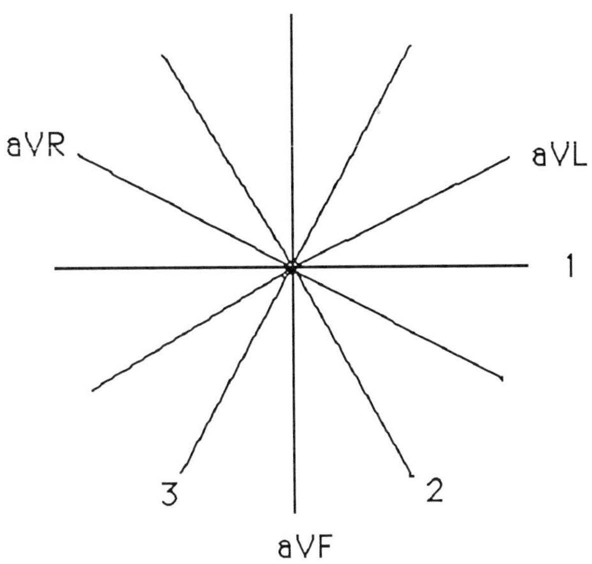

DIRECTIONS OF THE LEADS
AS SEEN FROM THE CENTRAL
TERMINAL

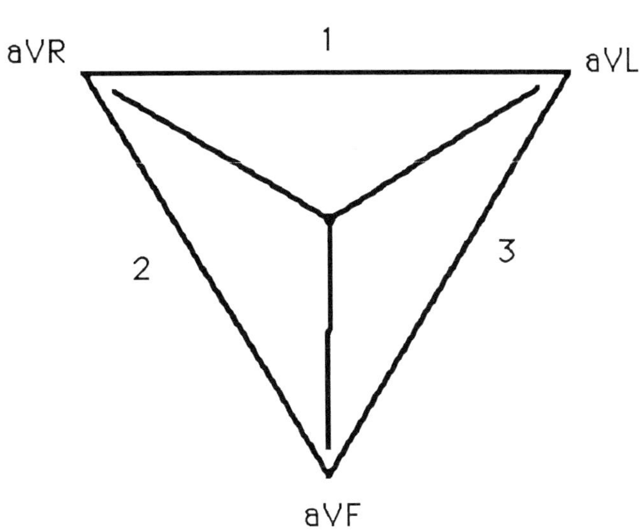

DIRECTIONS OF THE LEADS
AS SEEN FROM EINTHOVEN'S
TRIANGLE

<u>FIGURE 9</u>

<u>PLOTTING THE FRONTAL PLANE AXES: THE METHOD OF SEMICIRCLES OR HEMISPHERES.</u>

Most EKG machines today first take leads 1, 2, and 3 simultaneously, (from the top down on the page), then (without any pause), aVR, aVL, and aVF, then V1–V3, and finally V4–V6. Thus the EKG usually has 4 parts, from left to right: leads 1, 2, and 3, then leads aVR, aVL, and aVF, then V1–V3, and finally V4–V6.

Now look at Lead 1 (top left) of the normal EKG shown in Figure 10. The QRS is upward. This means that the QRS positivity is in the left semicircle (or hemisphere) surrounding the heart, in the center of the thorax. This semicircle is bounded by the vertical line (or plane) that is <u>perpendicular</u> to lead 1, as shown in Figure 11.

    This record shows regular sinus rhythm. The P-R, QRS, and Q-T durations are within normal limits. The frontal QRS axis is +20, the T axis is +15, and the P axis is +50 degrees. The horizontal QRS axis is -10, the T axis is +10, and the P axis is +15 degrees. No evidence of hypertrophy, infarction, or conduction disturbance is seen. The record is within normal limits.

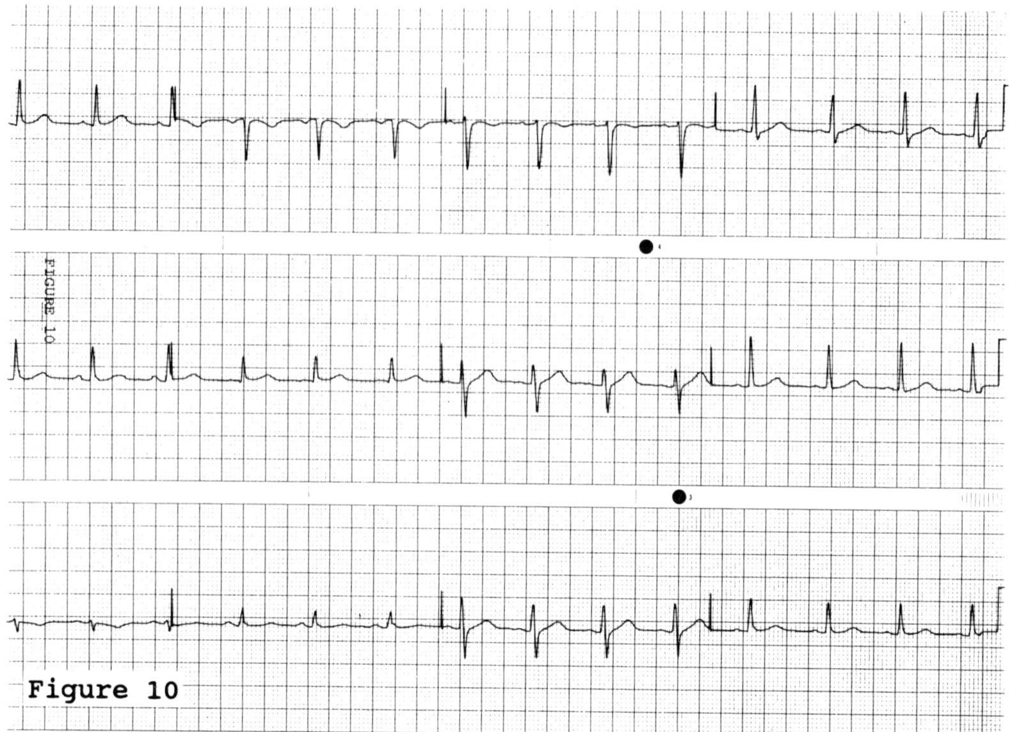

Figure 10

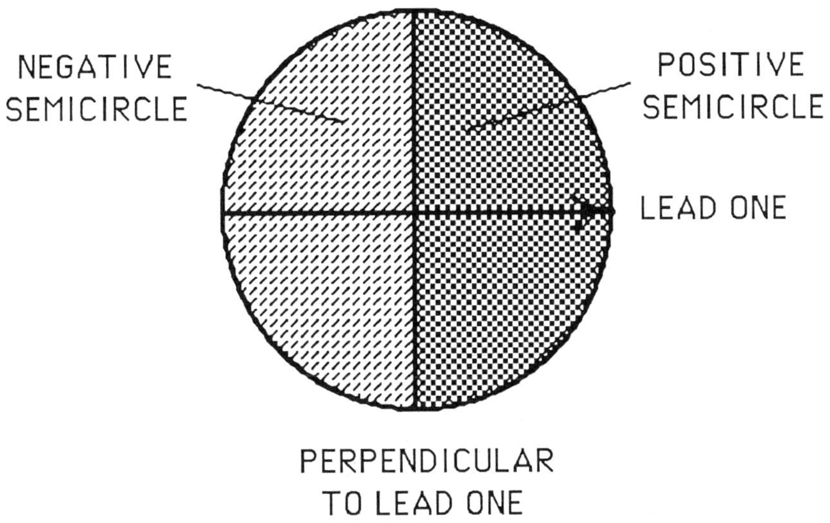

<u>FIGURE 11</u>

Now look at Lead aVF. The QRS is up here as well. Using the same approach as above, we see that the axis is also in the lower semicircle (or hemisphere) of aVF, and is bounded by the horizontal line (or plane) that is perpendicular to Lead aVF, as shown in Figure 12.

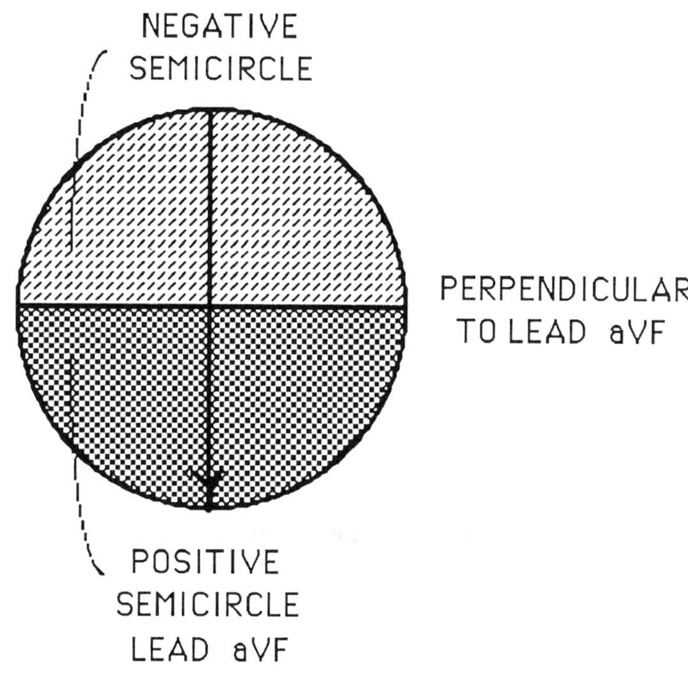

FIGURE 12

Putting these 2 sets of information together, we now know that the axis is in the patient's lower left quadrant, as shown in Figure 13.

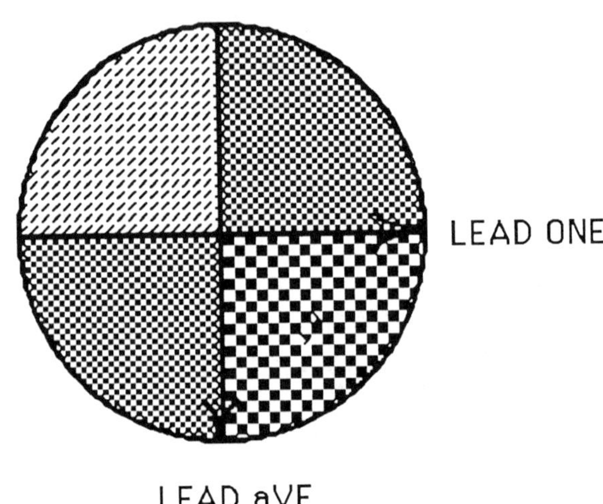

<u>FIGURE 13</u>

Now Leads 3 and aVL have perpendiculars which will help us cut up this quadrant (and the right superior quadrant also). Lead 3 has a perpendicular running from +30 to -150 degrees. In Figure 10, we see that the QRS complex is slightly down or negative in Lead 3. We also see that in Lead aVL, which has a perpendicular running from +60 to -120 degrees, the QRS complex is up or positive. Putting this all together, we see that the frontal QRS axis must lie between 0 and +30 degrees, (let us say about +20 degrees, as it is slightly more up in aVF than down in Lead 3), as shown in Figure 14.

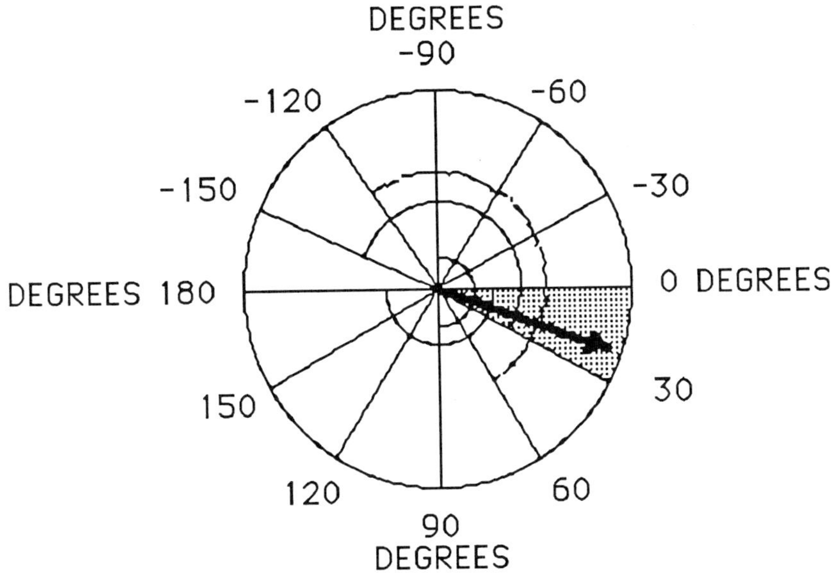

FRONTAL PLANE QRS AXIS
OF EKG IN FIGURE 10

FIGURE 14

In the same way, one can use Leads 2 and aVR to help cut up the left superior quadrant and the right inferior quadrant. Simply look at each lead and figure out which half of its field (which semicircle or hemisphere) the P, QRS, ST, or T axis or vector is in.

This method can also be used to plot the P and T axes (and the direction of the ST vector if there is an ST segment shift). We will do all of this later, and find it most useful. We will also do exactly the same thing, and with the same logic and application of the laws of physics, to plot the P, QRS, ST, and T vectors in the horizontal plane, which is related to the precordial leads, which we will consider soon.

<u>Normal</u> <u>Ranges</u>: <u>Frontal</u> <u>Plane</u> <u>Axes</u>

The normal range for the frontal plane P, QRS, and T axes are all from zero (or perhaps -30 degrees, some say) to +90 degrees (or perhaps +120 degrees, some say). <u>Right</u> <u>Axis</u> <u>Deviation</u> is present when the frontal QRS axis or vector is between +90 (or 120) and 180 degrees. <u>Left</u> <u>(or</u> <u>Superior)</u> <u>Axis</u> <u>Deviation</u> is present when the frontal QRS axis or vector is between zero (or -30, some say), and -90 degrees. The usual left lower quadrant includes about 95% of the normal frontal QRS axes. About 2 1/2 % of normal people will have a QRS axis superior to zero, and another 2 1/2% will have a QRS axis beyond +90 degrees.

The <u>angle</u> between the frontal QRS and T axes is normally <u>less</u> <u>than</u> <u>60</u> <u>degrees</u> in either direction, and is usually less than 30 degrees.

An abnormal P axis may suggest <u>right</u> <u>atrial</u> <u>enlargement</u> (if greater than +90 degrees), or an ectopic atrial focus causing an abnormally conducted P wave moving over the atria.

<u>Right</u> <u>Axis</u> <u>Deviation</u> may occur in a few normal ectomorphic people, but is usually produced by those conditions causing right ventricular hypertrophy, of which mitral stenosis, emphysema and cor pulmonale, and atrial or ventricular septal defects with pulmonary or right ventricular hypertension, and pulmonic stenosis are examples. Transient rightward shifts of the electrical QRS axis from a former position are often seen with the transient pulmonary hypertension and acute cor pulmonale caused by pulmonary emboli.

<u>Left</u> <u>(or</u> <u>Superior)</u> <u>Axis</u> <u>Deviation</u> may be seen in fat, squat people with transverse hearts on X-ray, with left ventricular hypertrophy, with various myocardial infarcts, and in some people with emphysema.

Precordial leads were then developed, where an exploring chest electrode was used. The "central terminal" was hooked to the other side of the galvanometer. The exploring electrode locations are as shown:

V1 - 4th intercostal space, to the right of the sternum.

V2 - 4th intercostal space, to the left of the sternum.

V3 - halfway between V2 and V4.

V4 - 5th intercostal space, in the mid-clavicular line.

V5 - 5th intercostal space, in the anterior axillary line.

V6 - 6th intercostal space, in the mid-axillary line.

Another lead, V3R, is also useful, especially to see P waves. It is in the same position as V3, but is on the right side of the chest. A lead on the ensiform process is also useful to see P waves.

An upward deflection is written when positivity is toward the exploring chest electrode, just as it was with aVR, aVL, and aVF.

The precordial leads approximate the electrical QRS activity as seen in the top view (horizontal plane). Actually, the plane is tilted about 30 degrees slightly downward to the left, as V5 and V6 are below the level of the heart, V1 and V2 are at the upper level of the heart, and V3 and V4 are in between. The "horizontal" plane, as perceived with the precordial leads, therefore actually slopes downward to the left when viewed from in front, at an angle of about +30 degrees on the frontal plane. More on this later.

<u>Plotting</u> <u>the</u> <u>Horizontal</u> <u>Plane</u> <u>Axes.</u> <u>Their</u> <u>Normal</u> <u>Ranges.</u>

Let us visualize ourselves looking down upon the heart in the thorax, as shown in Figure 15, with the precordial leads in place.

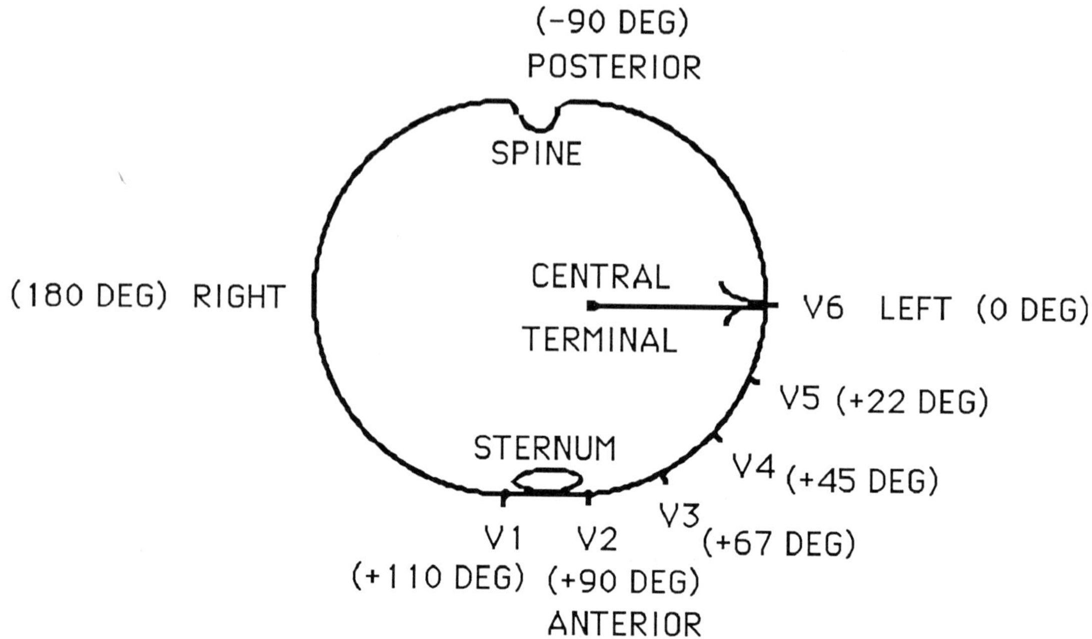

FIGURE 15

Using the same method of semicircles (or hemispheres) that we employed with the frontal plane P, QRS, ST, and T vectors or axes (the laws of physics are still the same!), let us similarly plot the horizontal plane QRS axis for the same EKG in Figure 10 (page 29). Here we see that the QRS is down in V1, and slightly down in V2. It is therefore in the semicircle away from V1 and V2. However, the QRS is slightly positive (upright) in V3, and therefore is in the semicircle toward V3. It is also in the semicircle toward V4, V5, and V6. Since it is away from V1 and V2 and toward V3-V6, the horizontal QRS axis is about minus 10 degrees.

The <u>Normal</u> <u>Horizontal</u> <u>Plane</u> <u>QRS</u> <u>Axis</u> usually ranges from about +15 degrees (perpendicular to V1) to about -80 degrees (having a perpendicular between V5 and V6, being away from V5 and toward V6).

Anterior displacement of the horizontal plane QRS axis or vector is usually caused by right ventricular hypertrophy or posterior infarction. Posterior displacement is usually caused by left ventricular hypertrophy, anteroseptal, anterolateral, or apical infarction, or by pulmonary disease.

The horizontal plane T axis in Figure 10 is away from V1 (inverted) and toward V2-V6 (upright). Its transition or isoelectric position is between V1 and V2, and its axis is perpendicular to that, or about +10 degrees.

The <u>Normal</u> <u>Horizontal</u> <u>Plane</u> <u>T</u> <u>Axis</u> is:

1. Slightly in front of (anterior to) the horizontal QRS axis, by about 5 or 10 degrees.

2. In any event, not more posterior than -15 degrees (having a perpendicular or isoelectric position between V2 and V3), and

3. Not more than 90 degrees anterior to the horizontal QRS axis.

The <u>Normal</u> <u>Horizontal</u> <u>Plane</u> <u>P</u> <u>Axis</u> is usually between about +10 degrees (perpendicular or isoelectric between V1 and V2) to about +50 degrees, but the horizontal P axis limits are not well-known, and the P axis is often hard to plot in this plane.

<u>Inconsistencies</u> between <u>the</u> <u>Frontal</u> and <u>Horizontal</u> <u>Axes</u>

Sometimes one will find a rightward frontal axis, more than +90, with a horizontal axis that is still leftward. One may also have a superior frontal axis, usually above -30 degrees, with a horizontal axis that appears to be rightward, with deep S waves and negative complexes in V5 and V6. These apparent contradictions can <u>usually</u> (but not always) be resolved by remembering that V5 and V6 are below the level of the heart, while V1 and V2 are slightly above it, thus tilting the "horizontal" plane downward toward the left by about 30 degrees. Now we can see that the "rightward" frontal axis is not really <u>yet</u> going <u>away</u> from V6, but is still toward it. Similarly, a very superior frontal axis, while still leftward, may actually be going <u>away</u> from V6.

In addition, one may see a "double transition" of the horizontal plane QRS axis in patients with excess anterior forces as with RBBB, posterior infarction, or right ventricular hypertrophy, as shown in Figure 38, for example. Here, the zigzag lead placement of the precordial lead electrodes may be a reason for this, with V1 and V2 placed high and level with each other, V3 and V4 zigzagging downward, and V5 and V6 going level again.

Lastly, local anomalies of the conductive field in the thorax do exist, and are probably the best explanations we can currently find for those EKG's we still see and do not know how to resolve with a better explanation.

<u>THE</u> <u>CUBE</u> <u>VECTOR</u> <u>SYSTEM</u> <u>LEADS</u>

Einthoven's triangle and the subsequent six-axis lead systems are cumbersome. So are the precordial lead systems. However, they are entrenched in the literature and are in common use.

Many workers have sought to simplify the EKG and at the same time to make it more informative. The Cube Vector System has been developed, in conjunction with the simultaneous display of 2 leads upon an oscilloscope. The leads (axes) used are as shown here in Figure 16.

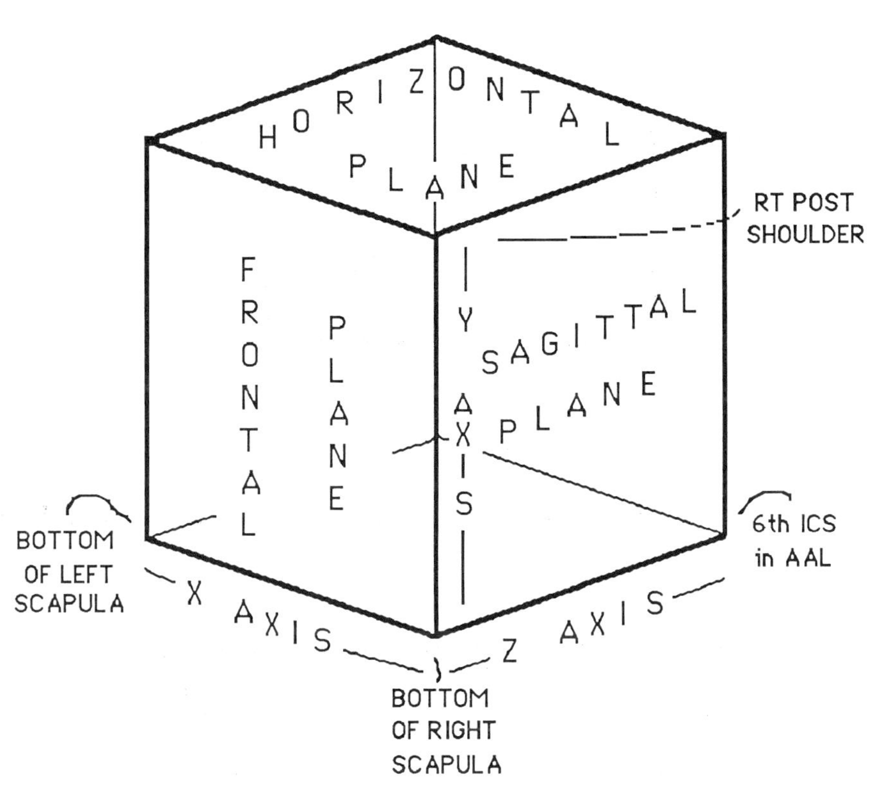

FIGURE 16

The 3 leads used reflect positive voltage along the X, Y, and Z axes.

Xaxis(right to left) - bottom of right scapula to bottom of left scapula.

Y axis (up and down) - bottom of right scapula to right posterior shoulder.

Z axis (front to back) - bottom of right scapula to 6th intercostal space in the right anterior axillary line.

31

The Frontal Plane (front view) consists of a simultaneous display on a scope of the X axis horizontally and the Y axis vertically. The scope as shown in Figure 17 below, then writes out the continuous recording of both the direction and magnitude of the positive voltage as seen in this plane.

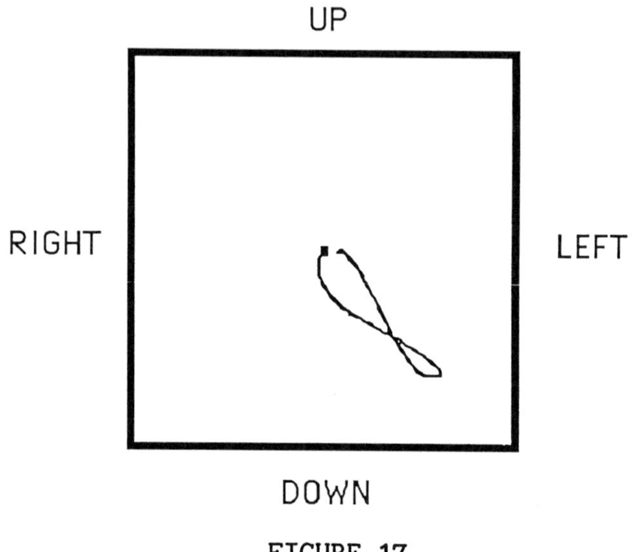

FIGURE 17

This is the frontal plane vector loop. This compares with Figure 18, below,

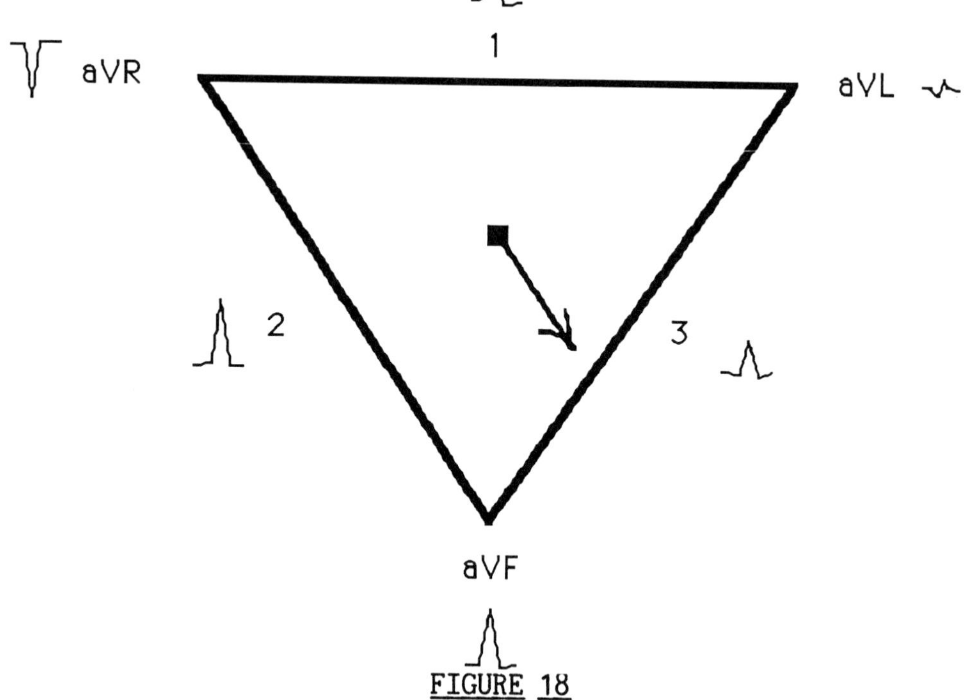

FIGURE 18

as laboriously plotted from the EKG limb leads.

32

The Horizontal Plane (top view) is shown by displaying

The X axis horizontally

The Z axis vertically, as shown in Figure 19.

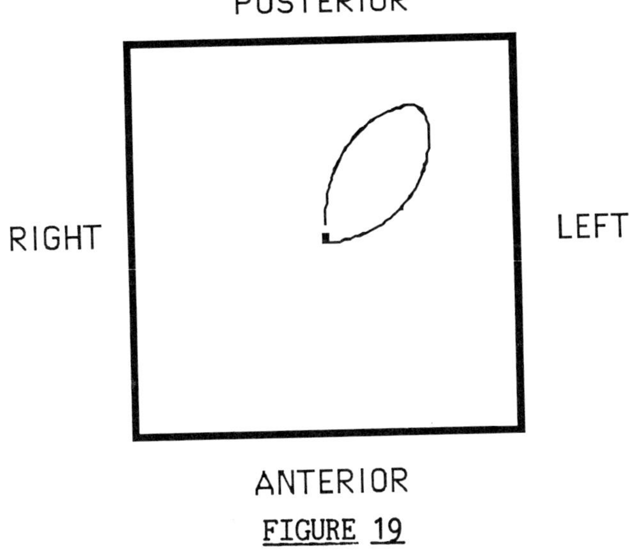

FIGURE 19

Whereas an analysis of precordial leads, as shown in Figure 20, will give the horizontal plane axis shown in Figure 20.

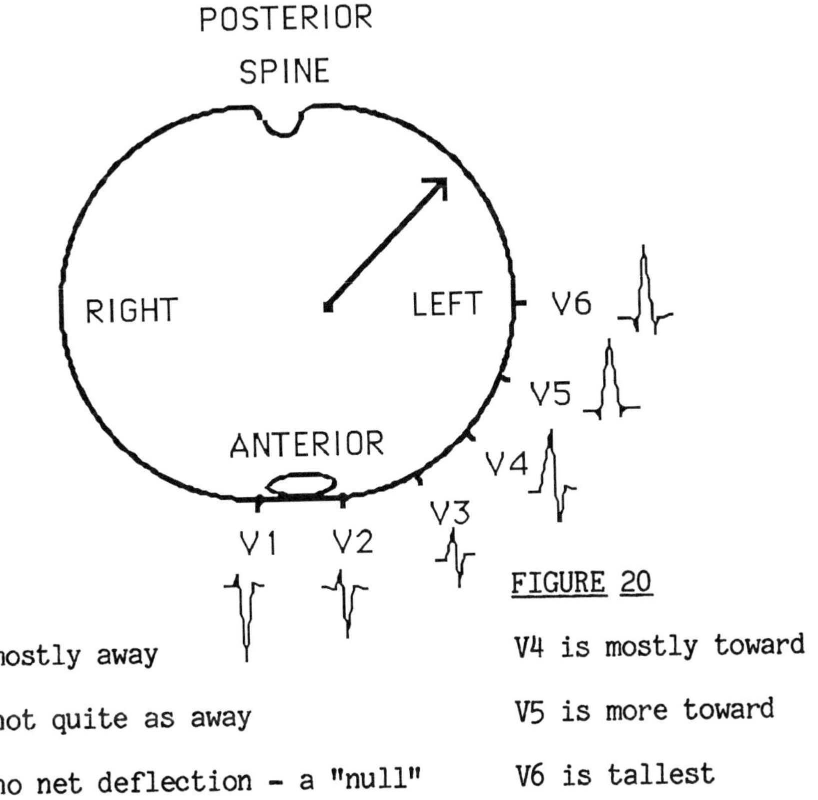

FIGURE 20

V1 is mostly away

V2 is not quite as away

V3 is no net deflection - a "null"

V4 is mostly toward

V5 is more toward

V6 is tallest

The <u>Right</u> <u>Saggital</u> <u>Plane</u> (right side view) is shown by displaying the Z axis horizontally and the Y axis vertically, as shown in Figure 21.

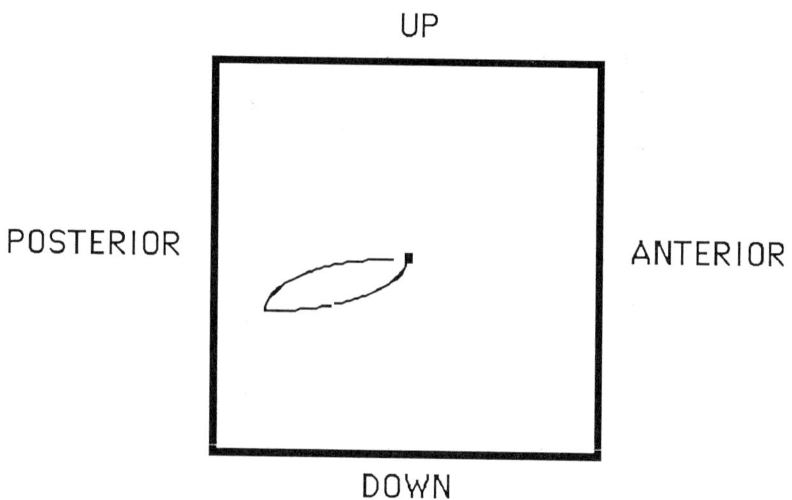

<u>FIGURE 21</u>

EKG leads have no data for this plane. Other vector lead systems (Frank, McFee, etc) have also been used. In a <u>timed</u> <u>vectorcardiogram</u>, as shown in Figure 22, the trace also sweeps from our left to our right with time.

<u>THE</u> <u>PATHWAY</u> <u>OF</u> <u>VENTRICULAR</u> <u>DEPOLARIZATION</u>

<u>The</u> <u>QRS</u> <u>Vector</u> <u>in</u> <u>More</u> <u>Detail</u>

The heart is not a strip of muscle in which depolarization only proceeds in one direction, as in our strip or core of myocardium. Rather, the wave front spreads down the Purkinje fibers to the ventricles, and then over the ventricles much like a stone makes a ripple in a pond. A knowledge of normal QRS patterns and axes is based on an accurate knowledge of the pathway of ventricular depolarization. Each portion of the ventricular myocardium is normally depolarized in a certain direction at a certain time. The sum total (positive voltage and direction) of such electrical activity

34

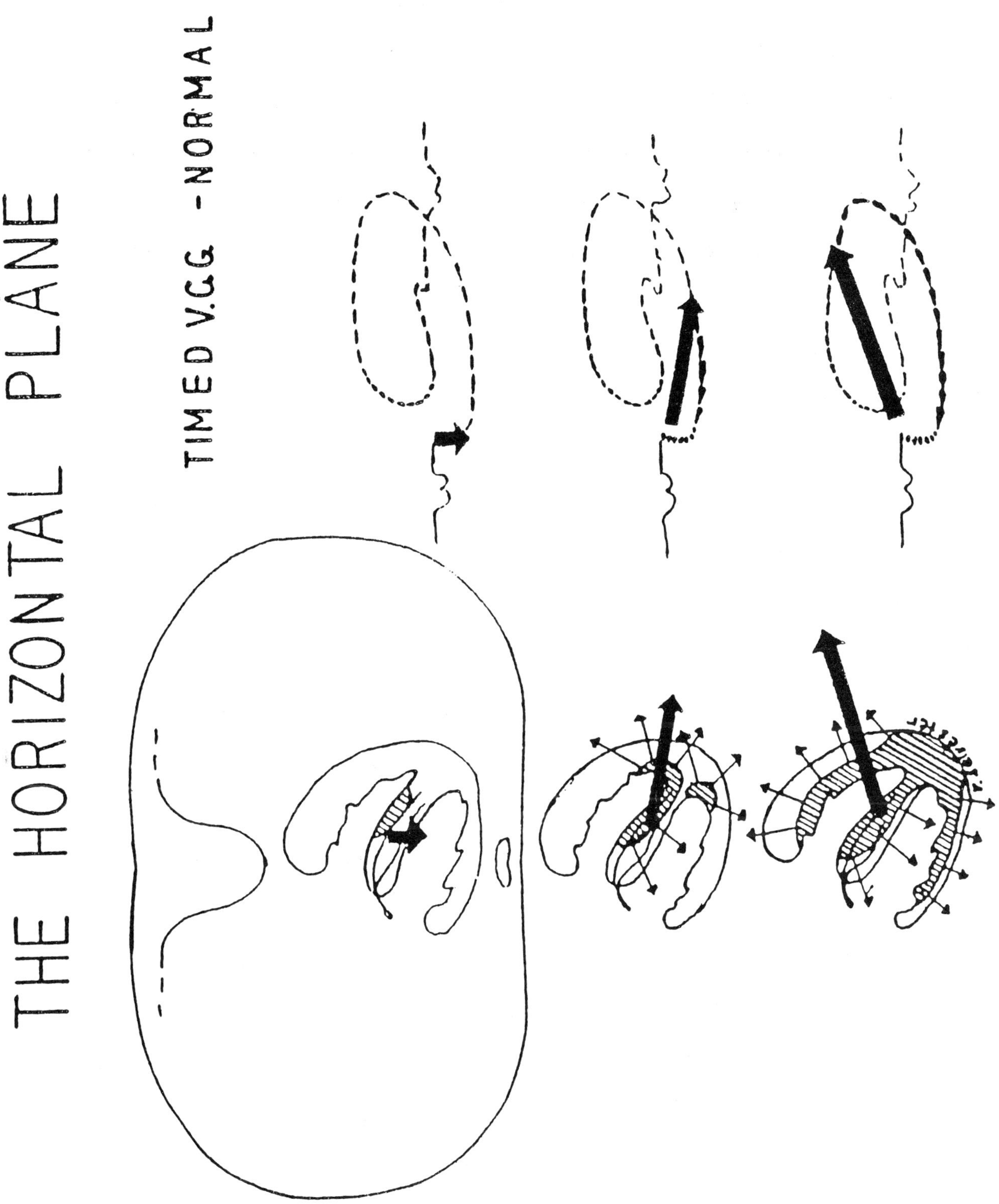
THE HORIZONTAL PLANE
TIMED V.C.G. -NORMAL

Normal Physiology
Courtesy of Dr. Ronald Selvester,
Rancho Los Amigos Hospital

FIGURE 22

in each place at each instant during the QRS complex causes the normal QRS patterns in the EKG and the normal QRS vector loops in the VCG.

Hypertrophy and infarction cause additions to and deletions from this normal loop. It is only through knowledge of the direction and the time of the changes in electrical activity thus produced that one can diagnose such lesions. Understanding the pathway of normal ventricular depolarization is therefore one cornerstone of EKG and vector interpretation. A knowledge of arrhythmias is the other.

The instantaneous electrical axis or vector at any given time in the QRS is the sum (in both magnitude and direction) of all the individual voltages in the wave front in the myocardium at that instant.

The wave of depolarization is brought by the left bundle to the lower part of the septum of the left ventricle. It moves rightward and anteriorly through the septum. Slightly later the inner part of the right ventricular apex is fired. Following these events, the impulse:

1. Spreads widely over the endocardial surface of both ventricles via the Purkinje cells at a speed of 3-4 meters/sec, and

2. Spreads from endocardium to epicardium as well, at a speed of about 1 meter/sec. What is now described below is a blend of these 2 basic modes of spread.

As shown in Figure 22, top, the first .01 seconds of QRS electrical activity is initiated by a wave of depolarization beginning in the lower left portion of the interventricular septum. The wave front (and the positive voltage) moves to the right and anteriorly, causing a small Q wave in Leads 1, V5, and V6, and usually a small R wave in Leads V3R, V1, and V2.

From .02 to .04 seconds, (Figure 22, middle), a cone of depolarization appears at the apex of each ventricle moving from inside outward. The sum of the positive vectors increases in amplitude and swings leftward and poster-

iorly. This usually causes a Q wave in aVR, an R wave in Leads 1, 2, aVL,

aVF, V5 and V6, and an S wave in leads V3R, V1, V2, and V3.

From .04 to .06 seconds (Figure 22, bottom), both ventricles are being

depolarized from inside out and the septum is being depolarized upward and

to the right. The sum of the vectors moves further leftward, posteriorly,

and slightly upward, due to the predominant muscle mass (more myofilaments

per cell) of the left ventricle.

From .06 to .08 seconds, the vector decreases to approximately isoelec-

tric, as the remaining portions of the ventricular myocardium have become

depolarized, and no significant voltage difference exists between the

cells. All ventricular cells are now in the plateau phase of their indi-

vidual action potentials. The QRS complex is over. The ST segment begins.

2
Hypertrophy, Strain, Ischemia, and Injury

<u>THE NORMAL P VECTOR OR AXIS, AND ATRIAL ENLARGEMENT</u>

As the propagated wave front spreads out from the SA node, it travels primarily over the right atrium first, and then later over the left atrium. The P vector or axis is therefore more anterior and downward at first, and later is more horizontal and posterior in its terminal portion. The overall normal frontal plane P vector is from horizontal (0 degrees) to somewhere between +60 and +90 degrees.

<u>Right Atrial Enlargement</u> or hypertrophy (Figure 23) is therefore revealed by tall vertical ("Pulmonale") P waves, over 2.5 mm tall, in Leads 2, 3, and aVF, and by a frontal plane axis greater than +60 degrees.

<u>Left Atrial Enlargement</u> or hypertrophy (Figure 23) is revealed by a wider P wave, with a P duration over about .12 seconds. It is often notched due to the accentuated posterior and leftward swing of the P vector or axis as it spreads over the dilated left atrium. This M – shaped "P mitrale" is often best seen in Lead 2. It is also seen as a downward deflection of the last half of the P wave in V3R and V1. In V1, the negative downward component stays down for at least .04 sec and reaches a depth of at least 1.0 mm. The terminal part is then said to be "down a box for a box" in V1.

<u>INTRACELLULAR EKG CHANGES WITH STRAIN, ISCHEMIA, HYPERTROPHY, AND INFARCTION</u>

The following explanation is not rigorously proven, but the available evidence suggests that all parts of it are based, in some way or other, on physiological data and on a reasonable consensus. This book combines them for the first time, to the author's knowledge, to provide a not unreasonable

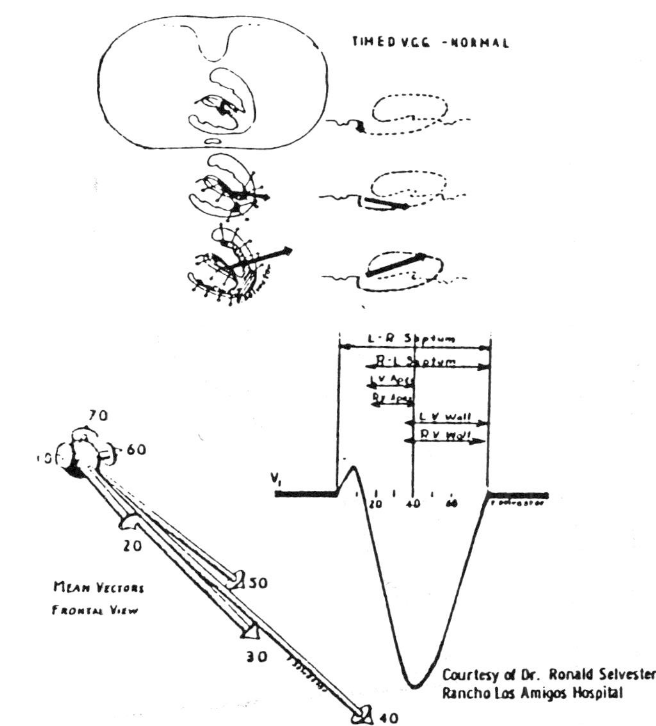

ATRIAL ENLARGEMENT
TIME RELATIONSHIPS

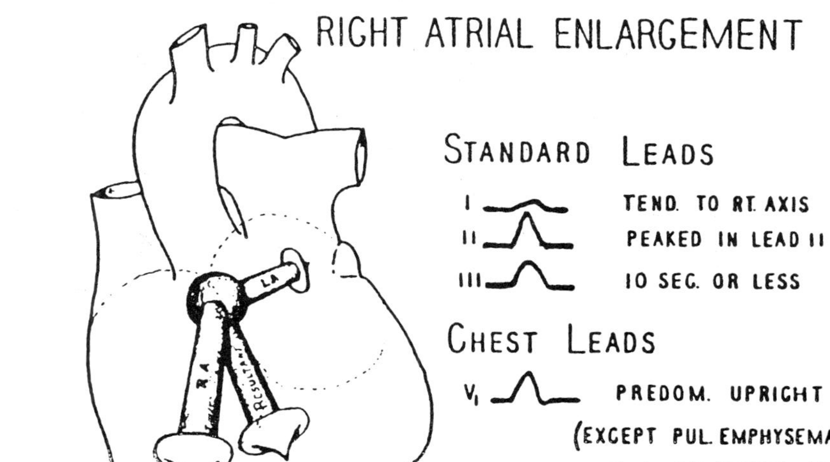

FIGURE 23

39

clinical explanation for the ST-T changes that occur with ischemia and "injury", and for the changes seen with hyper- and hypokalemia.

What we saw before, using the idea of "Cell A minus Cell B" and the action potentials, was first suggested to RJ in 1956 by Sperelakis (1). The subendocardial Purkinje cell was suggested by RJ to explain the upright T wave in people, as described earlier.

The following idea was also suggested to RJ by Sperelakis (1), and has been largely shown to be the case. When a myocardial cell must do a great deal of mechanical work (LV or RV "strain", for example), it consumes more ATP than usual, and its ATP stores will fall. The same thing happens during ischemia.

The reduced ATP stores cause a reduction of the usual Na-K ATPase activity, and myocardial K concentrations thus fall with "strain" or is- chemia. Because of this, since there is less K in the affected cell to take part in K outflow during phase 3 of the action potential, there is less deviation from the resting potential during this time, and the cell loses the "shoulder" off phase 3 of its action potential, as shown in Figure 24.

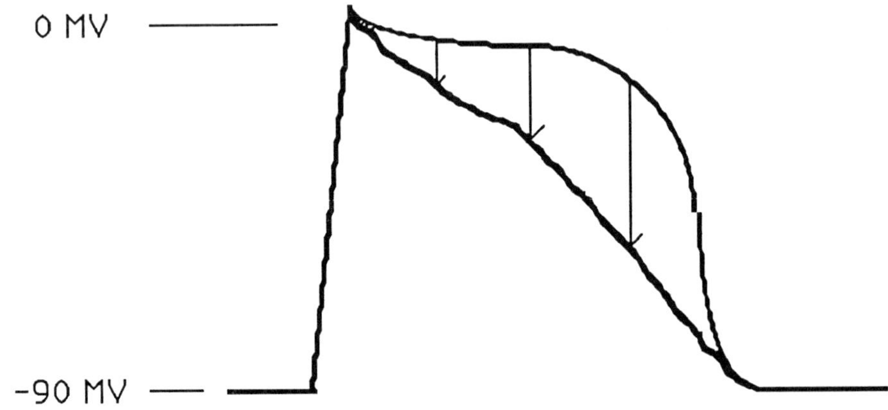

FIGURE 24

40

These changes are also discussed further by Noble (2). As also discussed by Noble (2), let us consider what next happens as the cell continues to
have its ATP stores reduced and continues to lose K. The resting potential
of the cell now falls. K is important in the maintenance of normal intracellular action potentials, and a diminished intracellular concentration
eventually becomes associated with a decrease in resting potential, as shown
in Figure 25.

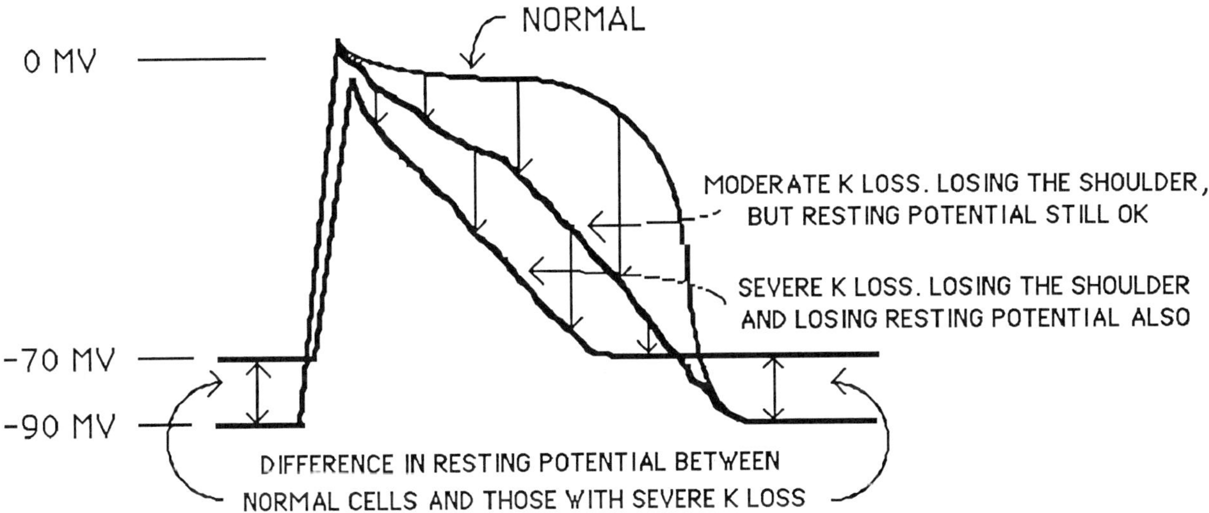

<u>FIGURE</u> <u>25</u>

Now, we have a sustained difference in potential between the normal
cells and the ischemic or hard-working cells. This difference is greatest
during diastole, and is least just after the spike potential, when the cells
are on the plateaus of their action potentials. This is why an "ST segment
shift" is really a <u>baseline</u> shift. We also see that it is not telling us
anything about the mystical word "injury", and we see no "current of injury". The EKG does not measure current. It is simply a voltmeter. An ST

41

segment shift therefore usually tells us that we have a significant group of
cells that is working under severe ischemia or under adverse mechanical
circumstances, and that the resting potentials of these cells are reduced
compared to that of the normal cells. That is the <u>way</u> that they are "injured".

Now, let us begin to put these things together. For our present
purposes, let us begin by neglecting the relatively small right ventricle.
Let us consider the heart as a single large (left) ventricle, as shown
in Figure 26.

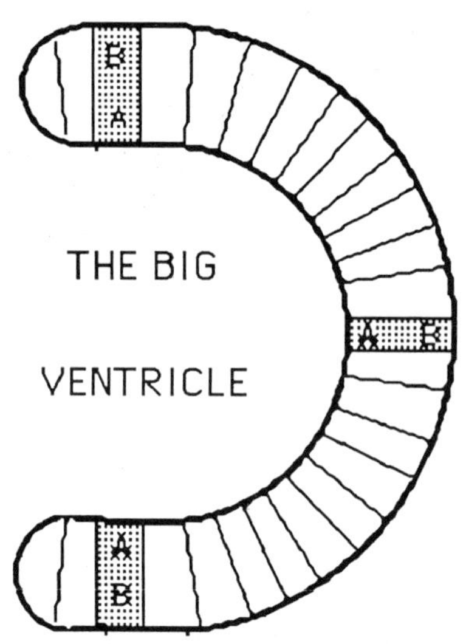

<u>FIGURE 26</u>

This ventricle is made up of an infinite number of the strips or cores
we discussed earlier, and each strip has its representative subendocardial
Cell A and subepicardial Cell B. To simplify matters, let us suppose that
the impulse conducted by the bundle of His is delivered simultaneously to
the entire endocardial surface of the single big ventricle, thus stimulating
the inner part of all the strips at exactly the same instant. If all the
strips are identical (and let us suppose this), then the voltage vectors of
the anterior strips will be identical in magnitude but opposite in direction
to those of the posterior strips, and will cancel them out, as shown in
Figure 27.

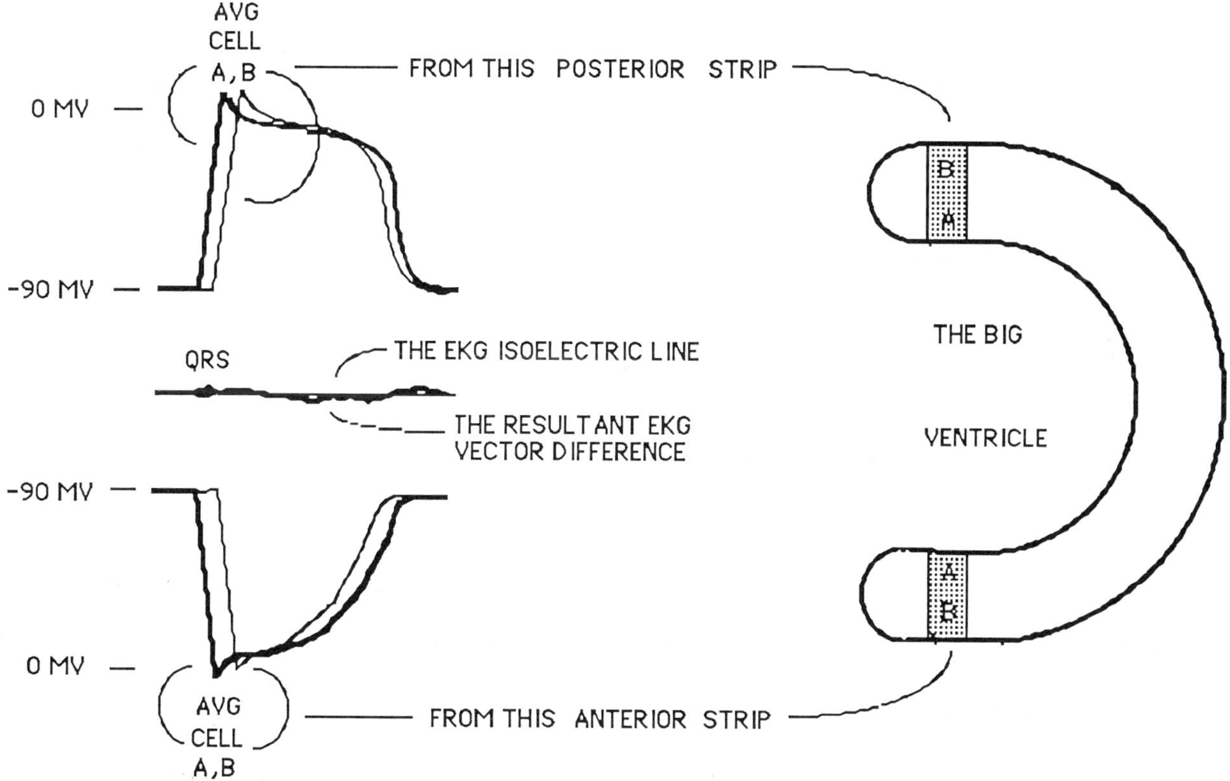

<u>FIGURE 27</u>

43

On the other hand, the unopposed strips toward the apex will _not_ be cancelled by the presence of strips opposite to them, as _only_ _the_ _atria_ are in the opposite direction. This part will resemble the _single_ strip of "Cell A minus Cell B".

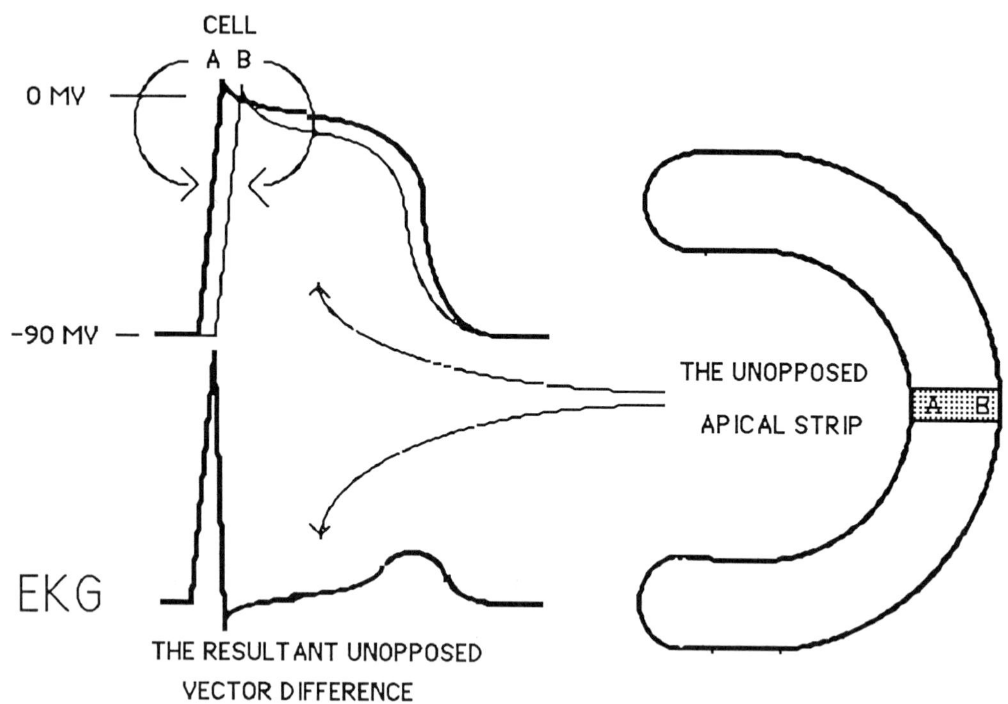

FIGURE <u>28</u>

The EKG is a blend of the overall result of the forces remaining unbalanced when they are all _added_ together _as_ _vectors_, their opposing directions being taken into account as differences.

The normal EKG consists of the differences in the the unbalanced parts of the heart (unopposed Cell A minus Cell B), as described in Figure 28 above, and the sums (Cell A plus Cell B) of cells in strips which are opposite in direction, so that the action potential of a Cell A in an

44

anterior strip is subtracted from that of a Cell A in a posterior strip, and that of an anterior Cell B is subtracted from that of a posterior Cell B, as shown in Figure 27 (Posterior Cell A - Anterior Cell A) + (Posterior Cell B - Anterior Cell B). Note that these opposed events take place only while the opposition actually exists, _during_ the action potentials. During diastole such opposition does _not_ exist, as no opposed events are taking place. These ideas also hold for the same events in all other directions - anteriorly, superiorly, inferiorly, and laterally.

<u>Changes with Strain, Ischemia and Injury: Opposed Muscle Strips.</u>

Let us now make a posterior Cell A go through the K losses seen with strain and/or ischemia. At first, the cell simply loses the shoulder off its action potential. This alters the balance of voltage so that the T wave vector or axis now swings away from the posterior (the involved) area, and moves anteriorly, as shown in Figure 29, away from the involved area.

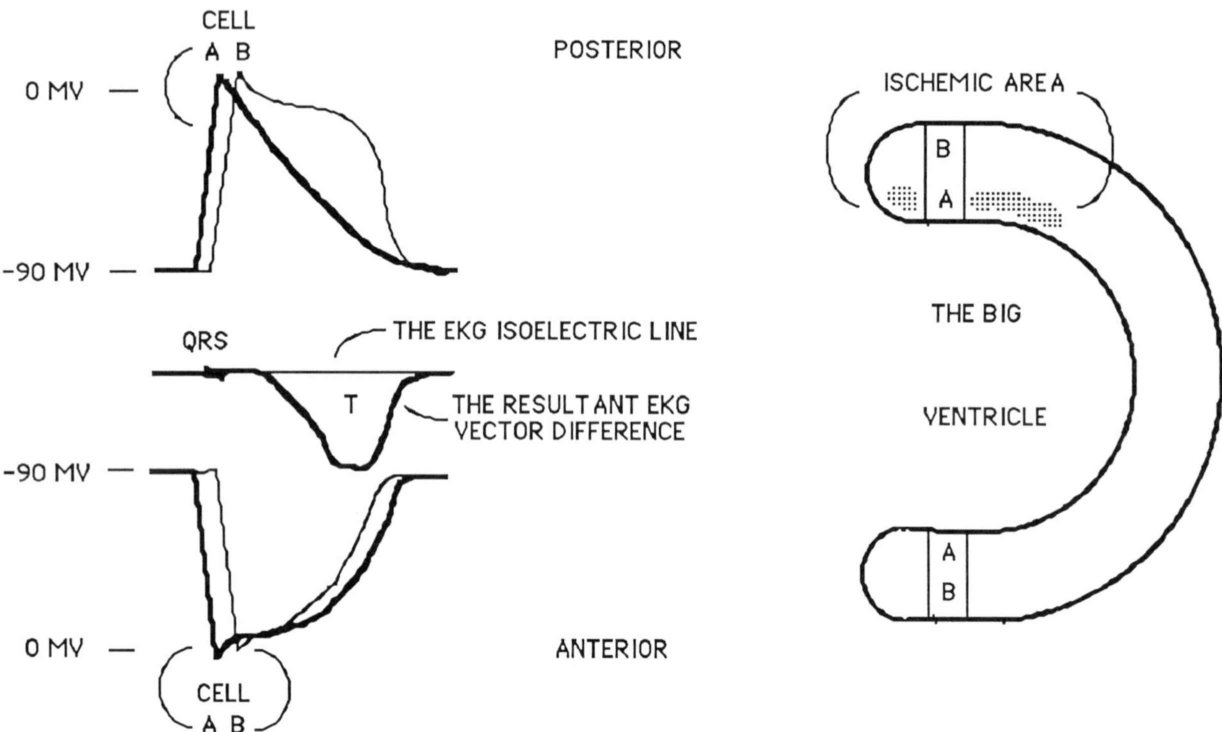

SUBENDOCARDIAL POSTERIOR ISCHEMIA

THE T VECTOR GOES AWAY FROM THE INVOLVED AREA

<u>FIGURE 29</u>

Now let posterior Cell A lose still more K, so that its resting potential falls. When the resting potential of Cell A is less negative with respect to Cell B, the baseline will move in the direction of Cell A. When Cell B is less negative (see later on) the EKG baseline is shifted in the opposite direction. Thus we are always taking the resting potential of Cell A into account <u>with respect to</u> the resting potential of Cell B. Remember that during diastole you could move that anterior or posterior ventricular strip <u>anywhere</u> anteriorly or posteriorly between the two EKG electrodes and the EKG would be basically unaffected, as no change in the basic positive and negative relationships has taken place.

Given Posterior Cell A's loss of resting potential, the EKG baseline will move posteriorly, as shown in Figure 30. An "EKG lead", the vector sum (A - A) + (B - B), will result, showing T inversion and ST depression. This is consistent with subendocardial ischemia, and the subendocardial Cell A (the early firing one) is the one with the pathology.

If these changes take place in Cell A (or B) of the opposite anterior strip, the direction of the positive and negative relationships and of the ST and T vector movement will be reversed. Notice that the <u>ST and T vectors both move away</u> from the involved area with <u>subendocardial ischemia or injury.</u>

In addition, remember that the ST depression and T inversion described here will look different when seen in other leads. For example, when viewed from leads on the opposite side of the body, they will show the reciprocal ST elevation with unusually upright T waves, closely resembling the "hyperacute ST-T changes seen with subepicardial ischemia and injury seen in the unopposed cores of ventricle which are discussed later on. It may well be difficult to tell the difference between the two processes.

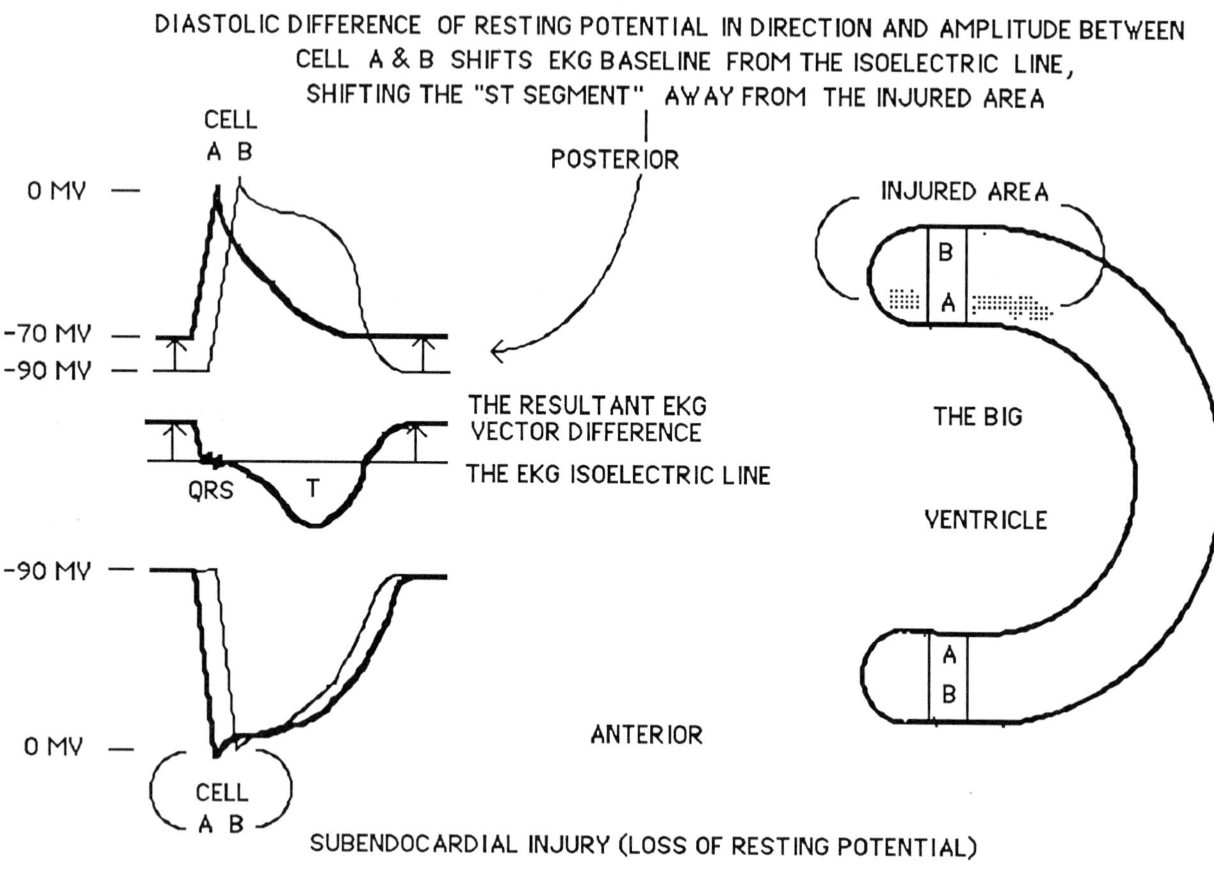

DIASTOLIC DIFFERENCE OF RESTING POTENTIAL IN DIRECTION AND AMPLITUDE BETWEEN
CELL A & B SHIFTS EKG BASELINE FROM THE ISOELECTRIC LINE,
SHIFTING THE "ST SEGMENT" AWAY FROM THE INJURED AREA
CELL
A B
POSTERIOR
0 MV
-70 MV
-90 MV
THE RESULTANT EKG
VECTOR DIFFERENCE
THE EKG ISOELECTRIC LINE
QRS
T
INJURED AREA
B
A
THE BIG
VENTRICLE
A
B
-90 MV
0 MV
ANTERIOR
CELL
A B
SUBENDOCARDIAL INJURY (LOSS OF RESTING POTENTIAL)
CAUSES BOTH THE ST AND T VECTORS TO GO AWAY
FROM THE INVOLVED AREA

FIGURE 30

Now, what about the posterior subepicardial Cell B? Let us do the same
for it. First, it loses the shoulder off its action potential, as shown in
Figure 31.

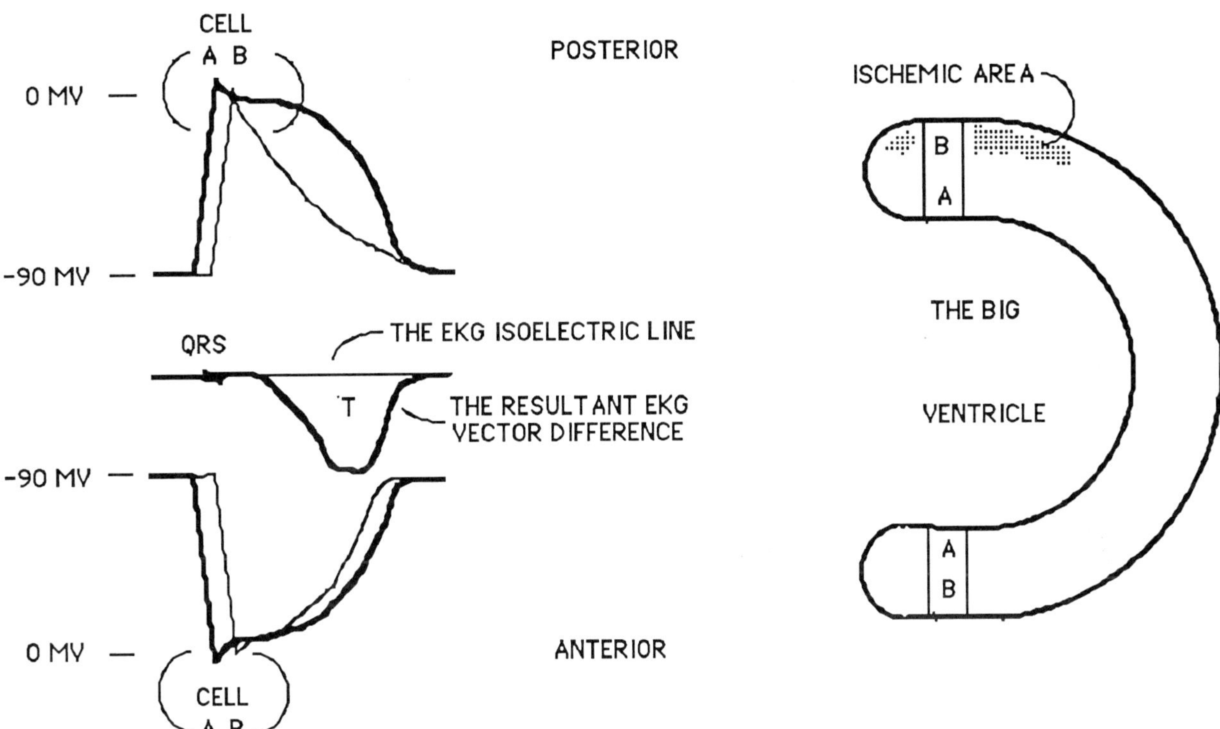

FIGURE 31

49

Once again, adding the opposing vectors, we see that the T wave vector moves away from the involved area, just as it did in Figure 29 when Cell A was ischemic.

Now, as Cell B further loses K so that its resting potential falls <u>with respect to Cell A,</u> the baseline now moves in the <u>opposite</u> direction, as the potential relationship of Cell A <u>with respect to that of Cell B</u> is reversed. This gives the result shown in Figure 32, a combination of ST <u>elevation</u> and T <u>inversion.</u>

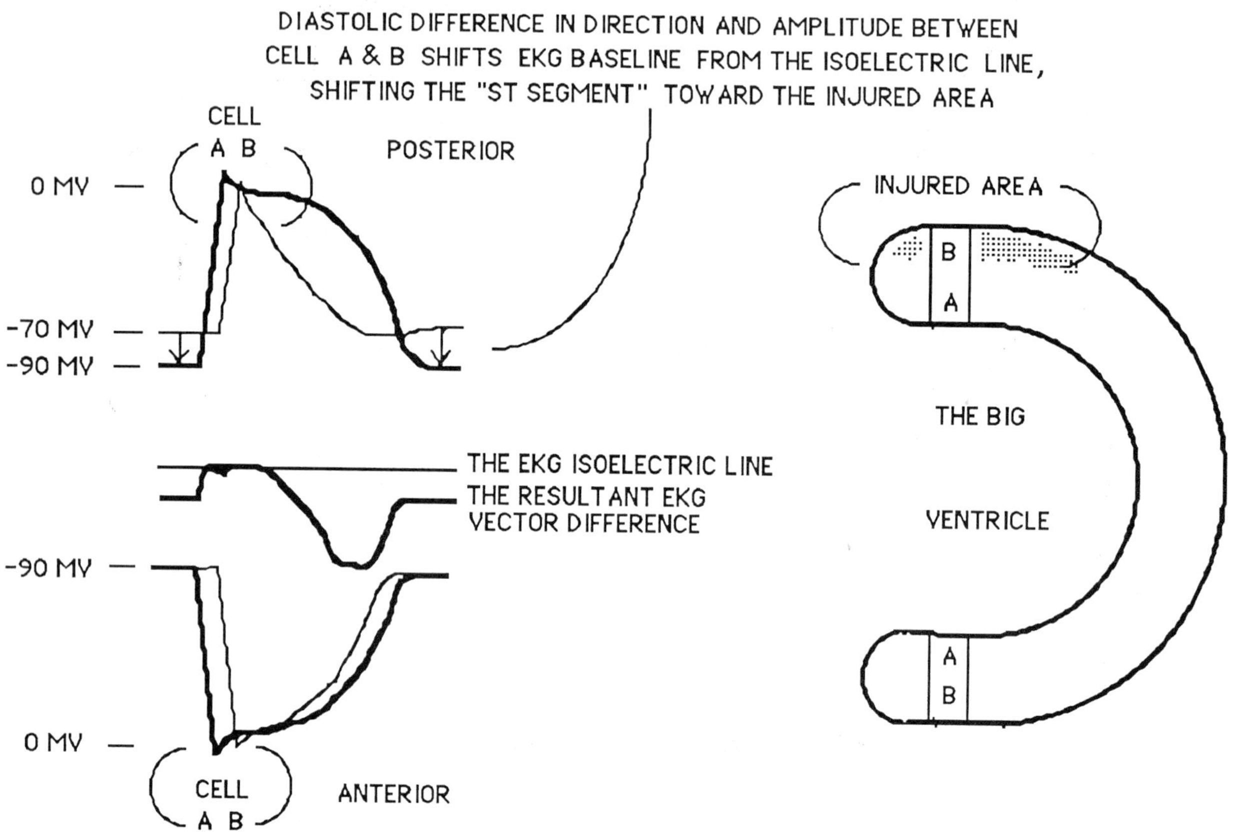

SUBEPICARDIAL INJURY (LOSS OF RESTING POTENTIAL) CAUSES THE ST SEGMENT VECTOR TO SHIFT TOWARD THE INVOLVED AREA, WHILE THE T VECTOR GOES AWAY FROM IT

<u>FIGURE 32</u>

Now, as viewed from the point of view of an exploring EKG electrode in the posterior region, the ST segment (or ST vector) is shifted <u>toward</u> the involved area, while the T wave vector is still shifted away, and we have the characteristic ST elevations seen with subepicardial ischemic pathology. Note that the T inversion may also be somewhat less here than with subendo-cardial pathology.

Summing all this up, we have:

Location of Pathology	ST Segment	T Wave
Subendocardial	Away	Away
Subepicardial	Toward	Away, but perhaps less so.

Here we have the basic relationship shown in Figure 28 for normally functioning cells. Now let us first have the typical Cell A undergo the K loss associated with strain or ischemia. It loses the shoulder off its action potential, causing the T wave to become inverted, as shown in Figure 33.

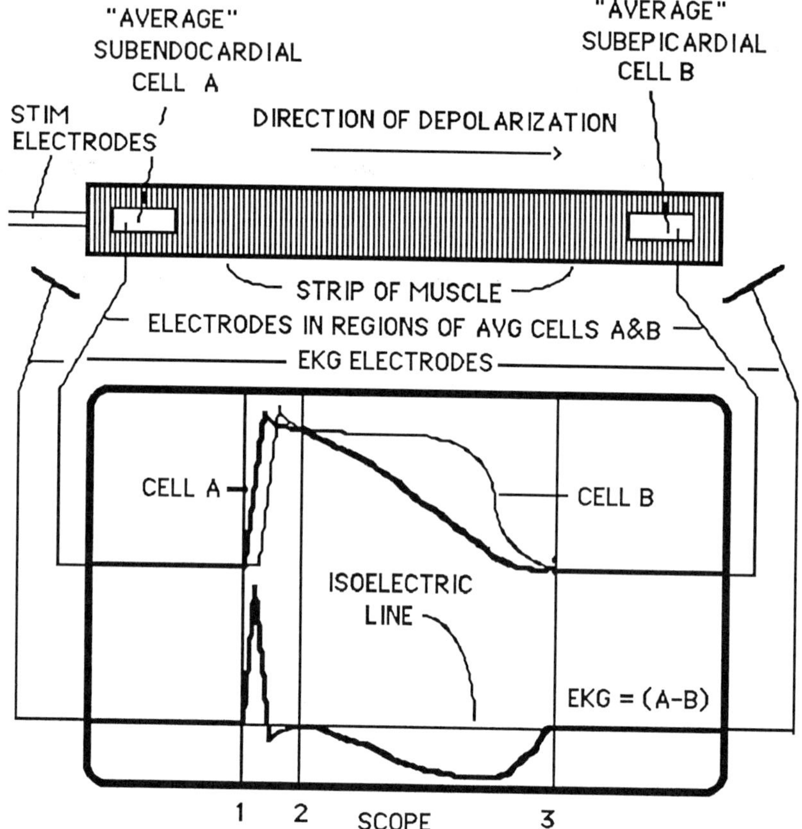

FIGURE 33

52

As the K loss progresses and Cell A's resting potential falls, we have the ST segment shift shown in Figure 34. Severe K loss in subendocardial Cell A causes an upward baseline shift which appears to our eyes as an ST segment depression.

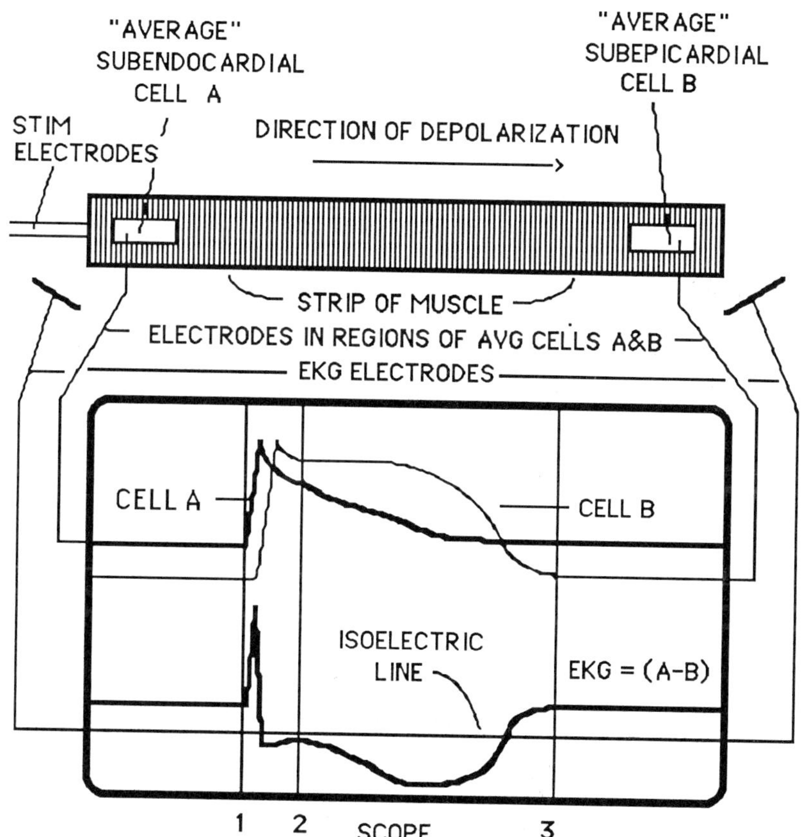

FIGURE 34

Now let us consider similar events in Cell B of the unopposed ventricular strip. Here things get a bit different. Note, as shown in Figure 35, that when strain or ischemia cause the K loss and the loss of the shoulder of the action potential of Cell B, this now results in a taller and broader T wave than we usually see in this lead. This is similar to some of the "hyperacute" T changes associated with anteroapical or inferoapical ischemia, where the ventricular tissue has no symmetrical corresponding ventricular tissue opposite to it.

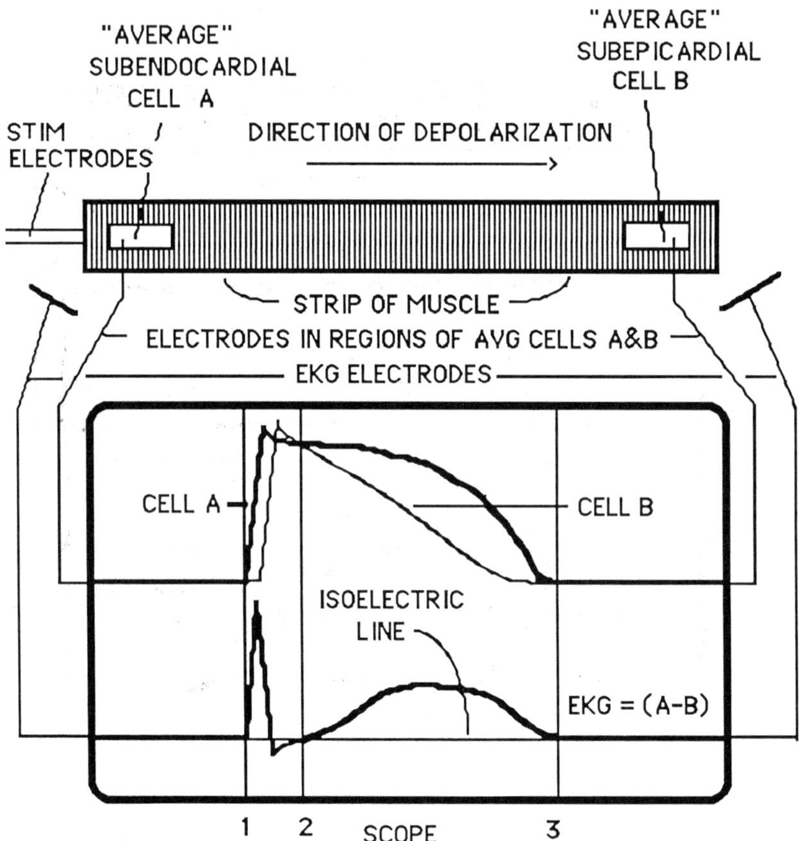

<u>FIGURE 35</u>

As this K loss progresses further and Cell B's resting potential falls, we now get ST segment elevation plus the taller and and broader T waves. Clinically, this reminds us again of the hyperacute ST-T changes we see in the anteroapical and inferoapical areas, where there is no corresponding opposite ventricular tissue. However, this explanation does not always work, as one may see such changes in several regions all at the same time, but perhaps losses in one area may leave others relatively unopposed.

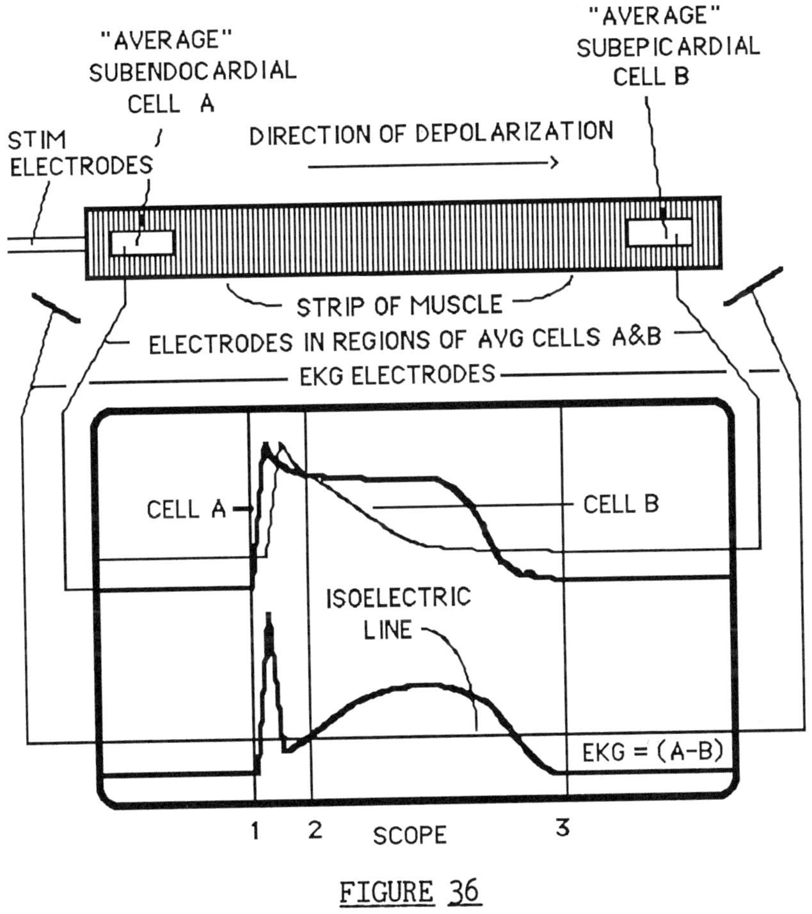

FIGURE 36

Summing this up, we have, for the unopposed ventricular strip:

Location of Pathology	ST Segment	T Wave
Subendocardial	Depression	Inverted
Subepicardial	Elevation	Taller + broader ("hyperacute")

55

An atrophied ventricle gives a QRS voltage of low amplitude, and a hypertrophied ventricle gives a QRS voltage of increased amplitude. These changes may relate to the number of myofibrils per cell, which can increase or diminish with a greater or smaller work load. These changes are reversible, as seen by the physical findings and EKG changes following successful treatment of hypertension, ligation of a patent ductus arteriosus, removal of a pheochromocytoma, mitral or aortic valvuloplasty or replacement, correction of septal defects, etc.

At birth the relative masses of right and left ventricles are about equal, because the right ventricle works under systemic pressure into a high-resistance, high-afterload pulmonary circulation. A normal newborn's EKG therefore has about the same appearance as does right ventricular hypertrophy in an adult.

Following birth, the lungs are inflated and pulmonary vascular resistance and right ventricular pressure fall. During the first two years of life the EKG and VCG gradually lose the appearance of right ventricular hypertrophy and gradually assume the configuration we are used to seeing and calling "normal" from then on. One might view this as disuse atrophy of the right ventricle following birth.

RIGHT VENTRICULAR HYPERTROPHY

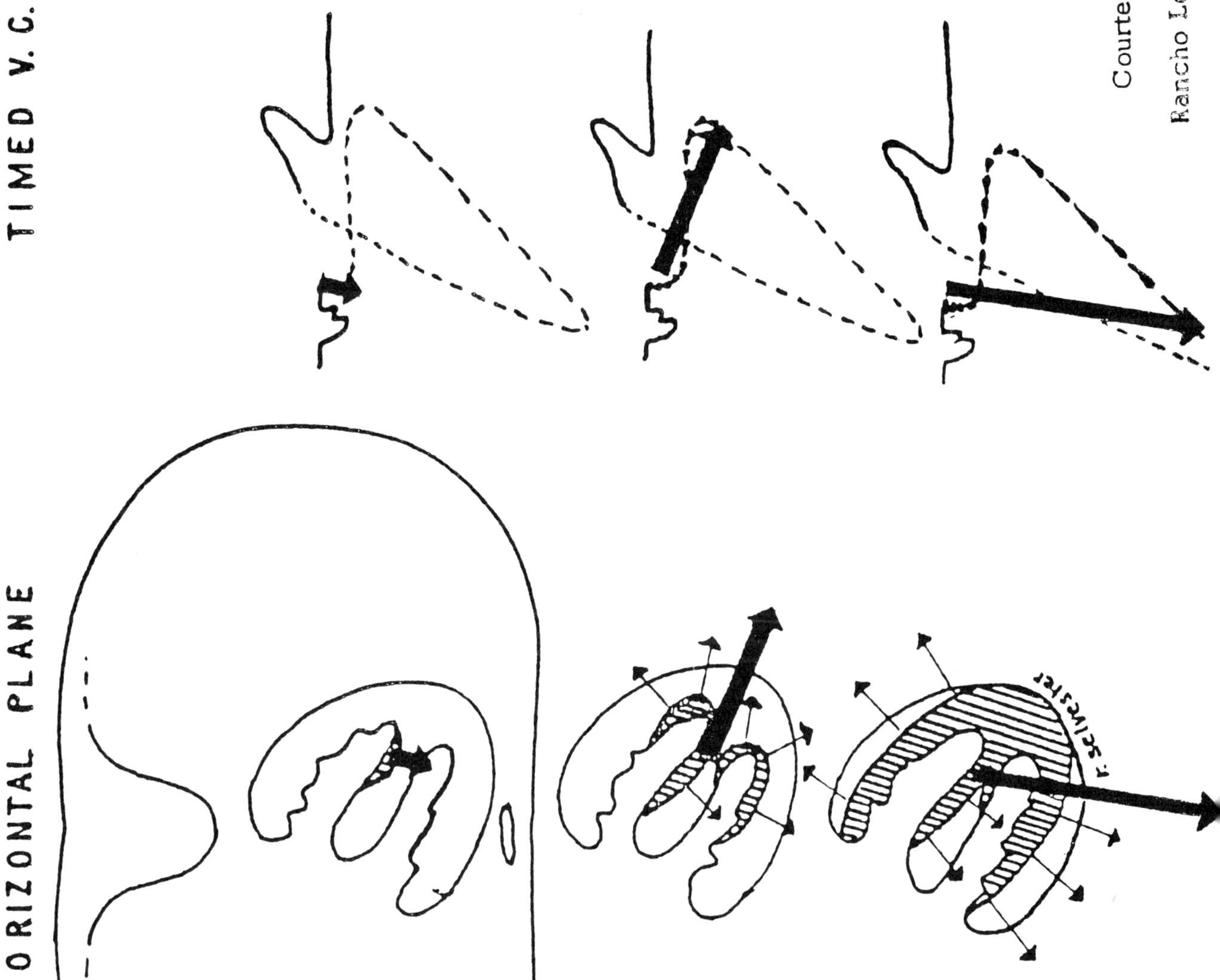

Courtesy of Dr. Ronald Selvester,
Rancho Los Amigos Hospital

FIGURE 37

This record shows regular sinus rhythm. The frontal QRS axis is +90, the T axis is +60, and the P axis is +75 degrees. The horizontal QRS axis has a double transition, one between V2 and V3, the other at V4-V6. There is clearly excess anterior force. The horizontal T axis is about -40, the P axis is about +10 degrees. There is evidence of left and possible right atrial enlargement. The rightward and anterior QRS forces suggest right ventricular hypertrophy, and the T changes suggest right ventricular strain (and/or anterior ischemia). Suggest repeat or serial records and clinical correlation.

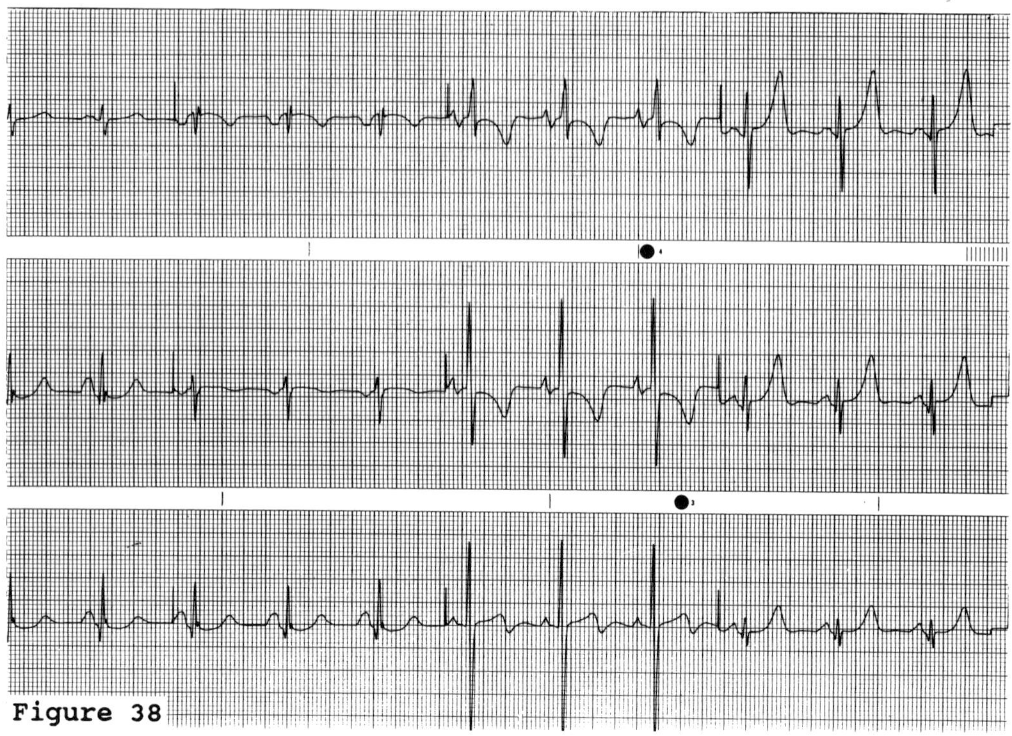

Figure 38

This record shows sinus tachycardia at 158/min. The frontal QRS axis is +105, the T axis is +60, the P axis is +80 degrees. The horizontal QRS axis has a double transition with excess anterior force, the T axis is -25, the P axis is -50 degrees. The right and anterior QRS forces and the posterior T and P forces suggest right ventricular hypertrophy, right ventricular strain (and/or anterior ischemia), and left atrial enlargement.

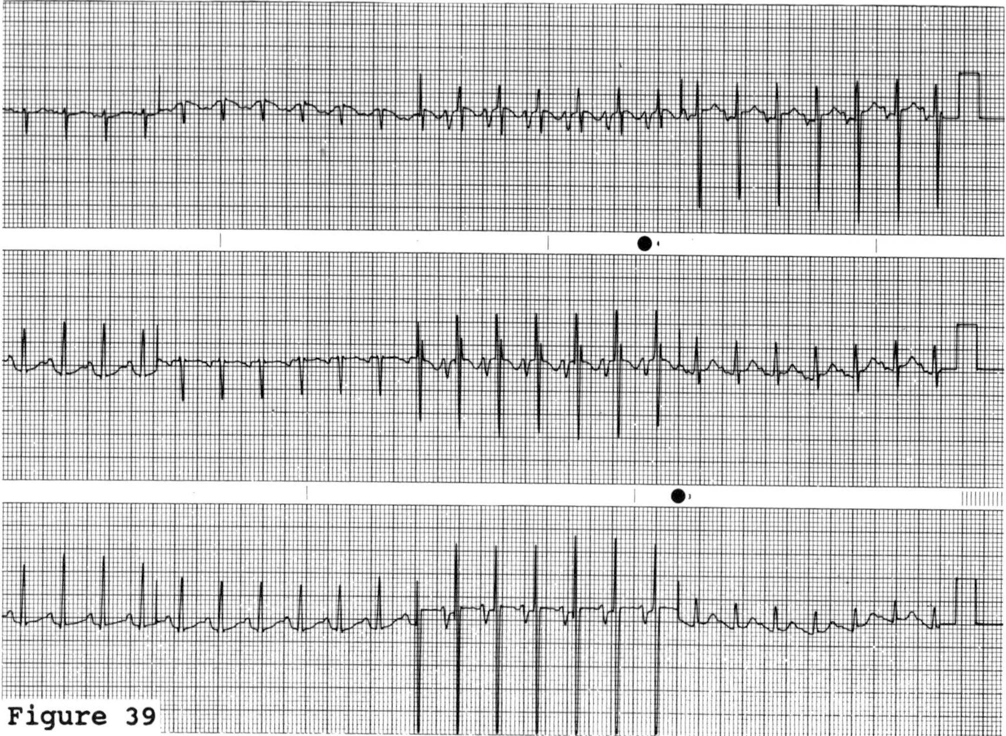

Figure 39

<u>RIGHT</u> <u>VENTRICULAR</u> <u>HYPERTROPHY</u> <u>(RVH)</u>: Figures 37 - 39.

When either ventricle hypertrophies, the <u>QRS</u> axis or vector is swung <u>toward</u> the direction of that ventricle and the <u>ST segment</u> and <u>T wave</u> axes are displaced or swung in the <u>opposite</u> <u>direction,</u> for the reasons we discussed in the previous chapter. As a result, RVH causes the terminal QRS complex to swing rightward, more vertically, and anteriorly in the frontal and horizontal plane. An RSR' complex (or a larger R) appears in lead V3R, V1 and V2, and a S wave appears in Lead 1 and V6.

The T vector swings posteriorly, and the T wave, which is normally inverted in V1, now becomes inverted in V2 and V3, as well, and possibly V4. With further increase in hypertrophy, the QRS vector swings further anteriorly until it assumes the form shown in Figures 37 - 39. There is a tall R' in V1, V2, and V3 with a depressed ST segment and an inverted T wave. In the limb leads the QRS vector becomes more vertical and may even swing beyond +120 degrees.

Clinically, RVH is often seen with mitral stenosis, pulmonary emphysema, cor pulmonale, and congenital lesions such as pulmonary stenosis, Tetralogy of Fallot, and atrial and ventricular septal defects.

<u>LEFT</u> <u>VENTRICULAR</u> <u>HYPERTROPHY</u> <u>(LVH)</u>: Figures 40 - 42.

Here the left ventricle (actually the left, posterior, and superior ventricle) swings the QRS vector in the above mentioned directions. Left axis deviation appears, and the terminal portion of the QRS loop is swung leftward, upward, and posteriorly, and the voltage is increased. LVH is recognized by deep S waves in V1 and V2, tall R waves in V5 and V6, and left axis deviation in the limb leads. Again, the ST segment and the T wave are swung in the opposite direction. The T waves become upright in V1,

LEFT VENTRICULAR HYPERTROPHY

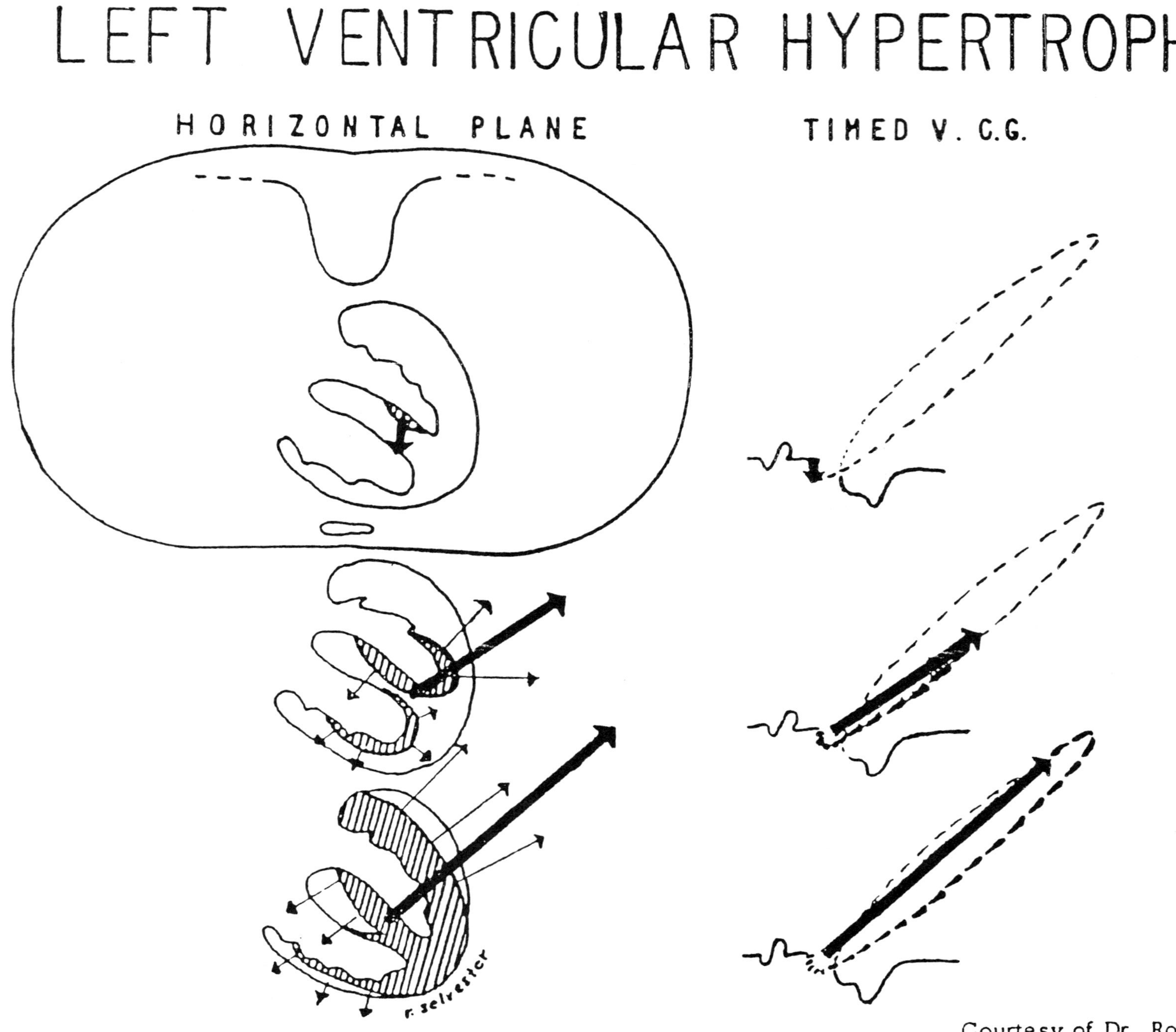

FIGURE 40

Courtesy of Dr. Ronald Selvester,
Rancho Los Amigos Hospital

This record shows regular sinus rhythm. The frontal QRS axis is +45, the T axis is -135, and the P axis is +35 degrees. The horizontal QRS axis is -15, the T axis is +160, and the P axis is zero degrees. The QRS duration is slightly wide. This EKG has 24 mm of voltage in lead 2 and evidence of left atrial enlargement, all of which are consistent with left ventricular hypertrophy. The T changes are consistent with left ventricular strain and/or inferior, posterior, and lateral ischemia. Suggest repeat or serial records and clinical correlation.

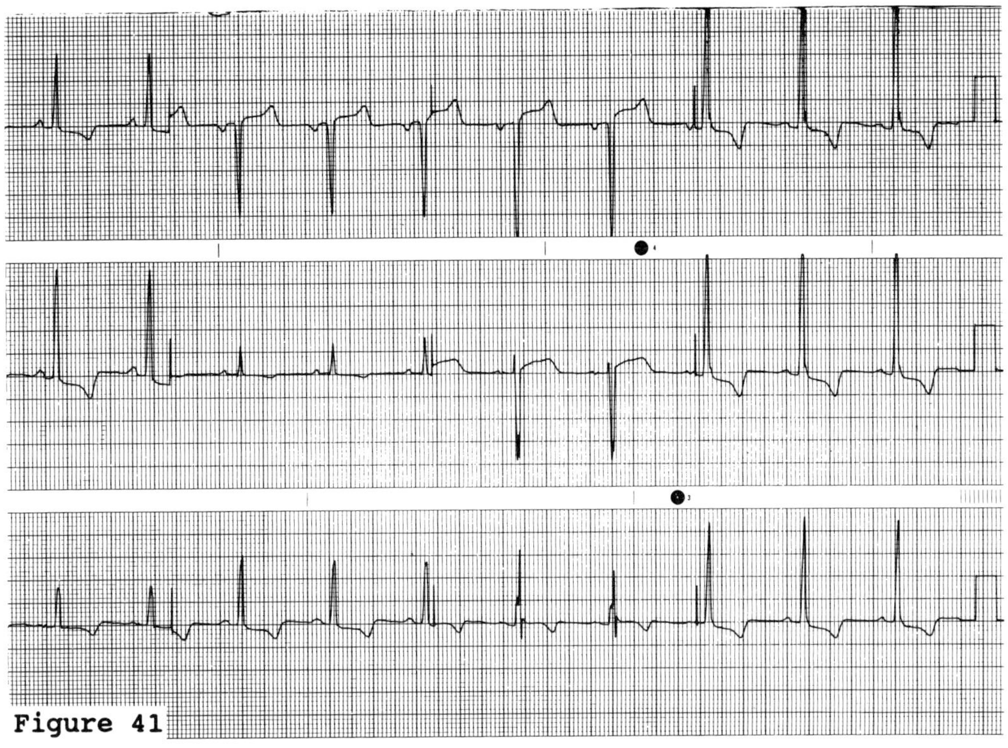

Figure 41

This record shows regular sinus rhythm. The QRS duration is slightly wide, .11 seconds. The frontal plane QRS axis is +75, the T axis is 180, and the P axis is +60 degrees. The horizontal plane QRS axis is -30, the T axis is +145, and the P axis is about +45 degrees. This record shows voltage in leads 2, 3, and aVF consistent with left ventricular hypertrophy, a slightly wide QRS consistent with the same, and T changes suggesting left ventricular strain and/or lateral ischemia. With LVH, the vertical frontal QRS axis suggests that combined LVH and RVH cannot be excluded. Suggest repeat or serial records and clinical correlation.

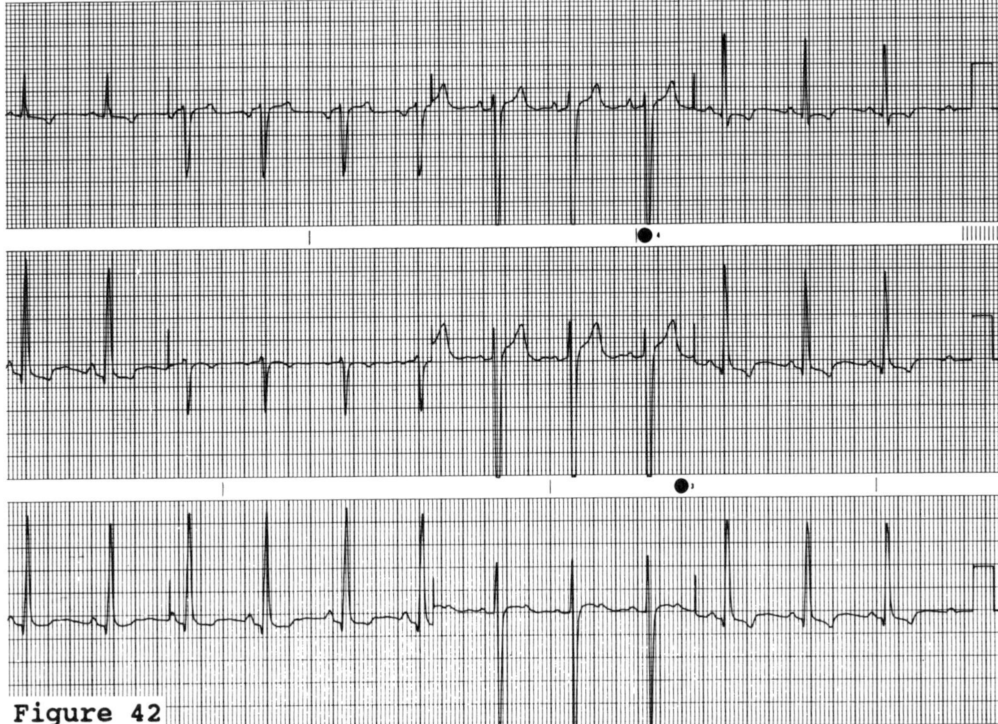

Figure 42

inverted in V6, and often inverted in leads 1 and aVL as well. The ST
segment is displaced in the direction of the T wave.

Clinically, LVH is often caused by arterial hypertension of any etiology, by aortic stenosis, aortic insufficiency, mitral insufficiency. etc..

Criteria for Left Ventricular Hypertrophy

Left ventricular hypertrophy has probably been one of the most
completely studied electrocardiographic entities. A plethora of criteria
are available with which to diagnose it, each with its own strengths and
weaknesses.

Sensitivity and Specificity

How do we evaluate such strengths and weaknesses? When we are seeking
a yes-or-no answer to a question, we can examine the sensitivity and specificity of a test, to evaluate the probability of a yes or no answer.
Sensitivity is defined as the percent of tests (EKG's) that are truly positive when the patients are known to be positive by some other "gold standard" criterion, such as heart weight as a percent of body weight, or some
similar expression. The percent of false-negative tests is 100% minus the
sensitivity. Specificity is defined as the percent of tests (EKG's) that are
truly negative by the "gold-standard" criterion. The percent of false-
positive tests or EKG's is 100% minus the specificity.

Bayes' Theorem

In 1763, the following work of the Reverend Thomas Bayes (1702-1761)
was posthumously submitted to and published by the Proceedings of the Royal
Society. It contains a theorem, now known by his name, which constitutes a
fundamental foundation of modern statistics and of the way we are now able
to perceive and understand reality. Reverend Bayes used this theorem to

help him "see through" the operations of chance, and to better understand the underlying structure of the world, and (to him at the time) the design of God for the universe.

This important theorem actually is used intuitively by all of us in making clinical judgments. It describes the _quantitative_ relationships between the "prior" probability of having some entity (LVH, etc.) _prior_ to obtaining some new relevant information such as an EKG, the quality (sensitivity and specificity) of that new information, and the revised, or "posterior", probability of having that entity (LVH, etc.) _after_ the new information has been obtained.

Bayes' Theorem is still more general. It also operates in a quantitative sense for entities that are continuous (pharmacokinetic parameter values, for example) in addition to discrete (yes/no) entities. Such pharmacokinetic applications, while important, will not concern us here.

Let us examine, using Bayes' Theorem, some of the common criteria used to recognize LVH. For example, the classical criteria of Sokolow and Lyon (3) have a sensitivity of 88% but a specificity of only 47%. The point score criteria of Romhilt and Estes have a sensitivity of only 58%, but a much higher specificity of 97% (4).

Let us use the following flow diagram to apply Bayes' theorem and to calculate the posterior probability of having LVH, supposing that the patient comes from a cardiology ward, where 25 percent (prior probability) of the patients there have LVH to begin with. Using the Sokolow & Lyon criteria:

Prior Probability	New Info (the EKG)	Positives & Negatives	
LVH 25	Sensitivity = .88 False Neg = .12	22 3	Prob pos/pos = $\frac{22}{(22+39.75)}$ = .36
No LVH 75	Specificity = .47 False Pos = .53	35.25 39.75	

If any 25 patients have LVH, then 88% of them, or 22, will be truly positive, and 12% of them, or 3, will be falsely negative. Similarly, of any 75 negative patients, 47% of them, or 35.25, will be truly negative, while 53% of them, or a whopping 39.75 patients, will be falsely positive.

Based on the above relationship, if the EKG is positive, the total number of positives generated (both true positives and false positives) is 22 + 39.75 = 61.75. Since the number of true positives is 22, the posterior probability of having LVH, given an EKG positive by the above criteria, is 22/61.75, or 36%. These criteria have <u>not</u> helped us much. If you think it is because the prior probability of 25% was already so high, redo the calculations using a prior probability of 5%, as in a shopping center family practice population, or a 1% probability, as might be the case in the Army. With these criteria, you can reliably be wrong much more often than right!!

Now let us do the same thing for the Romhilt and Estes criteria (a 5-point score or greater)

Prior Probability	New Info (the EKG)	Pos's & Neg's	
LVH 25	Sensitivity = .58 False Neg = .42	14.5 10.	Prob pos/pos = $\frac{14.5}{(14.5 + 2.25)}$ = .866
No LVH 75	Specificity = .97 False Pos = .03	72.75 2.25	

Here we see that these criteria will lead us to be correct far more often than those of Sokolow and Lyon. They also illustrate the power (and universality) of Bayes' Theorem throughout Medicine (and life!), and show us how using it, correctly taking into account both the prior probability and the quality of the test, can help us perceive things correctly much more often.

THE ROMHILT & ESTES CRITERIA - 1968 (4)

<u>Voltage</u> - R or S > 20mm in a limb lead, or

    - S in V1 or V2 > 30mm, or

    - R in V5 or V6 > 30mm --3 points

<u>ST-T</u> <u>Changes</u> - not on digitalis--3 points

        (on digitalis)----------------------------------1 point

<u>Left</u> <u>Atrial</u> <u>Enlargement</u>

    P in V1 down $\geq$ 1mm, with duration $\geq$.04 sec-----------------3 points

<u>Superior</u> <u>Axis</u> <u>Deviation</u>

    Frontal axis at least -30 deg------------------------------2 points

<u>Wide</u> <u>QRS</u> - $\geq$ .09 sec--1 point

<u>Late</u> <u>Intrinsicoid</u> <u>Deflection</u> (time from QRS onset to its last positive

    deflection in V5 or V6)

    $\geq$.05 sec in V5 or V6--1 point

Total of 5 points = LVH

Total of 4 points = Probable LVH

Sensitivity = 58 percent

Specificity = 97 percent

<u>ST Segment Changes with Left or Right Ventricular Hypertrophy</u>

Intramyocardial pressure is greatest in the subendocardial regions, and progressively decreases from endocardium to epicardium. Because of this, the systolic resistance to coronary blood flow is greatest in the subendocardial area. The blood supply to the myocardial cells is therefore worst in this area for the work that must be done.

It is probably for this reason that we see the ST depression (and T inversion) in V5 and V6 with LV strain, and its reciprocal ST and T elevation in V1 and V2. RV strain usually shows us ST depression and T inversion in V1, V2, and V3.

It is also likely that the usual ischemic ST depression seen with exercise and treadmill tests may also be for this reason. LV work is greatly increased, the subendocardial cells are most vulnerable, and most arterial lesions are in the larger coronary arteries which run over the surface of the heart, before its branches go inward to supply a certain region, to perfuse both its subendocardial and its subepicardial regions pretty much alike.

3
Intraventricular Conduction Defects

<u>LEFT</u> <u>BUNDLE</u> <u>BRANCH</u> <u>BLOCK</u> <u>(LBBB)</u>: Figures 43 - 46.

Here the apex of the right ventricle is depolarized first. Septal activation is now reversed (left and posterior). As a result, septal Q waves are not seen in V5 and V6, and only small R waves, if any, are seen in V1 and V2. The left ventricle then depolarizes, and the axis is displaced further posteriorly and leftward. The ST segment and T wave are displaced anteriorly (secondary ST-T changes). The lesion is best recognized by wide R waves in leads 1 and V5 and V6, usually with pronounced notching and an RSR' complex, followed by an inverted T wave and a depressed ST segment. The QRS duration is at least 0.12 seconds, and often is 0.14 or 0.16 seconds, as the left Purkinje system is bypassed, and the left ventricle depolarizes more slowly, primarily by the myocardial cells.

Clinically, LBBB correlates well with the presence of LVH and/or prior myocardial infarction, involving the left bundle branch system. <u>Incomplete</u> <u>left</u> <u>bundle</u> <u>branch</u> <u>block</u> is an uncommon form fruste which again correlates well with the presence of LVH or patchy myocardial fibrosis. It resembles LBBB but has a QRS duration between .09 and .12 seconds.

<u>RIGHT</u> <u>BUNDLE</u> <u>BRANCH</u> <u>BLOCK</u> <u>(RBBB)</u>: Figures 43 and 47-48.

When the conducted impulse cannot pass down the right bundle branch, the right ventricle cannot be activated by the normal pathway or at the usual time. As a result, the pathway of ventricular depolarization proceeds as shown in Figures 43 and 47-48. The left ventricle depolarizes in a normal manner, but the QRS vector at these times is probably displaced slightly posteriorly because of the absence of right ventricular participation. Following this, the right ventricle is depolarized more slowly, and the QRS

LEFT BUNDLE BRANCH BLOCK

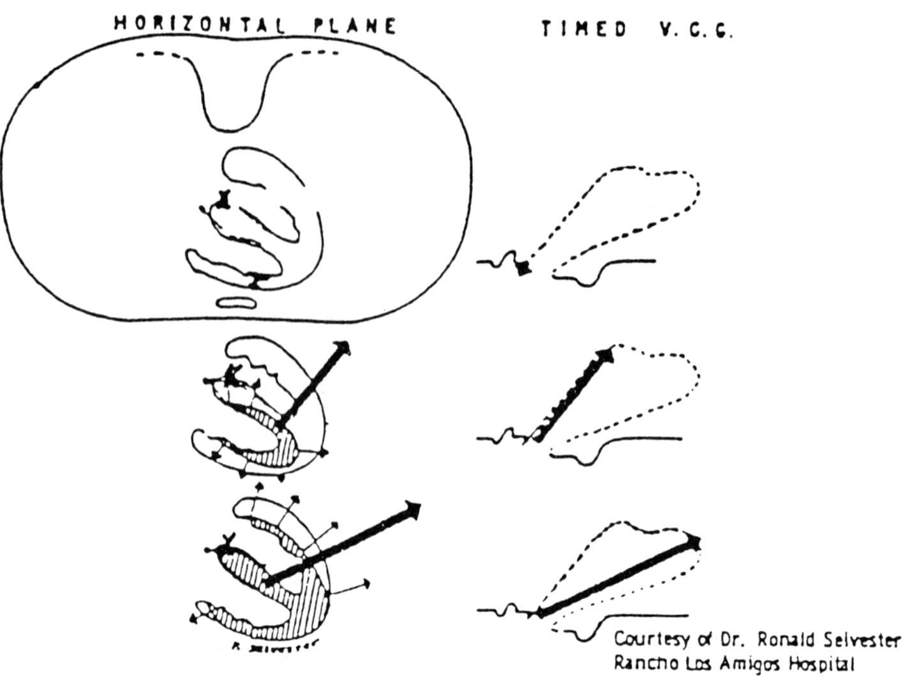

RIGHT BUNDLE BRANCH BLOCK

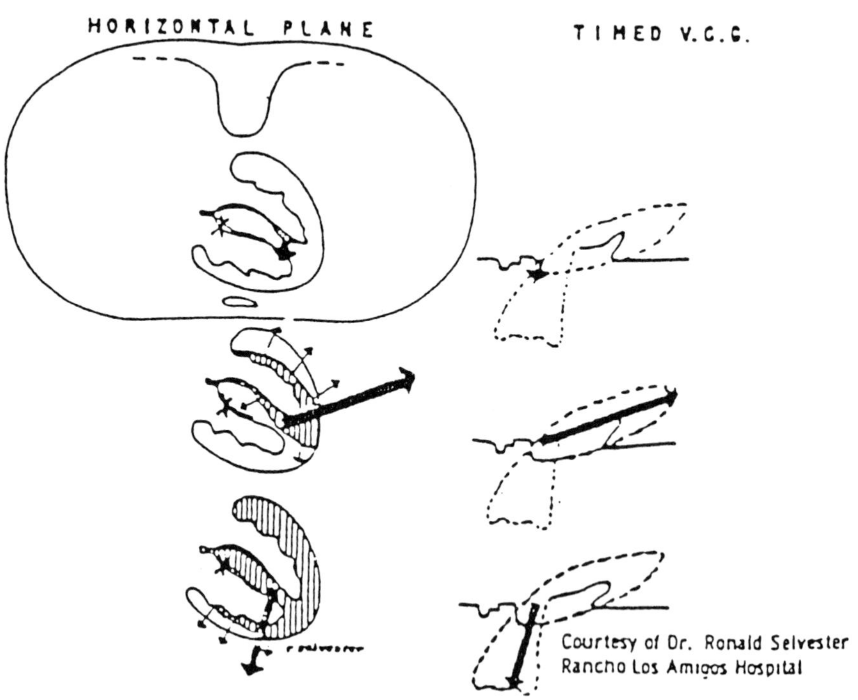

FIGURE 43

This record shows regular sinus rhythm and left bundle branch block. The QRS duration is .16 seconds. The frontal QRS axis is 0, the T axis is +135, and the P axis +40 degrees. The horizontal plane QRS axis is -50, the T axis is +130, and the P axis is probably about 0 degrees. Secondary ST-T changes associated with the left bundle branch block are seen.

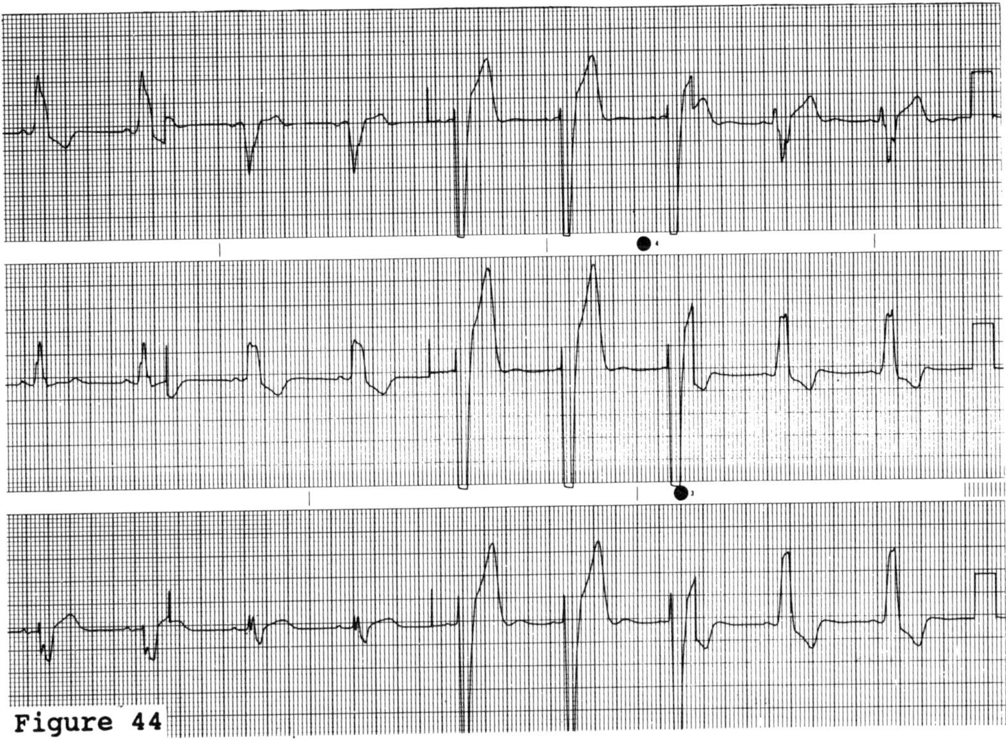

Figure 44

This record shows regular sinus rhythm and left bundle branch block. The QRS duration is .12 seconds. The frontal QRS axis is +15, the T axis is difficult to plot, and the P axis is +60 degrees. The horizontal plane QRS axis is -45, the T axis +105, and the P axis about +10 degrees. Typical secondary ST-T changes associated with left bundle branch block are present.

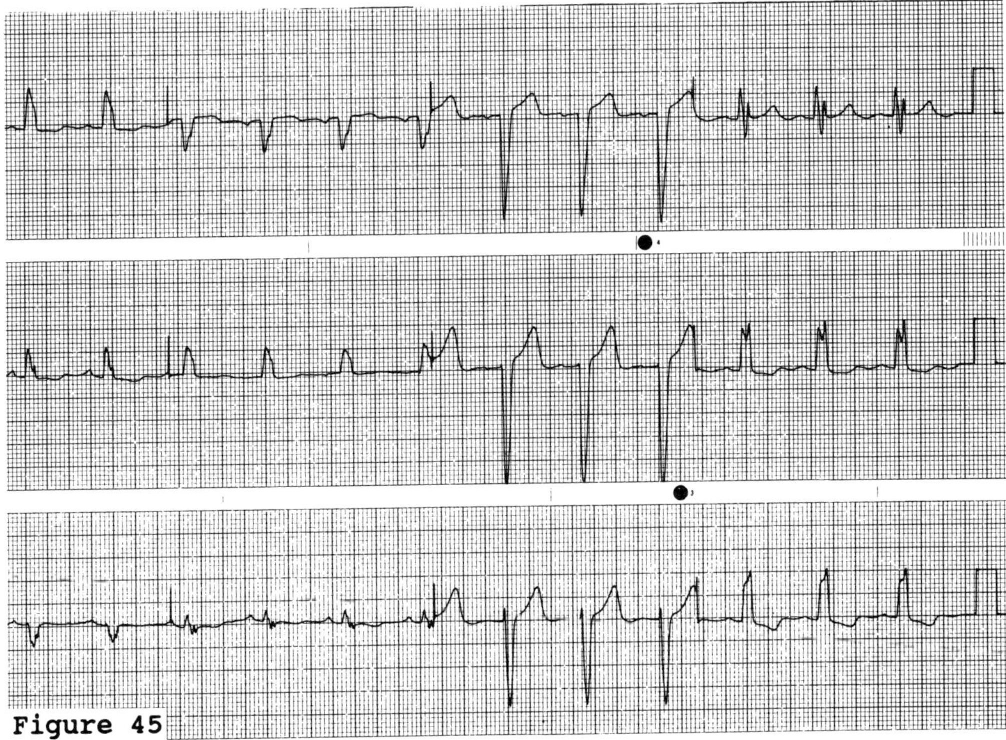

Figure 45

This record shows regular sinus rhythm and left bundle branch block. The frontal plane QRS axis is -10, the T axis is +120, and the P axis is +60 degrees. The horizontal QRS axis is -45, the T axis is +90, and the P axis is about +45 degrees. Typical secondary ST-T changes are present.

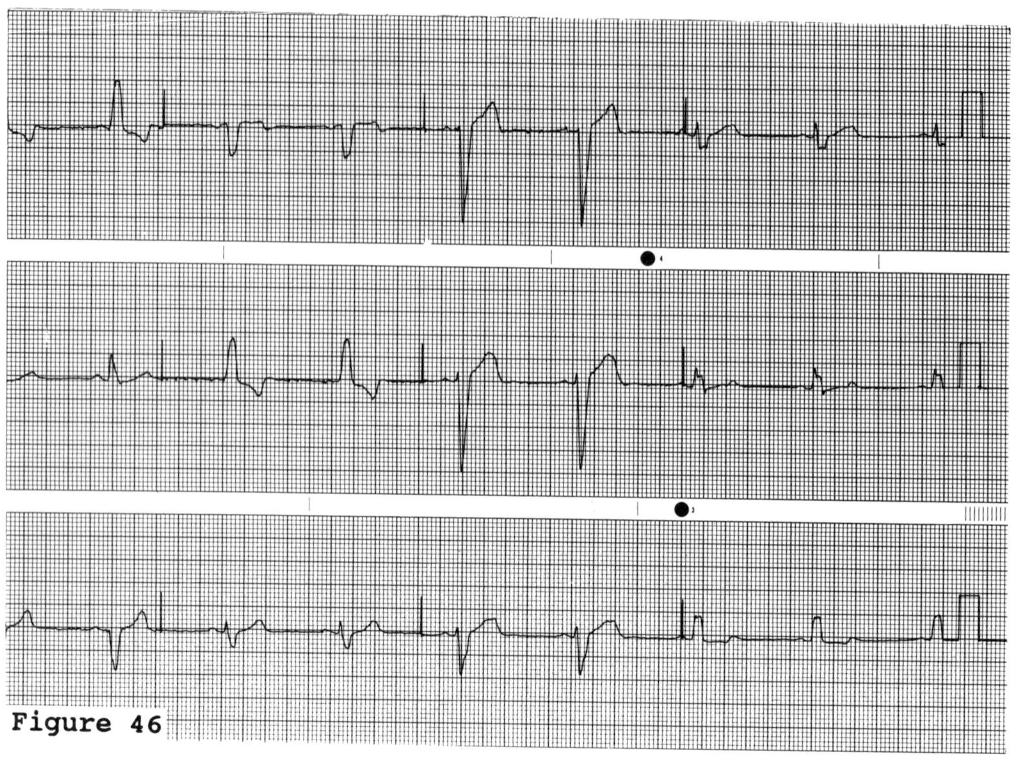

Figure 46

This record shows regular sinus rhythm and right bundle branch block. The frontal plane axis is about +30, the T axis is +60, and the P axis is about +45 degrees. The QRS duration is .12 seconds. The horizontal plane QRS axis is about +45, the T axis is about -30, and the P axis is about +45 degrees. Typical secondary ST-T changes associated with right bundle branch block are present, as the T is inverted in V1 through V3, but not in V4 through V6.

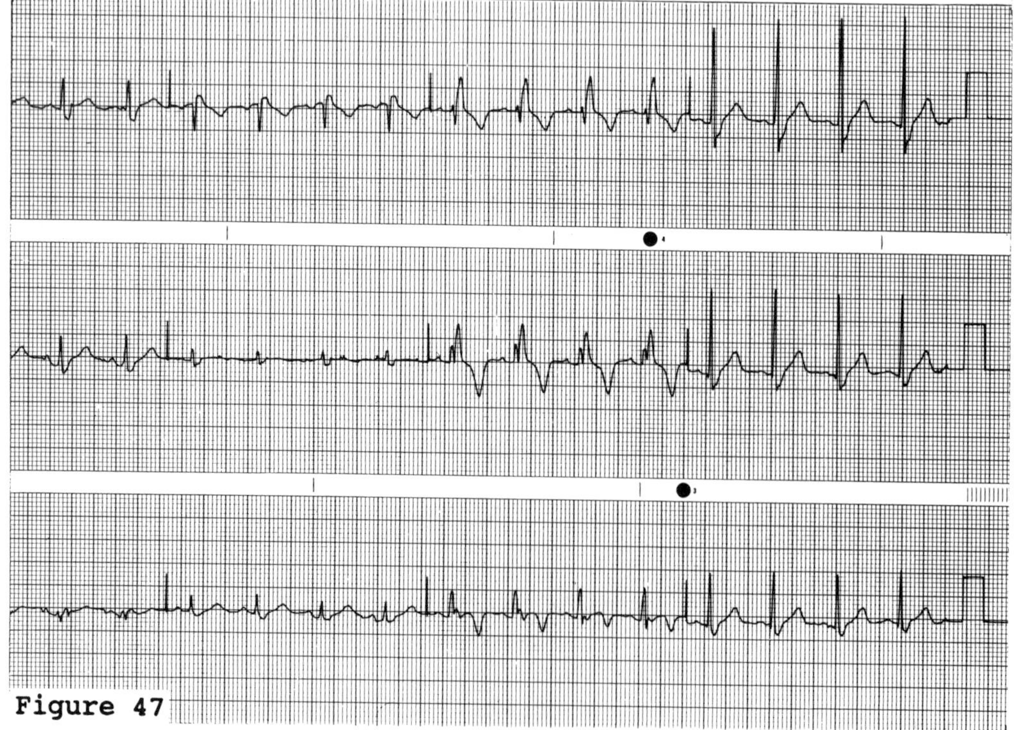

Figure 47

This record shows regular sinus rhythm and right bundle branch block. The QRS duration is .12 seconds. The frontal plane QRS axis is +100, the T axis is +60, and the P axis is about +80 degrees. A double transition is seen in the horizontal plane. One is between V1 and V2, and the other is between V2 and V4. Excess anterior forces are present in V1. The horizontal plane T axis is +5, and the P axis about +45 degrees. Posterior inferior hemiblock cannot be excluded.

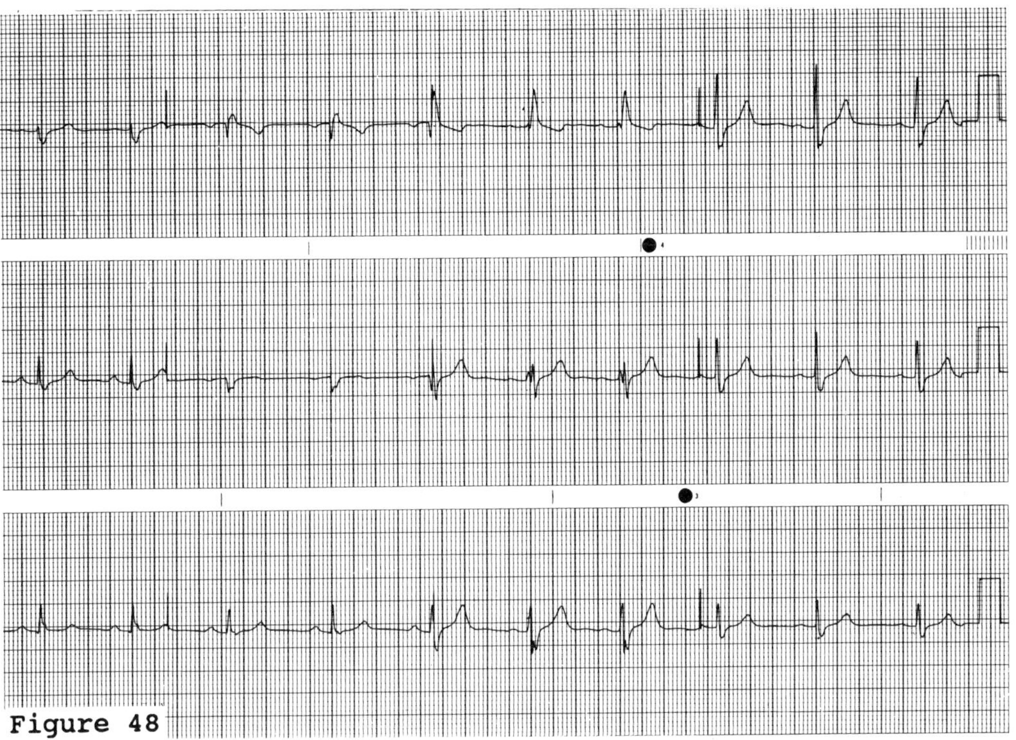

Figure 48

vector, now relatively unopposed, swings around anteriorly and to the right.
QRS duration in RBBB is longer than 0.12 seconds. RBBB causes a deep,
round, wide S wave in leads 1, V5, and V6, and a tall, round, wide R wave in
V1 and V2. These are the hallmarks by which this lesion is recognized.
<u>Incomplete</u> RBBB is a fairly uncommon intermediate form in which the shape of
the EKG leads and vector loop is similar, but the QRS duration is shorter,
between .09 and .12 seconds.

Clinically, RBBB is caused by myocardial lesions, by surgical pro-
cedures affecting the right bundle branch system, and by arteriosclerotic
heart disease or myocardial infarction involving the RBBB. It has been said
that transient "incomplete RBBB" may accompany acute cor pulmonale due to
pulmonary emboli. However, much of this information was gathered prior to
the days of the vectorcardiogram, and it is very likely that much "incomplete RBBB" may actually represent right ventricular enlargement.

The Hemiblocks

The left bundle branch itself divides into 2 (or more) branches, known
as the left anterior superior fascicle and the left posterior inferior
fascicle respectively. Either of these fascicles may be blocked. The main
manifestations of the hemiblocks are in the superior-inferior directions.
Little significant happens in a right-left or anterior-posterior direction.

<u>Left (Anterior) Superior Hemiblock (or Fascicular Block) LASHB</u>

Here the superior (or anterior and superior) fascicle is blocked, as
shown in Figure 49.

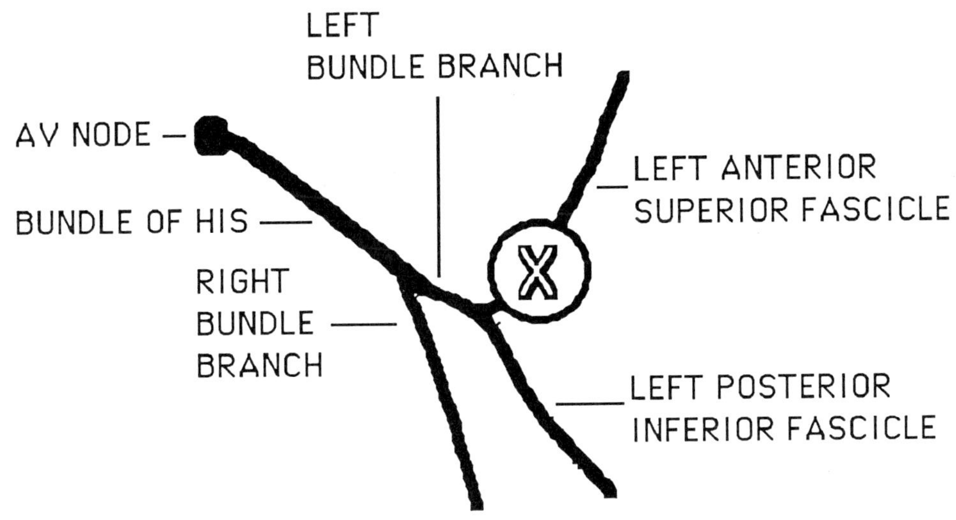

FIGURE 49

As a result the conducted impulse first goes inferiorly, causing R waves in Leads 2,3, and AVF. Then, spreading through the myocardial fibers (at about 1 meter/sec) instead of through the Purkinje system (at about 3-4 meters/sec), the wave of depolarization spreads superiorly, causing an R wave in AVL and S waves in 2,3, and AVF. In addition, the overall frontal axis is superior to -30 degrees, and the QRS complex is slightly wider than normal, usually wider than .09 or .095 sec, but not as wide as a full bundle branch block.

In general, then, LASHB is recognized by a frontal axis superior to -30 degrees, a slightly wide QRS complex (evidence for slow conduction outside the Purkinje system) and rS complexes in 2,3, and AVF. Examples are shown in Figures 50 - 53.

This record shows regular sinus rhythm, left atrial enlargement, left anterior superior hemi-block, and anteroapical myocardial infarction. The QRS duration is .11 seconds. The frontal plane QRS axis is -45, the T axis is +150, the P axis is +70 degrees. The horizontal plane QRS axis is -90, the T axis is +45, and the P axis is approximately -30 degrees, also consistent with left atrial enlargement. The abnormal R progression in V3 and the Q in V4 reflect anteroapical infarction. The absence of acute ST-T changes suggests that it might perhaps be old. The rightward and inferior frontal T axis may well represent secondary ST-T changes associated with the hemiblock, although left ventricular strain and/or superior ischemia cannot be excluded. Left ventricular hypertrophy is probably present. Suggest serial records and clinical correlation.

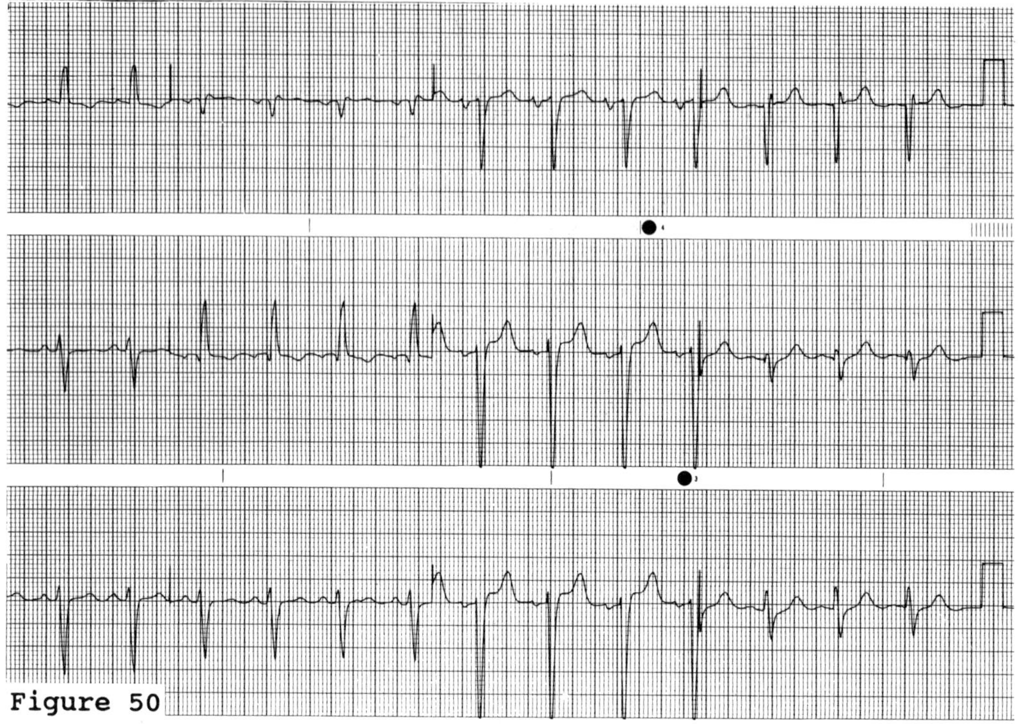

Figure 50

This record shows regular sinus rhythm, left atrial enlargement, probable left ventricular hypertrophy, probable left anterior superior hemiblock, and anteroseptal and anteroapical in-farction, possibly recent, with ST-T changes consistent with left ventricular strain and/or lateral ischemia with subendocardial injury. The frontal plane QRS axis is -30, the T axis is +120, and the P axis is +75 degrees. The horizontal plane QRS axis is -60, the T axis is +120, and the P axis is -20 degrees, also consistent with left atrial enlargement. Suggest repeat or serial records and clinical correlation.

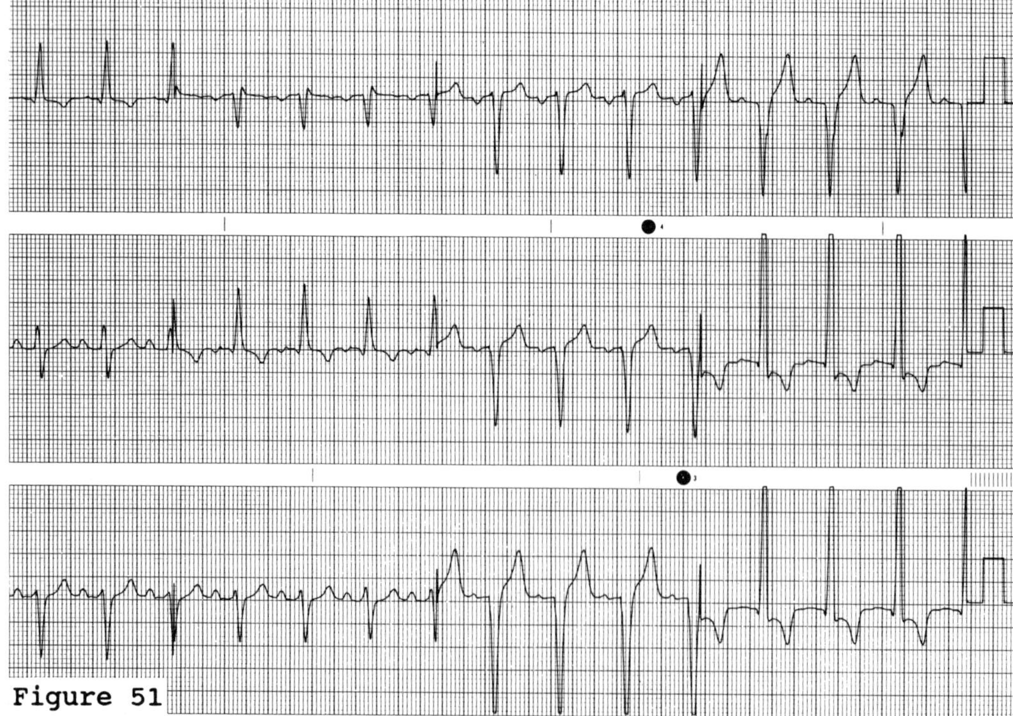

Figure 51

This record shows regular sinus rhythm, left atrial enlargement, anteroseptal infarction, left anterior superior hemiblock, probable left ventricular hypertrophy, and T changes consistent with lateral ischemia and/or left ventricular strain. The frontal plane QRS axis is -50, the T axis is +135, and the P axis is +60 degrees. The horizontal plane QRS axis is -40, the T axis +140, and the P axis is -15 degrees, consistent with left atrial enlargement.

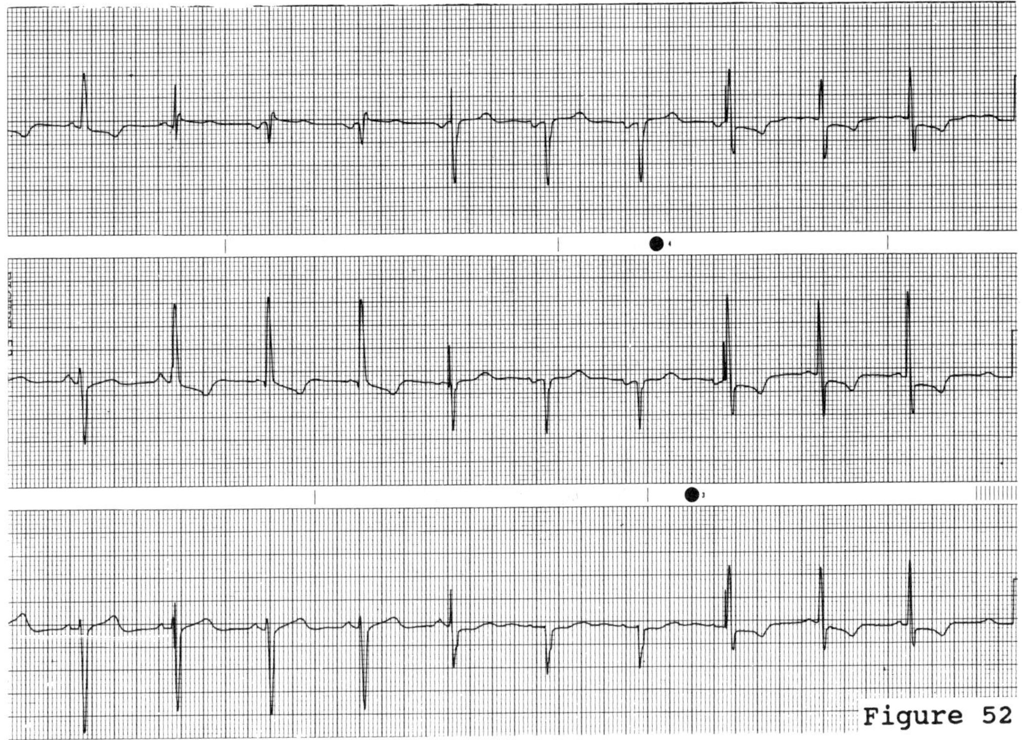

Figure 52

This record shows regular sinus rhythm, left atrial enlargement, left anterior superior hemiblock, and probable left ventricular hypertrophy. T changes consistent with left ventricular strain and/or lateral ischemia are present. The broad Q in AVL suggests that superior infarction cannot be excluded, although this may be part of the hemiblock. The frontal plane QRS axis is -60, the T axis +120, and the P axis +60 degrees. The horizontal plane QRS axis has a double transition at V2 and V5, and may be about -40, the T axis also has a double transition and may be about 180, and the P axis is -15 degrees, consistent with left atrial enlargement.

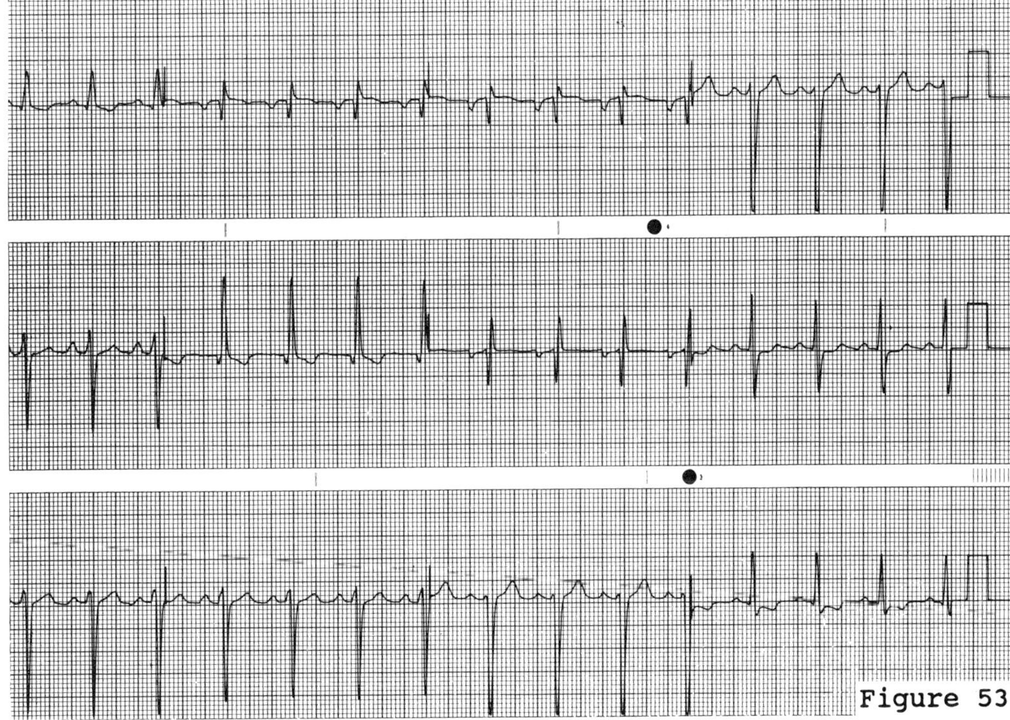

Figure 53

<u>Left (Posterior) Inferior Hemiblock (or Fascicular Block)</u>

Here the inferior fascicle is blocked, as shown in Figure 54.

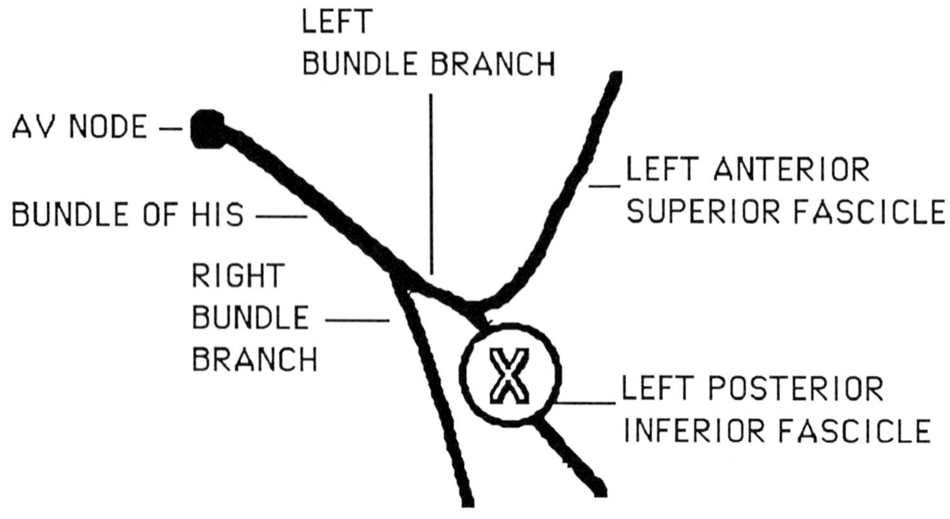

<u>FIGURE 54</u>

As a result, the wave of depolarization first proceeds superiorly, causing Q waves in 2,3, and AVF (just like those of an inferior myocardial infarct! - see later on). Then, spreading through the myocardial cells from above down, the wave of depolarization spreads inferiorly, causing S waves in AVL and R waves in 2,3, and AVF. In addition, the frontal axis is vertical, usually greater than +60 degrees, and the QRS complex is again slightly wider than normal, usually wider than .09 sec. In general, then, left posterior inferior hemiblock is recognized by a frontal axis more rightward than +60 degrees, by qR waves in 2,3, and AVF (the Q waves are indistinguishable from those seen with inferior infarction), and by a slightly wide QRS complex. Examples are shown in Figures 55 - 57.

This record shows sinus tachycardia, probable left posterior inferior hemiblock, left atrial enlargement, and T changes consistent with left ventricular strain and/or lateral and inferior ischemia. An inferior infarct cannot be ruled out. The frontal plane QRS axis is +115, the T axis is -60, and the P axis is +75 degrees. The horizontal plane QRS axis is -60 degrees, the T axis is about +45 degrees, and the P axis is -30 degrees. Suggest serial records and clinical correlation.

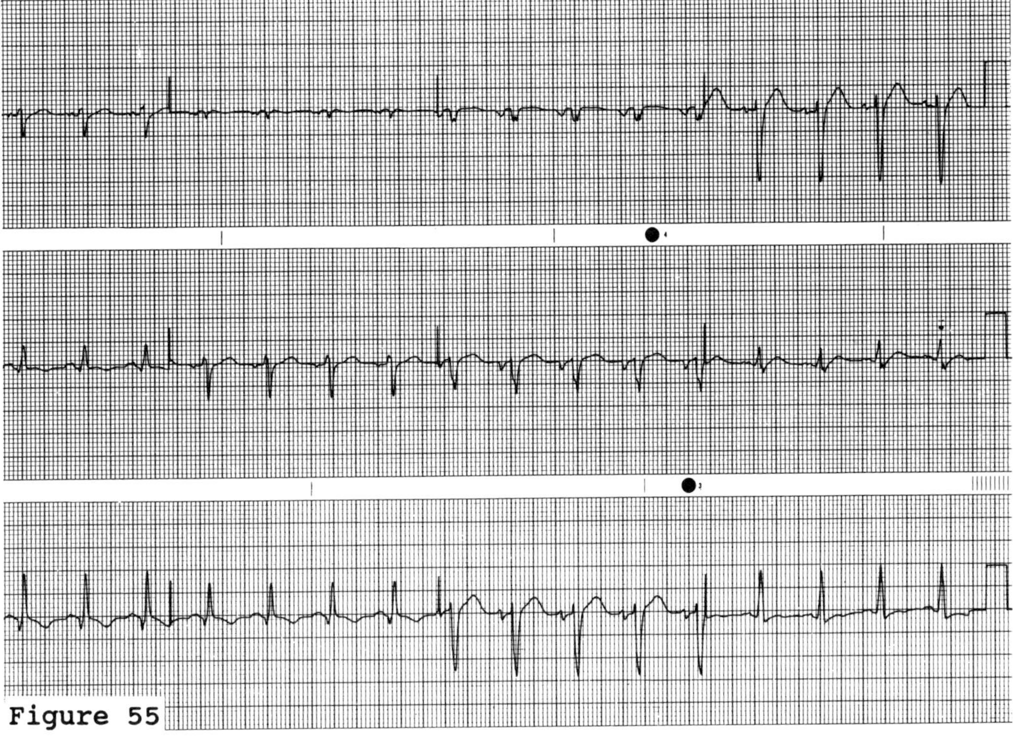

Figure 55

This record shows sinus rhythm, probable posterior inferior branch hemiblock, possible inferior infarction, possible left atrial enlargement, and an anteroapical infarct, possibly recent, with T changes consistent with lateral ischemia and/or left ventricular strain. The frontal plane QRS axis is +60, the T axis is +120, and the P axis is +75 degrees. The horizontal plane QRS axis is -45, the T axis is +150, and the P axis is -15 degrees. Suggest serial records.

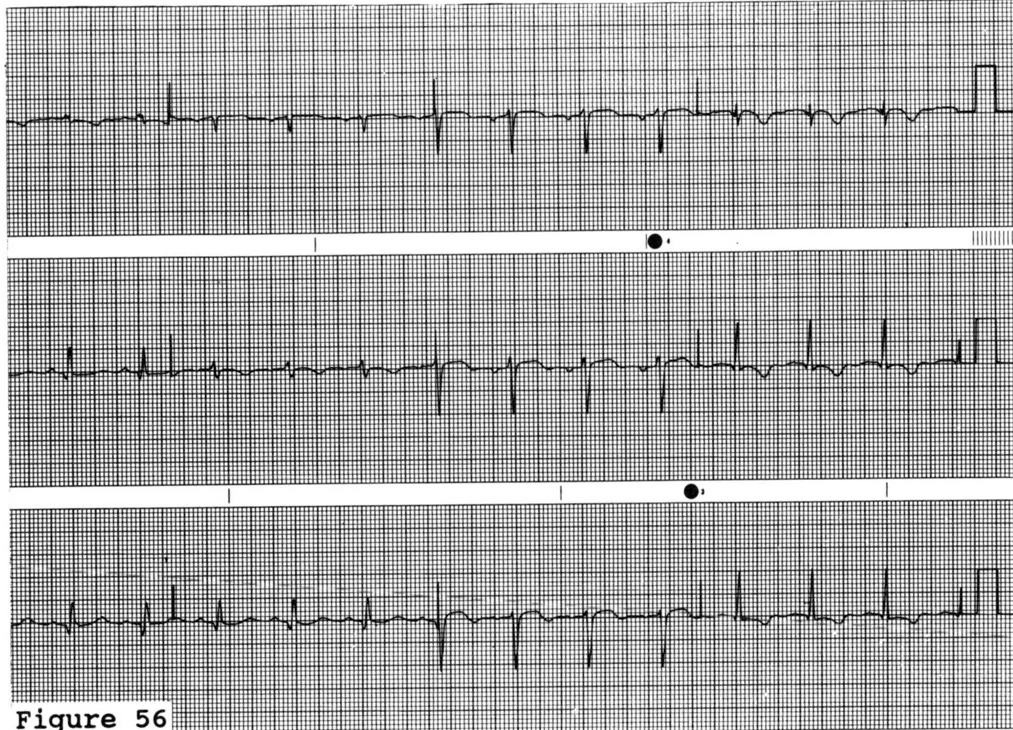

Figure 56

    This record shows regular sinus rhythm, first degree AV block, probable right bundle branch block, left anterior superior hemiblock, and a possible anteroseptal infarct. T changes consistent with left ventricular strain and/or lateral ischemia are present. The frontal plane QRS axis is -75, the T axis is +115, and the P axis is +45 degrees. The horizontal plane QRS axis is +90, the T axis is -90, and the P axis is difficult to plot, but may possibly be -20 degrees. Suggest serial records and clinical correlation.

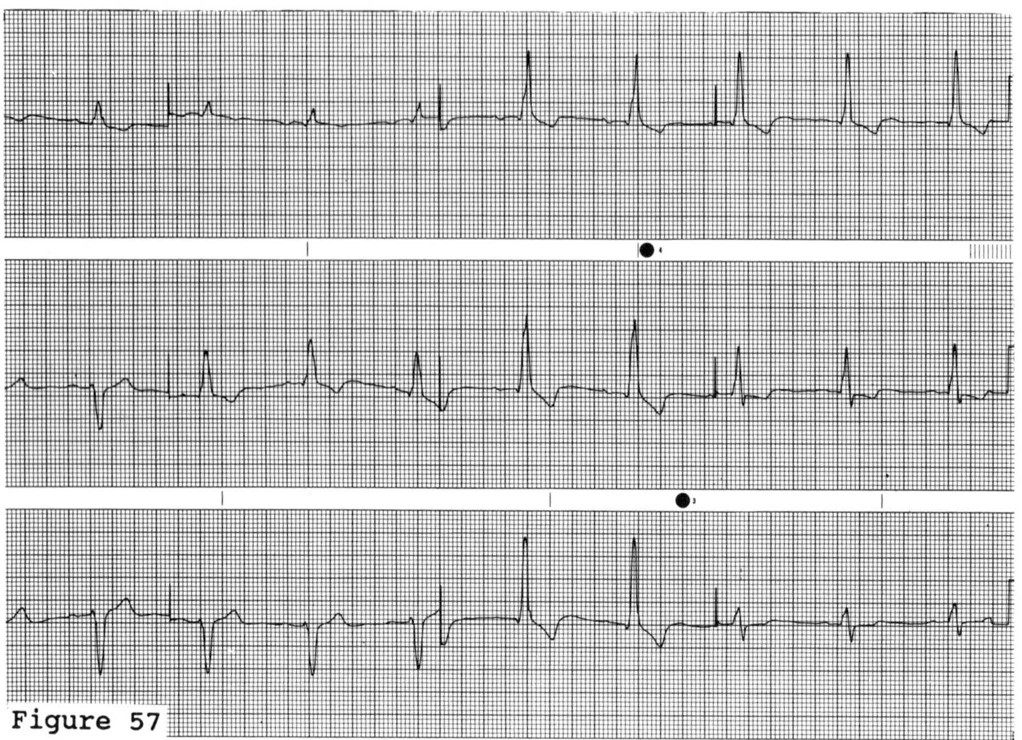

Figure 57

<u>Coexisting</u> <u>BBB</u> <u>and</u> <u>Hemiblocks</u>

Theoretically, all combinations of BBB and hemiblock may coexist in the same EKG. Common examples are RBBB and either LASHB or left inferior hemiblock. Less common is LBBB and LASHB. We have not yet seen LBBB and left inferior hemiblock together.

<u>Right</u> <u>Bundle</u> <u>Branch</u> <u>Block</u> <u>and</u> <u>LASHB</u>

Remember that RBBB usually has a normal frontal plane axis. When RBBB and LASHB coexist, the frontal axis shows the LASHB as well, with its superior axis deviation, the rS in 2,3, and AVF, and the slight further widening of the QRS complex. Examples are shown in Figures 58 - 60.

<u>Right</u> <u>Bundle</u> <u>Branch</u> <u>Block</u> <u>and</u> <u>Left</u> <u>Inferior</u> <u>Hemiblock</u>

When RBBB and Left Inferior Hemiblock coexist, the frontal axis (greater than +90 degrees), the Q waves in 2,3, and AVF, and the slight further widening of the QRS complex will reveal the lesion. This rare lesion must be distinguished (if possible) from an inferior infarct. A probable example is shown in Figure 61.

This record shows regular sinus rhythm, right bundle branch block, and left anterior superior
hemiblock. An anteroseptal infarct of undetermined age cannot be excluded. Typical secondary ST-T
changes associated with right bundle branch block are present. The frontal plane QRS axis is -90,
the T axis is +15, and the P axis is +45 degrees. The horizontal plane QRS axis is +90, the T axis
is -15, and the P axis is +5 degrees. Suggest repeat or serial records and clinical correlation.

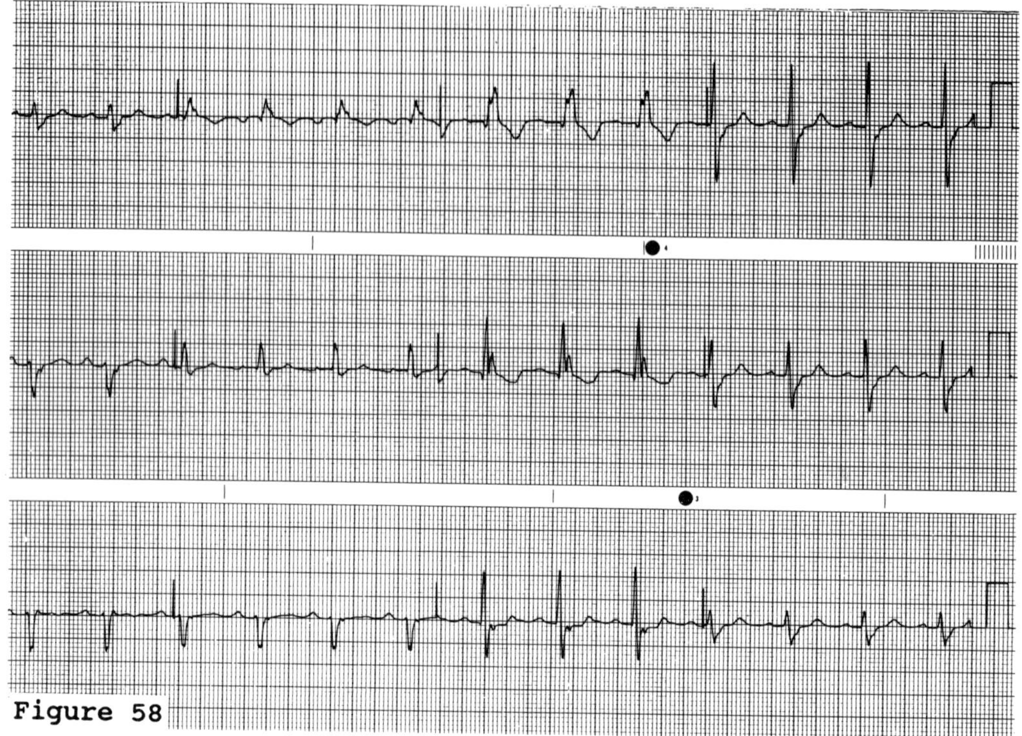

Figure 58

This record shows sinus tachycardia, possible left atrial enlargement, right bundle branch
block, left superior branch hemiblock, and a possible acute anteroseptal and apical infarct. ST
elevations are present in V3 thru V5, consistent with anteroapical subepicardial injury, and T
inversions in V4 and V5 suggest apical ischemia. The frontal plane QRS axis is about -90, the T
axis is +75, and the P axis is +90 degrees. The QRS duration is .16 seconds. The horizontal plane
QRS axis is about +110, the T axis is -80, and the P axis is about -40 degrees. Suggest serial
records.

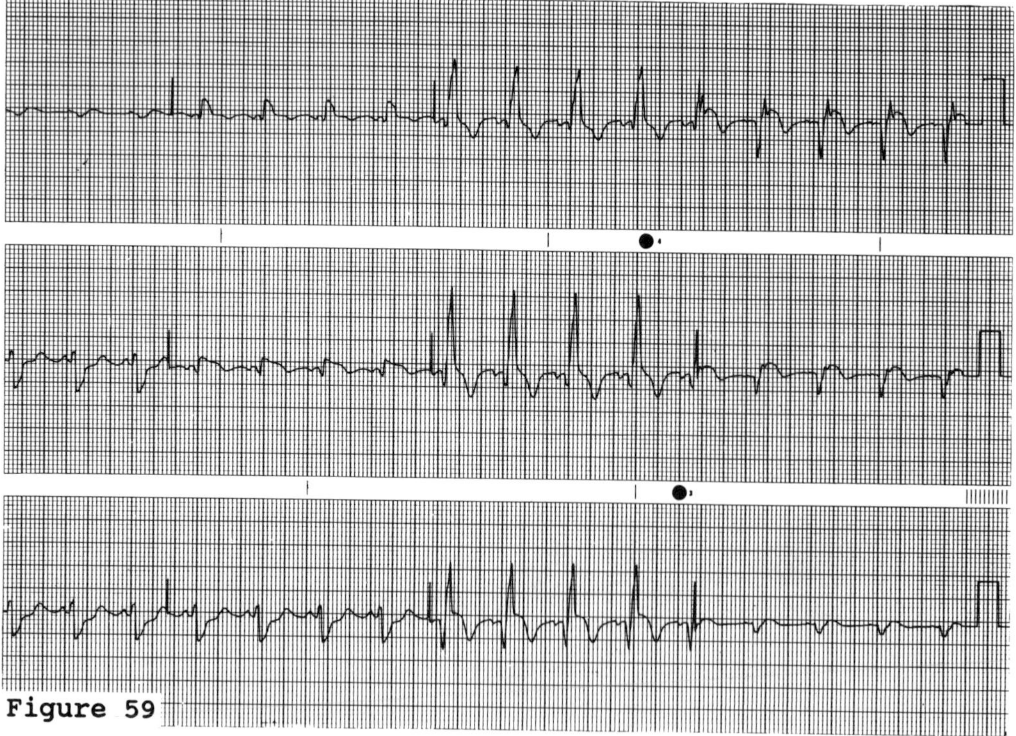

Figure 59

This record shows sinus rhythm, first degree AV block, possible left atrial enlargement, right bundle branch block, and left superior branch hemiblock. Inferior forces are minimal, and an inferior infarct cannot be excluded. The frontal plane QRS axis is -80, the T axis is +75, and the P axis is +45 degrees. The horizontal plane QRS axis is about +100, the T axis is 0, and the P axis is -10 degrees.

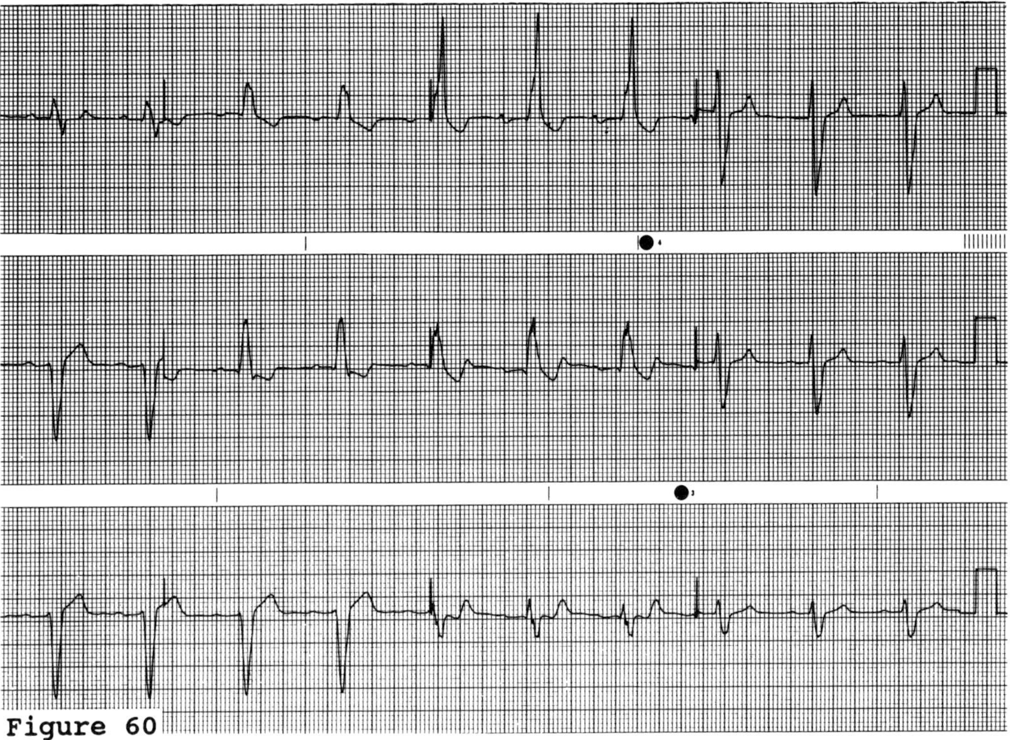

Figure 60

This record shows sinus tachycardia, right bundle branch block, and possible left posterior inferior hemiblock. The frontal plane QRS axis is +105, the T axis is -5, and the P axis is about +55 degrees. The QRS duration is .13 seconds. The horizontal plane QRS axis is about +60, the T axis is -70 degrees, and the P axis is difficult to plot. T changes associated with inferior and apical ischemia cannot be excluded. Suggest repeat or serial records and clinical correlation.

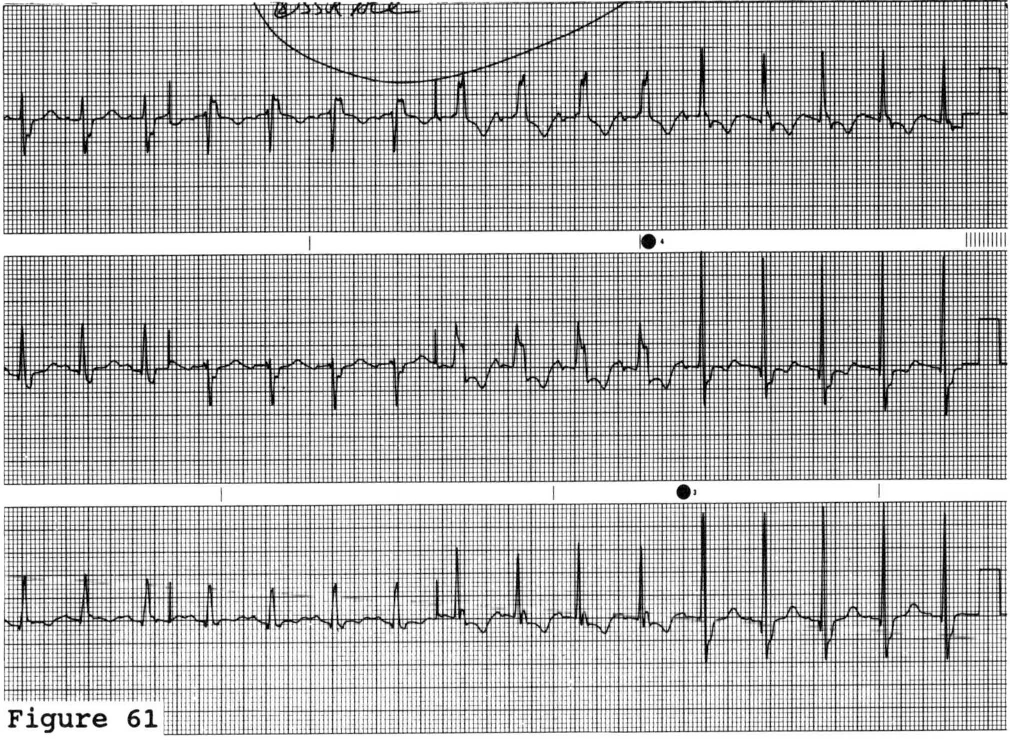

Figure 61

How can this be? If the patient already has LBBB, which blocks the whole left bundle branch, how can he have LASHB as well? He can, as shown in Figure 62.

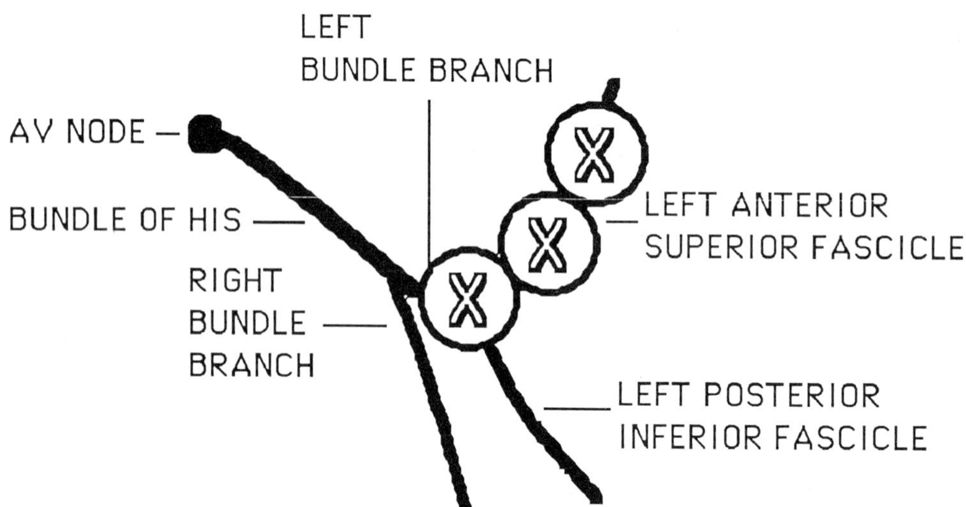

FIGURE 62

Note how the lesion not only involves the bundle, but also <u>extends</u> <u>up</u> the superior fascicle, including both.   As the impulse proceeds down the right bundle and then moves leftward, it will first encounter the functioning inferior fascicle which will rapidly depolarize the inferior portion, only later spreading more slowly to the superior portion, because of the LASHB.

LBBB, like RBBB, usually has a normal frontal plane QRS axis by itself, as shown earlier in Figures 43 and 44 - 46. LBBB with LASHB is recognized by the presence of both lesions together. The QRS is usually slightly wider than with LBBB alone, and the superior axis and rS complexes in 2,3, and AVF also give the hemiblock away. Sometimes, with LBBB, the LASHB may come and go in a day or so, clearly revealing its presence and absence. An example of LBBB and LASHB is shown in Figure 63.

<u>Left</u> <u>Bundle</u> <u>Branch</u> <u>Block</u> <u>and</u> <u>Left</u> <u>Inferior</u> <u>Hemiblock</u>

Theoretically, this lesion should also exist, showing LBBB with a vertical frontal axis and Q waves in 2,3, and AVF. However, we have not seen an example yet. It must also be distinguished from an inferior infarct.

<u>WOLFF-PARKINSON-WHITE</u> <u>SYNDROME</u>:   Figure 64 - 66.

The Wolff-Parkinson-White syndrome consists of a short PR interval (less than .12 sec) and a wide QRS complex (longer than .12 seconds). This is a "false" bundle branch block. The wide QRS is due to early depolarization of the ventricles via an accessory Bundle of Kent that does not insert the usual AV delay (P-R interval) that the AV nodal cells do. Usually a sharp delta wave initiates the QRS complex which then is replaced by the more normal main portion of the QRS complex.

        This record shows sinus rhythm, occasional atrial extrasystoles, left atrial enlargement, left
bundle branch block, and left anterior superior hemiblock. The QRS duration is .15 seconds. The
frontal QRS axis is -50, the T axis +120, and the P axis is +60 degrees. The horizontal plane QRS
axis is -85, the T axis is +110, and the P axis is -10 degrees. An apical infarct of undetermined
age cannot be excluded, as suggested by the possible abnormal R progression from V2 thru V5. Suggest
repeat or serial records and clinical correlation.

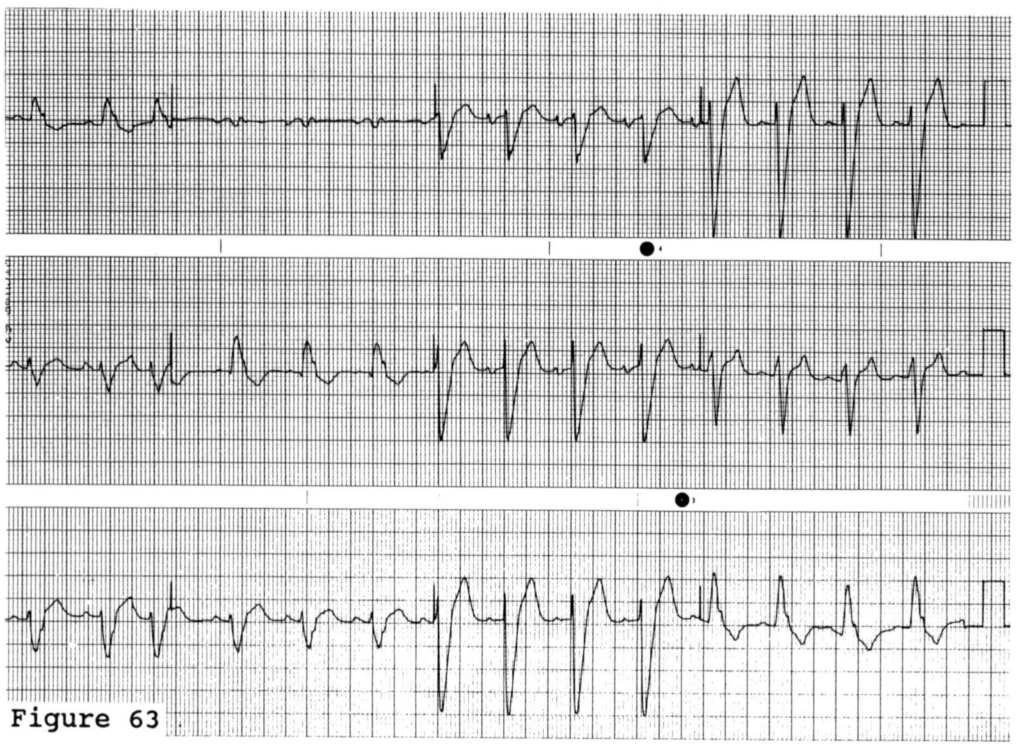

Figure 63

This record shows regular sinus rhythm and the Wolff-Parkinson-White Syndrome. The frontal
plane QRS axis is -15, the T axis is +15, and the P axis is +45 degrees. The frontal plane axis of
the Delta wave is about -60 degrees. The horizontal plane QRS axis is about +30, the T axis is +30,
the P axis is +45, and the horizontal plane delta axis is about +45 degrees. The Bundle of Kent may
be located inferiorly and posteriorly. An inferior infarct cannot be completely excluded. The
relatively normal PR interval is longer than is usually seen with WPW, but, as shown, this can
occur.

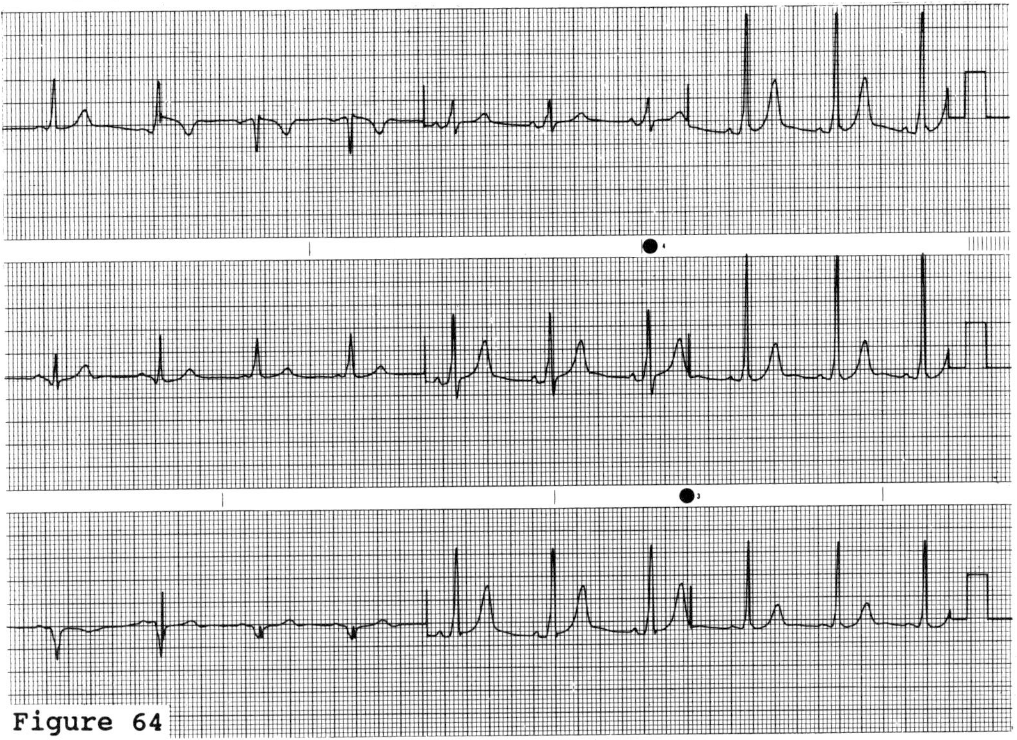

Figure 64

This record shows regular sinus rhythm and the Wolff-Parkinson- White Syndrome. The frontal
plane QRS axis is -15, the T axis is +105, and the P axis is +15 degrees. The QRS duration is .12
seconds. The horizontal plane QRS axis is +5, and the T axis has a double transition between V1 and
V2 and between V3 and V4, but may be about +30 degrees. The P axis is about +45 degrees. The
frontal plane delta axis is -15, and its horizontal plane axis is +10 degrees. The Bundle of Kent
appears to be located primarily inferiorly. Lateral and anterior ischemia and/or left ventricular
strain must be considered, although T changes from the WPW syndrome cannot be excluded. Suggest
serial records and clinical correlation.

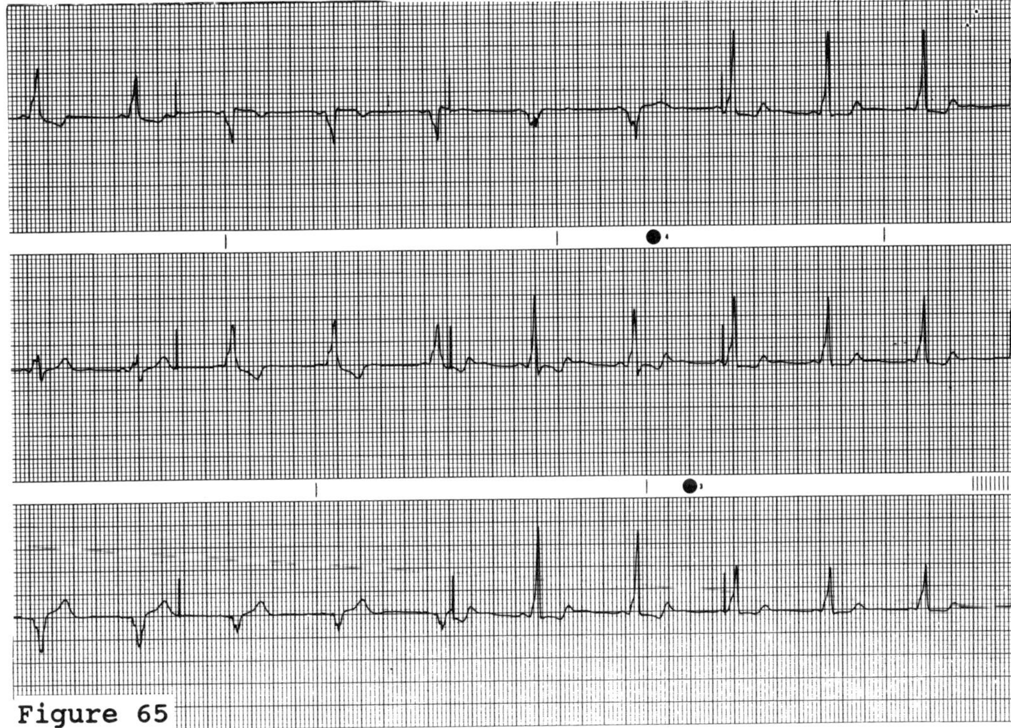

Figure 65

This interesting record shows regular sinus rhythm and frequent appearance of the Wolff-
Parkinson-White Syndrome with almost every other beat. In the normal complexes the frontal plane
QRS axis is +45, the T axis is +30, and the P axis +70 degrees. The horizontal plane QRS axis of a
normally conducted beat is +5, the T axis is +50 or 60, and the P axis is +45 degrees. The frontal
plane delta axis is +70, and its horizontal plane axis may be +90 degrees. The Bundle of Kent may
be located posteriorly and superior.

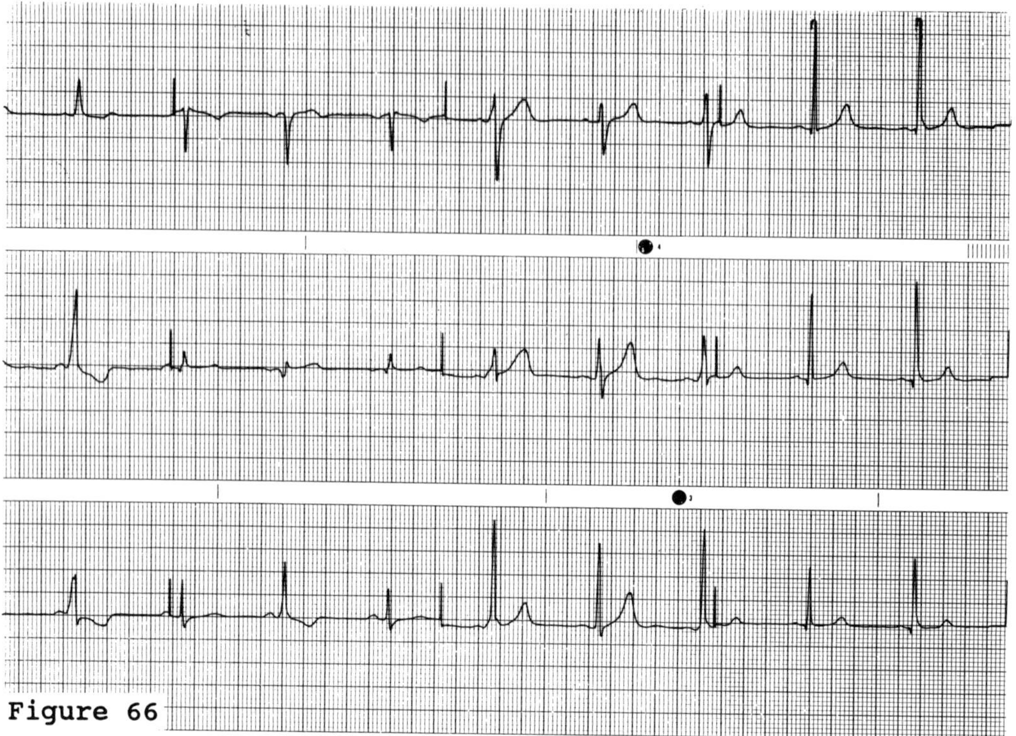

Figure 66

One can tentatively try to locate the bundle of Kent by plotting the axis of the delta wave in the frontal and horizontal planes. For example, a delta that is upright in 2,3, and AVF (the wave is traveling downward) has a Kent bundle that probably is located on the superior part of the heart. A delta that is upright in V1 and V2 (going anteriorly) has a Kent bundle that is probably located posteriorly. One that is negative or downward in V1 and V2 has one that is probably located anteriorly. An inferior Kent bundle will have negative delta waves (Q waves) in 2,3, and AVF. One can put together information of this type to obtain a tentative idea of where the bundle of Kent may be located in patients with WPW. Some patients, however, may have more than just one bundle of Kent.

Clinically, this syndrome may come and go spontaneously and may be seen on the EKG to appear and disappear from beat to beat, as shown in Figure 66. It is often abolished by exercise. Frequently, though, these otherwise healthy patients are prone to episodes of paroxysmal arrythmias, the cause of which is thought to involve ventricular impulses re-entering the atria by way of the Bundle of Kent and setting up an ectopic tachycardia by a circus movement involving such re-entry, followed by travel down the usual Bundle of His, hiding the WPW. However, the circus movement also may go in the other direction, showing the WPW. If these episodes become serious and are refractory to therapy with various drugs, then surgery, guided by careful electrical mapping to locate the accessory bundle (or bundles) may be successful in finding and cutting it (or them), eliminating the WPW and the resultant re-entry arrhythmias.

Patients with WPW may also develop atrial fibrillation with very fast ventricular rates and wide QRS complexes. This may be very hard to distinguish from a ventricular tachycardia. Their generally young age and the absence of a history or evidence of other types of heart disease may help to recognize them. Cardioversion, not lidocaine, is usually what they need, and lidocaine, by shortening the refractory period, may sometimes make them worse, with a faster ventricular rate.

THE LOWN-GANONG-LEVINE SYNDROME

Sometimes one will see a short PR interval (less than .12 sec) with a normal P axis, so there is no evidence of an ectopic atrial rhythm, and a normal QRS duration (less than .09 sec). This occurs when there is accelerated AV conduction, but the _whole_ process is accelerated, without the usual delay produced by the slow (about 1 cm/sec) conduction velocity produced by the cells of the atrial crest of the AV node. This has been called the Lown-Ganong-Levine syndrome.

This syndrome may be produced by a postulated fast extra pathway lying close to the bundle of His and communicating with it, or possibly by a congenital hole in the layer of cells of the atrial crest of the AV node, so that the atrial impulse can come right down to the bundle of His without the usual AV nodal delay inserted by these cells.

The clinical significance of such accelerated AV conduction (the LGL syndrome) is similar to that of patients with the WPW syndrome. Both may have supraventricular arrhythmias. In addition, LGL patients may also be troubled by extremely fast rates if they develop atrial fibrillation, just as with WPW patients.

Electrical alternans consists of a normal QRS followed by an abnormal QRS complex in an alternating fashion. It is most commonly seen with diffuse myocardial disease and may often be a grave prognostic sign. It is probably caused by groups of myocardial cells being unable to recover adequately during diastole and consequently being unable to initiate a propagated spike when next stimulated. These groups of cells, therefore, are lost from the EKG and the QRS pattern is thus altered. These QRS complexes cannot be classified as either a right or left bundle branch block, but have forms mid-way between normal and those of bundle branch blocks, due to patchy losses of myocardial cells which cannot participate in the electrical events of that particular electrical systole.

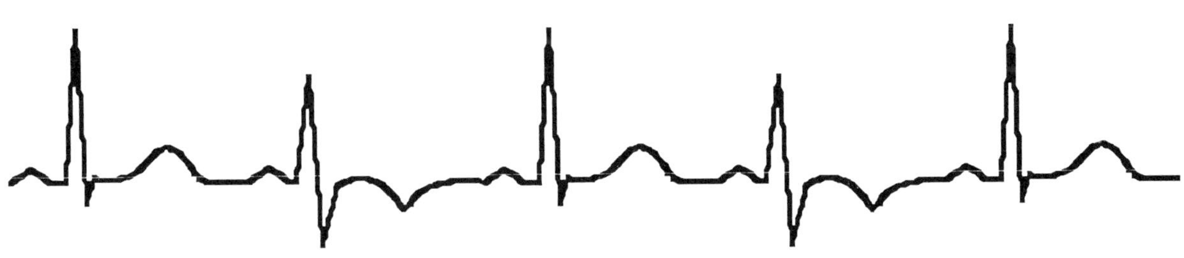

ELECTRICAL ALTERNANS

FIGURE 67

4
The Infarcts

<u>MYOCARDIAL INFARCTION</u>

<u>Ischemia, Injury Currents, and EKG Evolution Following Infarction</u>

When the heart is made ischemic or hypoxic, the action potential duration of the involved cells is shortened, as the cell loses the shoulder off phase 3 of its action potential (the moderate K loss), and the net result is that the T wave vector swings away from the involved area, as discussed earlier. If the ischemia is relieved, the T wave returns to normal.

If ischemia persists, however, more severe K losses occur. Because of the K loss and the importance of K to intracellular resting potential (the Nernst equation), the involved cells become unable to maintain their normal resting potential, and it then falls from -90 mv to something less, as we discussed earlier. Furthermore, these cells fire less well upon stimulation, and thus contribute only poor spike potentials to the EKG or VCG, which may or may not be conducted, or which may be conducted decrementally only for a short distance, to contribute to aberrant intraventricular conduction. It is these "injured" cells with <u>reduced resting potentials</u> that cause the ST segment shifts usually seen in the EKG. Furthermore, as cells die and do not fire any more, these dead unfired cells cause deletions from the normal QRS complex. Thus the changes seen with myocardial "injury" are ST segment shifts <u>toward</u> or <u>away</u> from the involved area, if <u>subepicardial</u> or <u>subendocardial</u> respectively, and the <u>T wave usually shifts away</u> from the involved area, unless the changes are "hyperacute", as discussed earlier. <u>Infarction</u> (dead cells) causes <u>deletions from the QRS</u> complex.

It is by such deletions in the QRS vector that we recognize and localize myocardial infarcts. Generally, unfired cells are dead cells.

As injured cells die, the QRS deletions appear, the ST shifts usually disappear, and the T waves usually move further away from the involved area. The time required for these changes to occur varies from hours to a few (4-7) days.

From the onset on, over perhaps the next 2 weeks, the T vector often moves further away from the involved area ("waxing T changes"). Then, after the dead cells are digested by polys, and after hypertrophy of the remaining myocardium has taken place, with less stress on each individual myofibril, the T waves often move somewhat back toward normal ("waning T changes"). The waxing T changes may well be due to the transfer of the work load formerly handled by the infarcted cells to the cells of adjacent areas, greatly increasing the tension they must develop to generate a reasonable systolic pressure. Later on, as these cells hypertrophy and add new myofibrils, the tension and work per myofibril will decrease. This decreased work per myofibril, with its decreased ATP consumption and decreasing intracellular K loss, may be responsible for the waning T changes later on. Sometimes, however, the hypertrophy of the remaining myocardial cells is not sufficient. This is commonly the case when the infarct is so large that it causes a ventricular aneurysm. In that case, ST-T changes resembling those seen with acute infarction will persist chronically, due to the chronic severe work load these cells must endure.

<u>Anteroseptal</u> <u>Myocardial</u> <u>Infarction</u>- Figures 68 - 70.

When the lesion is in the anterior or the apical portion of the intraventricular septum, the normal left to right septal activation process cannot occur. The early R wave in V1, V2, V3, and sometimes V4 is lost or diminished and/or is replaced by a Q wave. This is the hallmark of this lesion. The <u>normal</u> R wave early in the QRS complex wave should increase or <u>progress</u> steadily as one moves or progresses steadily from V1 to V6, because the angle of the exploring electrode becomes progressively less and less in relation to the direction of the main QRS axis or vector. An <u>abnormal R progression</u> is seen if the height of the R wave in any precordial lead from V1 through V4 is less than that in the <u>preceding</u> lead. One should then suspect the presence of an infarct in that area.

The R wave may normally decrease somewhat as one progresses from V4 to V5 or V6, possibly due to intervening lung tissue between the heart and the chest wall (air does not conduct as well as normal saline or tissue). The appearance of a Q wave in a precordial lead when there is an R in a <u>preceding</u> precordial lead usually reflects an infarct. The exception is the small normal "septal Q" in V5 and/or V6 mentioned earlier. Remember that those small septal Q's in V5 and V6 (less than .025 sec wide) are also the "septal R's" in V1 and V2, and the "septal Q" in lead 1, all of which show the rightward and anterior direction of the normal septal depolarization in the first 10 to 25 msec of depolarization (see Figure 22 again).

If a Q wave or an abnormal R progression occurs in V1, and V2, or V3, one should strongly suspect the presence of an anteroseptal infarct. It is normal to have a Q in V1, and <u>sometimes</u> in V2 as well, but rarely. A Q in V3 is almost never normal.

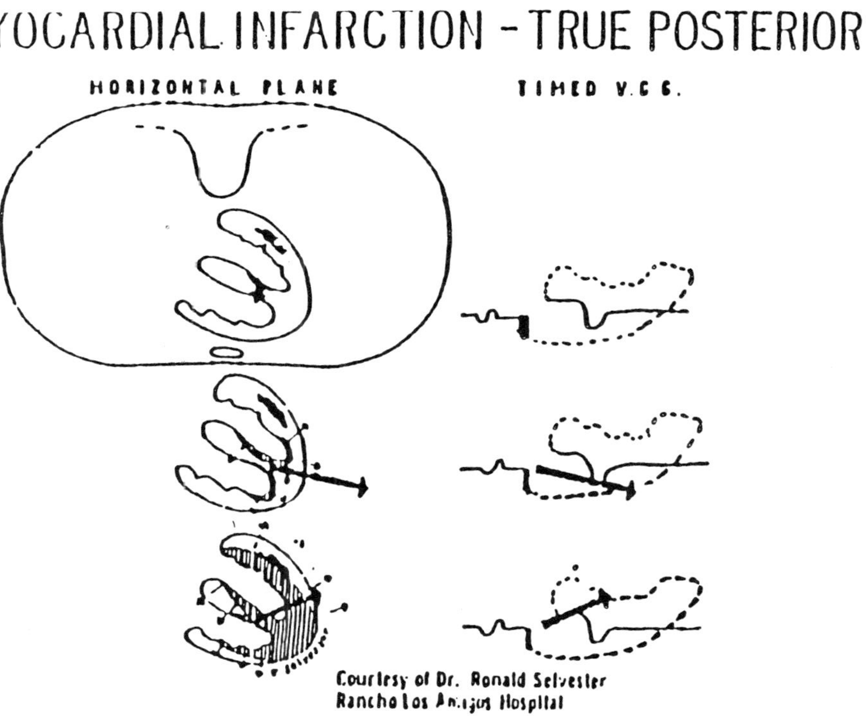
MYOCARDIAL INFARCTION - TRUE POSTERIOR
HORIZONTAL PLANE
TIMED V.C.G.
Courtesy of Dr. Ronald Selvester
Rancho Los Amigos Hospital

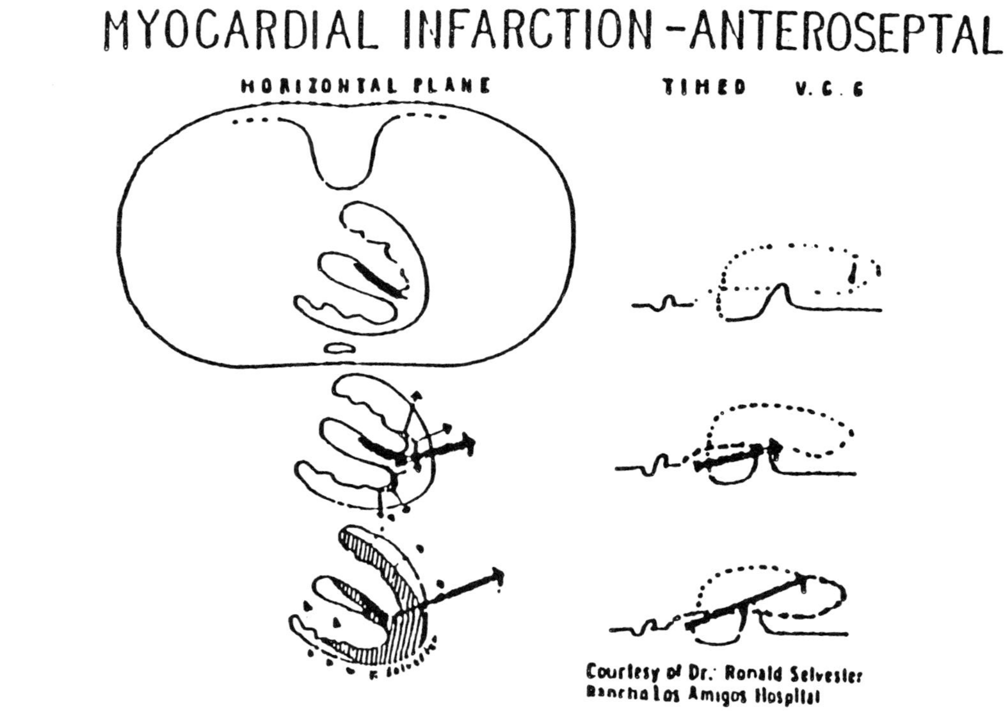
MYOCARDIAL INFARCTION - ANTEROSEPTAL
HORIZONTAL PLANE
TIMED V.C.G
Courtesy of Dr. Ronald Selvester
Rancho Los Amigos Hospital

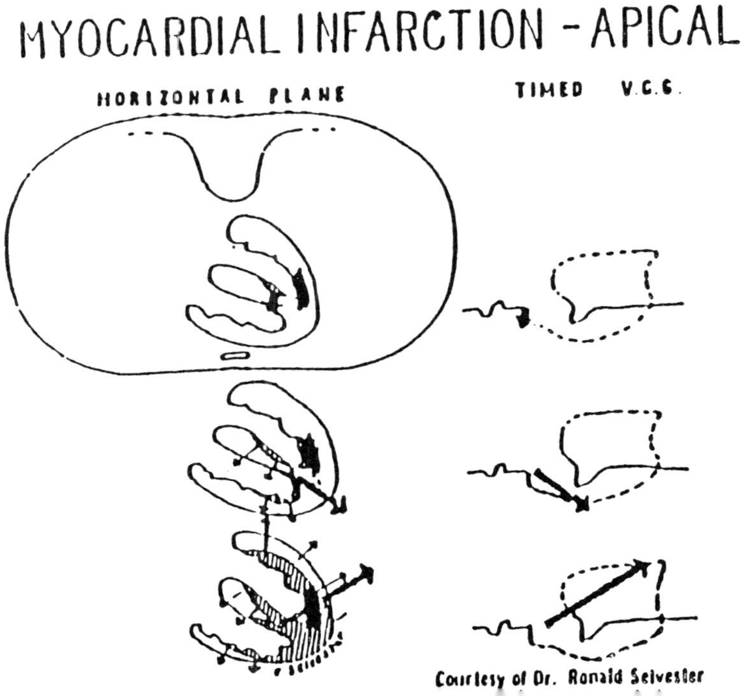
MYOCARDIAL INFARCTION - APICAL
HORIZONTAL PLANE
TIMED V.C.G.
Courtesy of Dr. Ronald Selvester

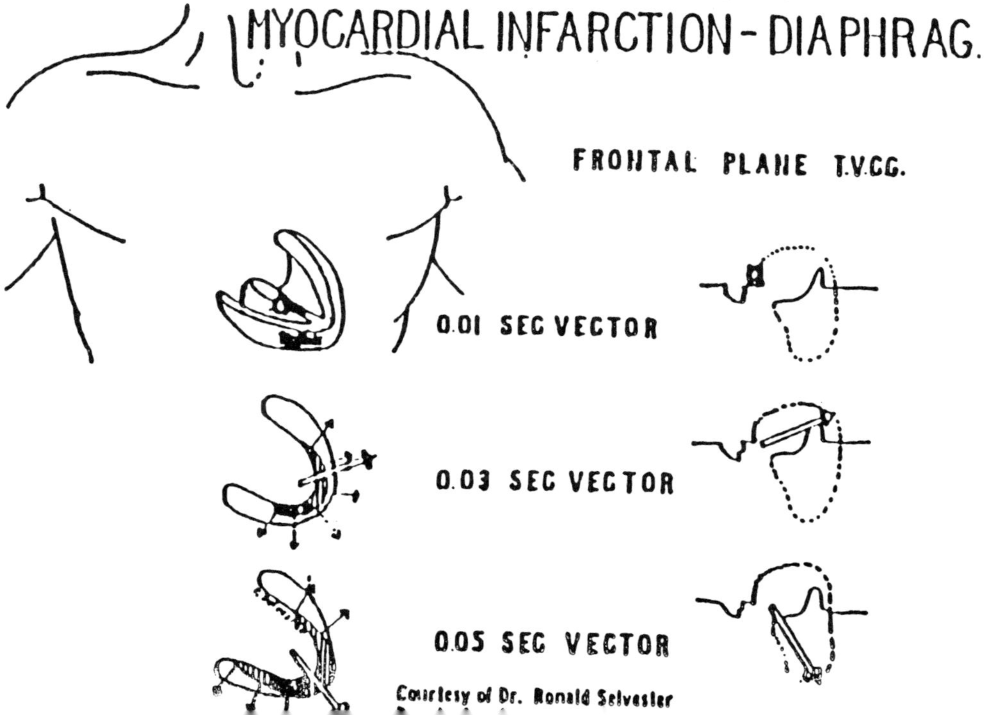
MYOCARDIAL INFARCTION - DIAPHRAG.
FRONTAL PLANE T.V.C.G.
0.01 SEC VECTOR
0.03 SEC VECTOR
0.05 SEC VECTOR
Courtesy of Dr. Ronald Selvester

FIGURE 68

This record shows regular sinus rhythm and an acute anteroseptal infarct. The frontal plane QRS axis is 0, the T axis is +45, and the P axis +70 degrees. The horizontal plane QRS axis is difficult to plot because of the ST elevations in V2 and V3, but may be about -10 degrees. The horizontal T axis is +45, the P axis is +45, and the horizontal plane ST segment axis is about +50 degrees. The failure to find inverted T waves in the presence of the ST segment elevation suggests that these changes may be hyperacute, reflecting unopposed myocardial cores having anteroapical subepicardial ischemia and injury.

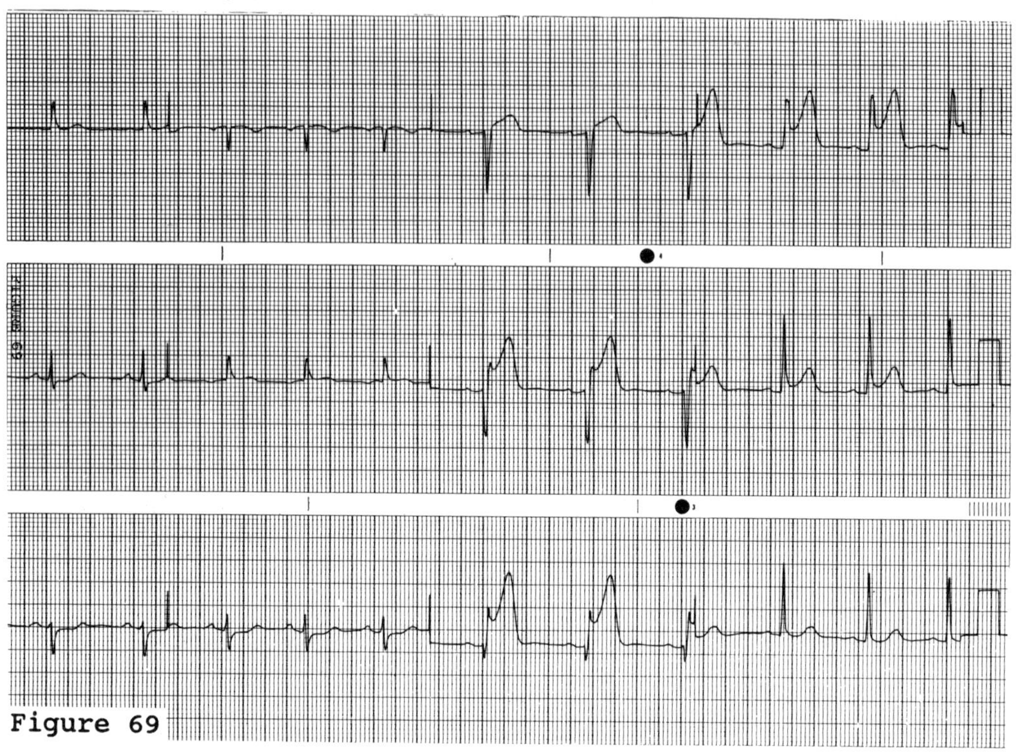

Figure 69

This record shows regular sinus rhythm, a probable anteroseptal infarct, possible left atrial enlargement, and T changes consistent with anterior, apical, and lateral ischemia with apical subepicardial injury. The frontal plane QRS axis is +15, the T axis is +160, and the P axis is +50 degrees. The horizontal plane QRS axis is -50, the T axis is 180, and the P axis is about -15 degrees. Suggest serial records.

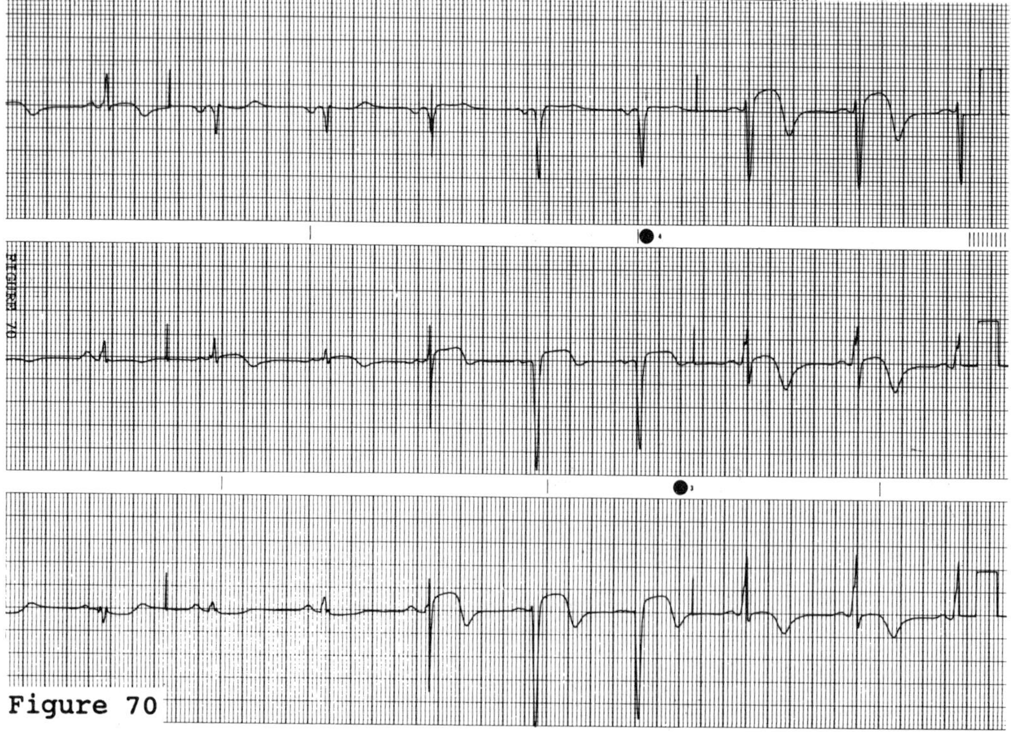

Figure 70

The ST segment is usually displaced either toward or away from those same leads, showing subepicardial or subendocardial injury (abnormal resting potentials), and the T wave is swung away posteriorly (anterior ischemia). Consequently, the hallmark of acute anteroseptal infarction is Q waves in V1, V2, and perhaps also V3. ST elevations or depressions and T wave inversions in those leads may also be present.

<u>Apical</u> <u>or</u> <u>Lateral</u> <u>Myocardial</u> <u>Infarction</u>- Figures 68 and 71 - 74.

When the infarct involves the apex, most of the septal depolarization is normal, and the QRS deletion occurs slightly more laterally (in V4, V5, and/or V6. Apical infarction is recognized by a loss of lateral positivity ("force"), with Q's in V4, V5, and/or V6, and sometimes in Lead 1 as well. In contrast to normal septal Q's, these Q's are usually greater than .025 seconds in duration.

The ST segment may be either elevated or depressed, reflecting either subepicardial or subendocardial location, and the T waves are inverted, the T vector usually being pushed away from the lesion.

<u>Inferior</u> <u>or</u> <u>Diaphragmatic</u> <u>Myocardial</u> <u>Infarction</u>- Figures 68 and 75 - 78.

Here the lesion involves the bottom surface of the myocardium near the diaphragm. This portion of the myocardium usually contributes its downward force fairly early in the QRS complex, and a loss of such force results in an upward displacement of the early portion of the QRS vector in the frontal plane, causing Q waves to appear in leads 2, 3, and aVF. Especially, look for a Q in aVF that is wider than .025sec, regardless of its amplitude. The QRS vector simply should be going inferiorly by .025 sec, and if it isn't, something is wrong. The ST segment is often displaced toward the foot and

This record shows regular sinus rhythm and anteroseptal and apical infarction of undetermined age, possibly recent. The ST elevations in V1 through V5 and T inversions in V2 through V5 suggest anterior and apical subepicardial injury and superior and lateral ischemia. The frontal plane QRS axis is +50, the T axis is +120, the P axis + 60 degrees. The horizontal plane QRS axis is -80, the T axis is about -170, and the P axis is about +45 degrees. A small Q is noted in front of the R in both V1 and V2, in addition to the larger Q in V4. There is a minimal R in V3. Suggest serial records.

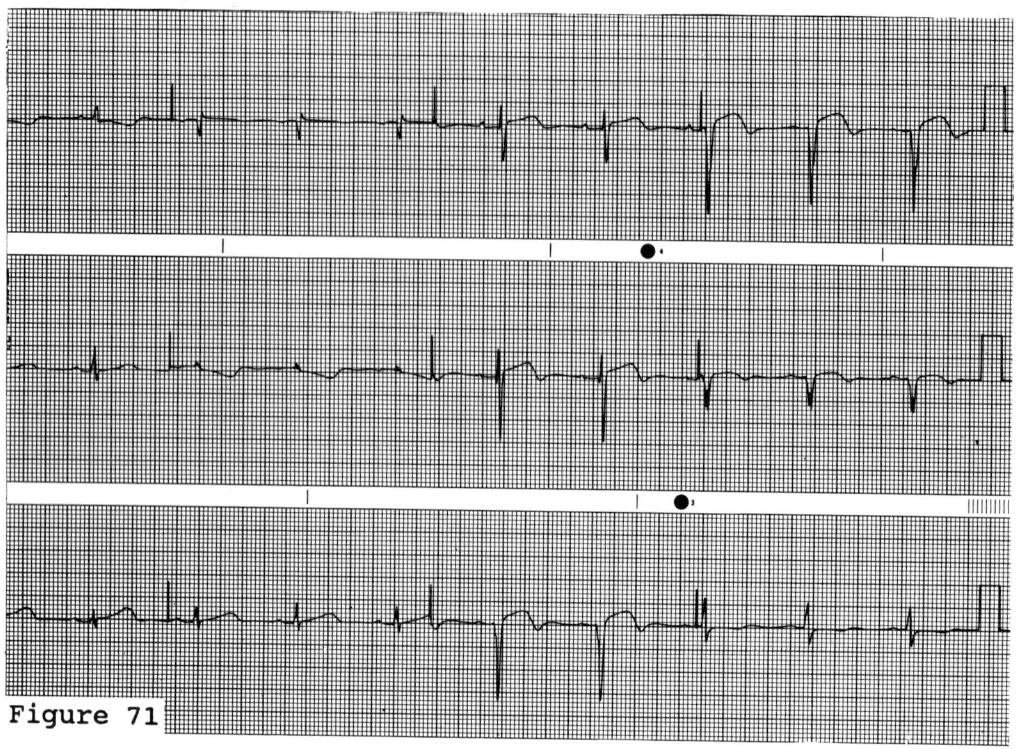

Figure 71

This record shows sinus tachycardia, left atrial enlargement, and anteroseptal and anterolateral infarction, probably acute. S-T elevations consistent with lateral subepicardial injury and hyperacute T changes are seen, which may reflect ischemic and injured unopposed subepicardial myocardial cores in the apical region. The frontal plane QRS axis is +80, the T axis +100, and the P axis +75 degrees. The horizontal plane QRS axis is -70, the T axis about +80, and the P axis -15 degrees. The horizontal plane ST segment vector is about +30 degrees. Suggest serial records.

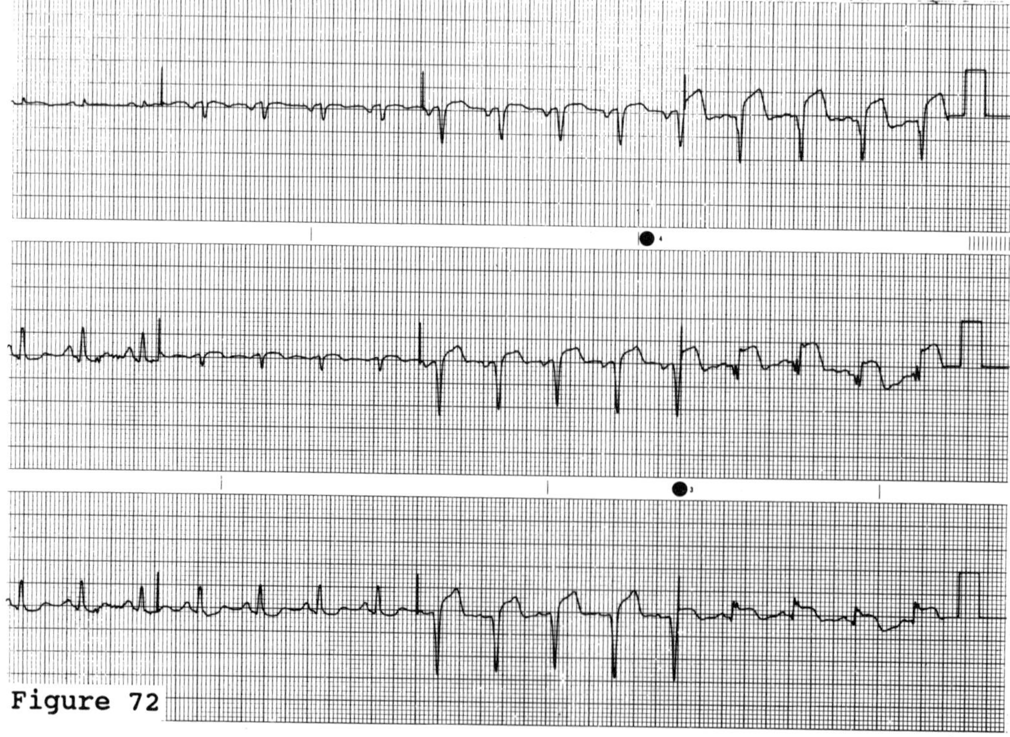

Figure 72

This record shows regular sinus rhythm and anteroapical infarction, with T changes consistent with lateral ischemia and/or left ventricular strain. The frontal plane QRS axis is +15, the T axis +160, and the P axis is 0 degrees. The horizontal plane QRS axis is -50, the T axis is +130, and the P axis is about 0 degrees. Suggest repeat or serial records and clinical correlation.

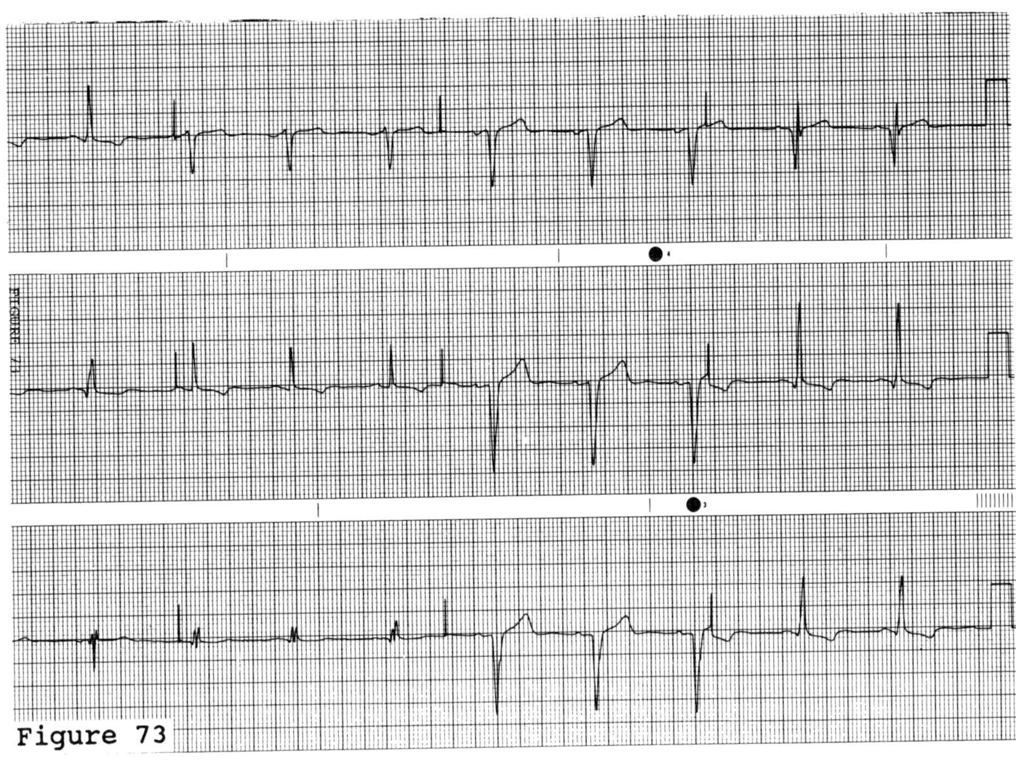

Figure 73

This record shows sinus tachycardia, low frontal plane voltage, and posterior displacement of the horizontal plane QRS axis, consistent with pulmonary disease. In addition, an abnormal R progression is noted in V2-V6, consistent with apical and lateral infarction. Occasional PVC's are present. ST elevations and T inversions in V5 and V6 are consistent with lateral subepicardial ischemia and injury. The frontal plane QRS axis is +60, the T axis is +90, and the P axis is +60 degrees. The horizontal QRS axis is about -110, the T axis is about +100, and the P axis is about 0 degrees. The lateral infarct may be acute. Suggest serial records.

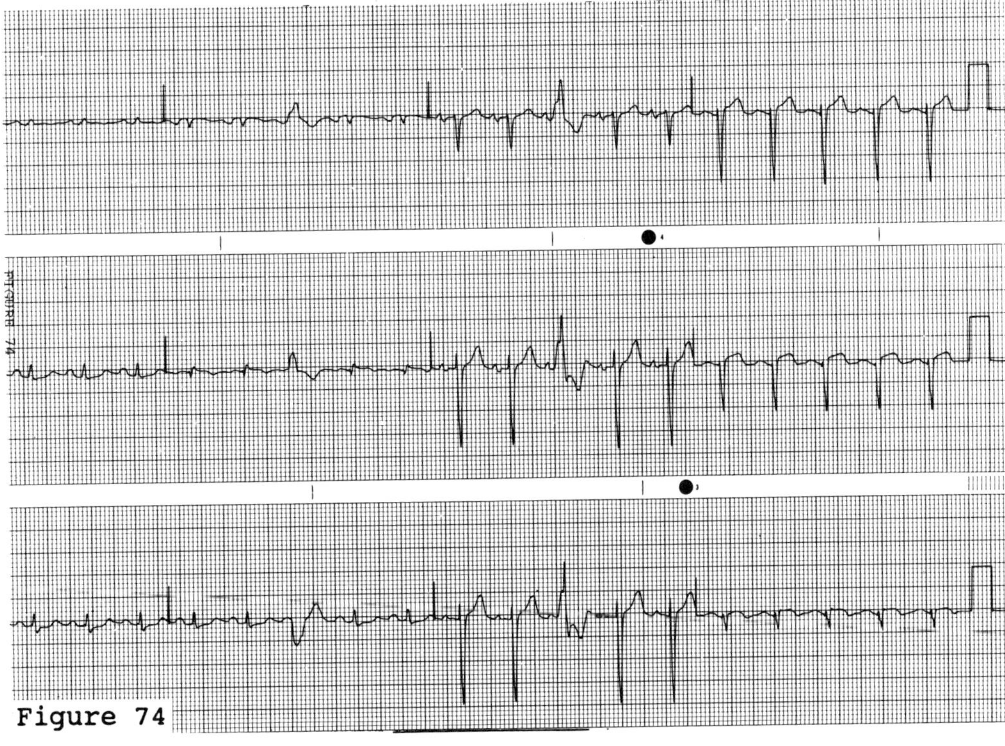

Figure 74

This record shows regular sinus rhythm and inferior infarction, with T changes consistent with inferior, anterior, and apical ischemia. Reliable tracings of lead 2 are not present. The frontal plane QRS axis is between 0 and -60, perhaps about -30 degrees. The T axis is similar. The P axis is difficult to plot. The horizontal plane QRS axis is -50, the T axis is -100, the P axis is 0 degrees. Suggest serial records.

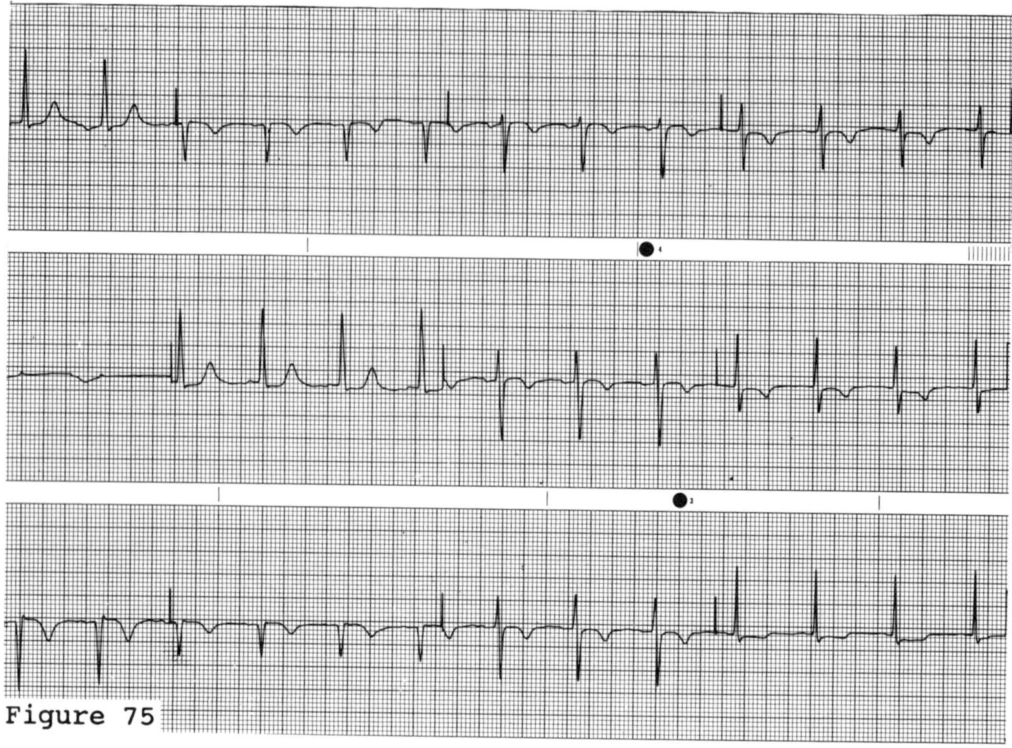

Figure 75

This record shows regular sinus rhythm and inferior infarction, with inferior and possible lateral ischemia. The frontal plane QRS axis is 0, the T axis is -50, and the P axis is +40 degrees. The horizontal plane QRS axis is +20, the T axis is +45, and the P axis is about +30 degrees. Posteroapical infarction cannot be excluded. Suggest serial records.

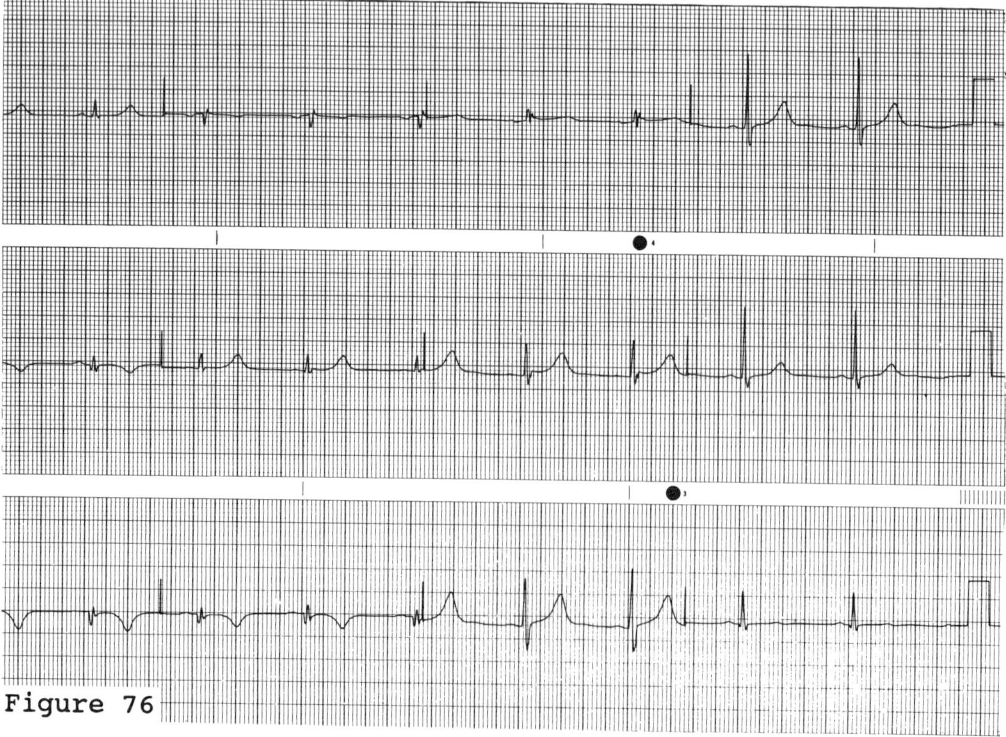

Figure 76

This record shows an ectopic atrial rhythm. The frontal and horizontal P axes are -100 and -135 degrees respectively, clearly indicating that the atrial focus is ectopic. The P-R interval is normal, not short as in a junctional rhythm. The record also shows evidence of probable acute inferior infarction with inferior ischemia and subepicardial injury. The frontal QRS axis is -15 and the T axis is minus -30 degrees. The horizontal plane QRS axis is -45 and the T axis is +50 degrees. Suggest serial records.

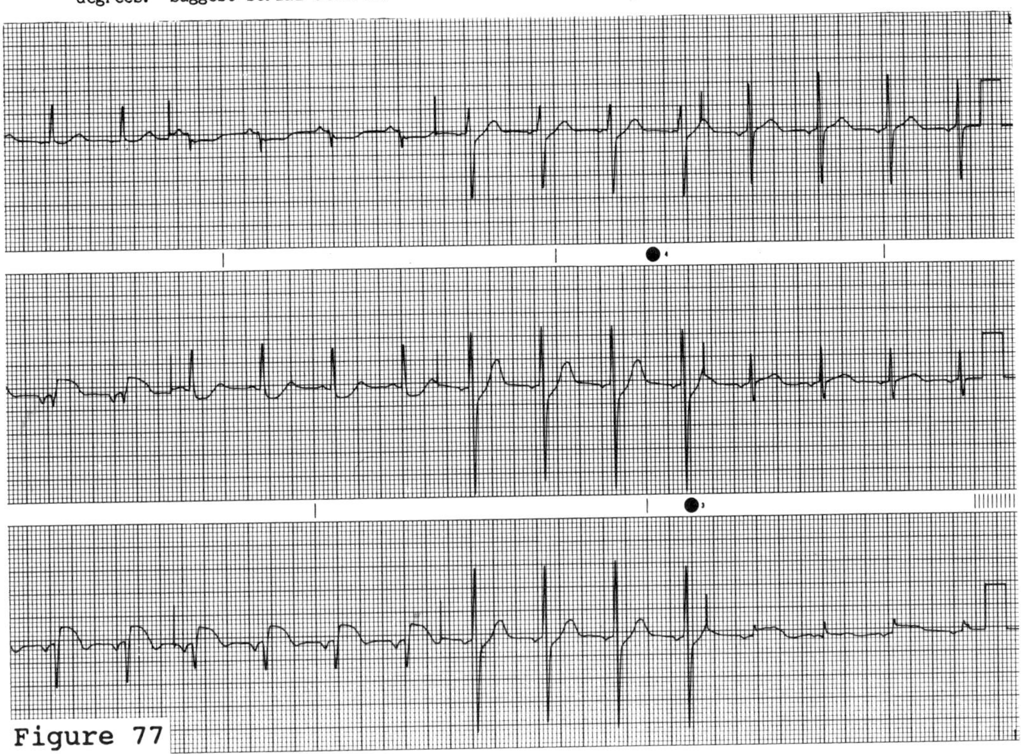

Figure 77

This record shows regular sinus rhythm and an inferior infarct, probably acute. The frontal plane QRS axis is 0 degrees, the T axis is -15, and the P axis +45 degrees. The horizontal plane QRS axis is -30, the T axis +5, and the P axis is about +20 degrees. Suggest serial records.

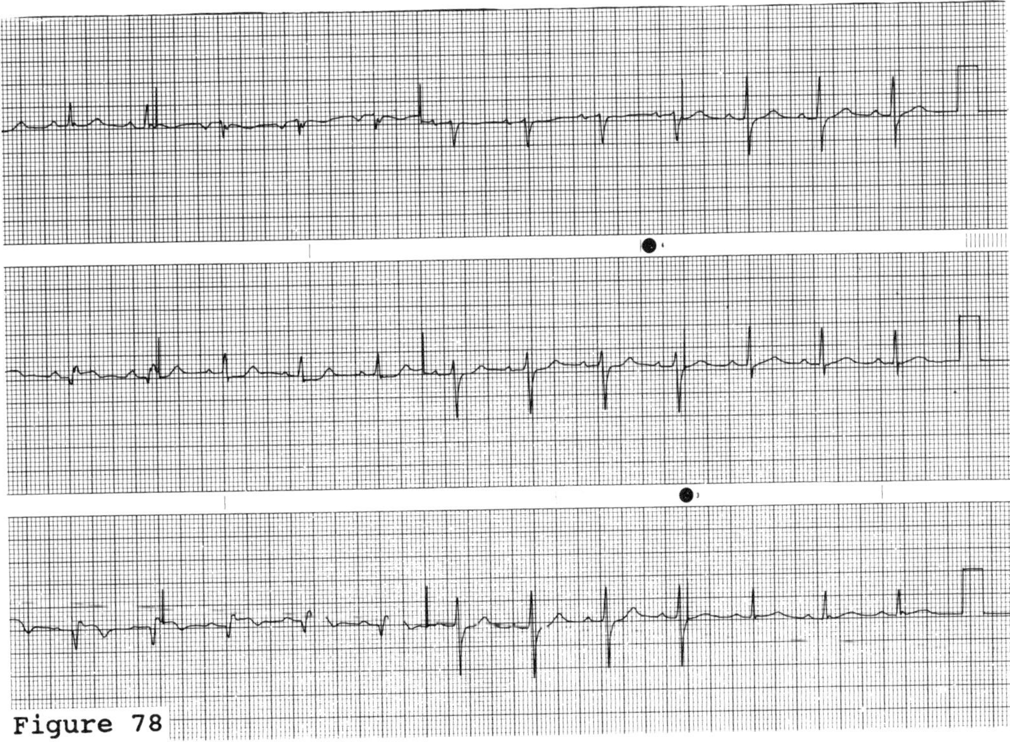

Figure 78

the T wave toward the head, causing ST elevations and T wave inversions in leads 2, 3, and aVF.

Inferior Infarction and/or Inferior Hemiblock?

Dead men tell no tales, and dead myocardial cells don't fire, ever again. For example, if one has an anterior infarct, its EKG location usually correlates well with the location of the poorly-functioning area of the ventricle as seen with a left ventriculogram, and the EKG evidence of infarction stays there forever.

However, this is _not_ true of a number of patients with inferior infarcts. Often they will show poor LV function _not_ in the apex of the left ventricle, as suggested by the initial Q waves in leads 2, 3, and aVF, but rather in the mesial or basal regions, under the papillary muscle or up near the A-V groove. There is _no way_ that such mesial or basal myocardial cells can be fired in the first 40 msec of the depolarization sequence. There is _no way_ those cells can have any relation to the above Q waves. In addition, some of these patients will later go on to _lose_ their Q waves!

How can this be? If we remember that the inferior fascicle (and often the AV node as well) are supplied by a dominant right coronary artery, we can see how common it is for patients with inferior infarcts to develop AV blocks, inferior hemiblock, and other combinations of AV and IV conduction defects. Frequently, if one examines the vectorcardiogram of such patients, their lesion is seen to be the combination of an inferior hemiblock, causing the smooth wide Q waves in 2, 3, and aVF, plus an infero_mesial_ or infero-_basal_ infarct, resulting in a _loss of inferior positivity_ during the middle or later portions of the QRS. That loss of inferior positivity brings the

This record shows sinus rhythm, an inferior infarct of undetermined age, possibly recent, and a slightly wide QRS complex. Coexisting inferior hemiblock cannot be excluded. The T changes suggest inferior ischemia. The frontal plane QRS axis is +20, the T axis is -45, and the P axis is +15 degrees. The horizontal plane QRS axis is -30, the T axis is about +60, and the P axis is about +5 degrees. Suggest serial records.

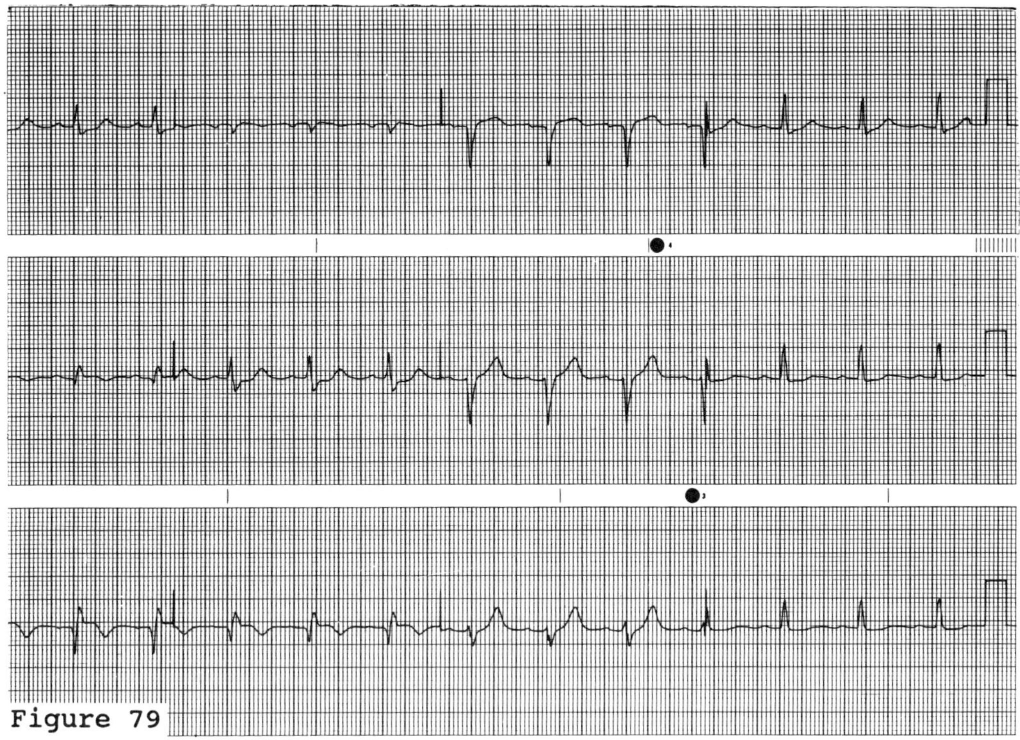

Figure 79

This record shows regular sinus rhythm, left atrial enlargement, anteroapical infarction of undetermined age, possibly recent, and inferior infarction and/or coexisting inferior branch hemiblock. The QRS duration is .11 seconds. The frontal plane QRS axis is +50, the T axis is +15, and the P axis +60 degrees. The horizontal plane QRS axis is -60, the T axis is +5, and the P axis is 0 degrees. ST elevations in V4, consistent with apical subepicardial injury, and hyperacute T changes, are present. Suggest serial records.

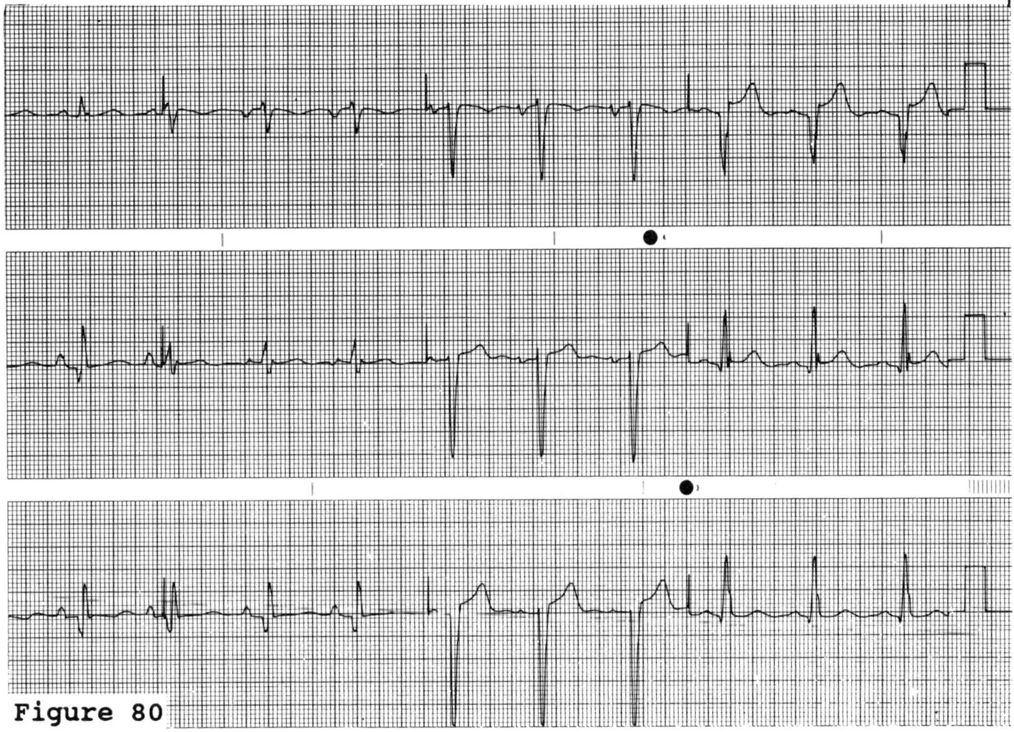

Figure 80

This record shows regular sinus rhythm, left atrial enlargement, inferior infarction (possibly inferomesial), with probable coexisting inferior branch hemiblock. T changes consistent with left ventricular strain and/or lateral ischemia are present, and left ventricular hypertrophy is probably present. The QRS duration is .11 seconds. The frontal plane QRS axis is +15, and the T axis is difficult to plot, but may be almost straight anterior, with little projection into the frontal plane. The P axis is +70 degrees. The horizontal plane QRS axis is -35, the T axis is +120, and the P axis is +10 degrees. Suggest serial records.

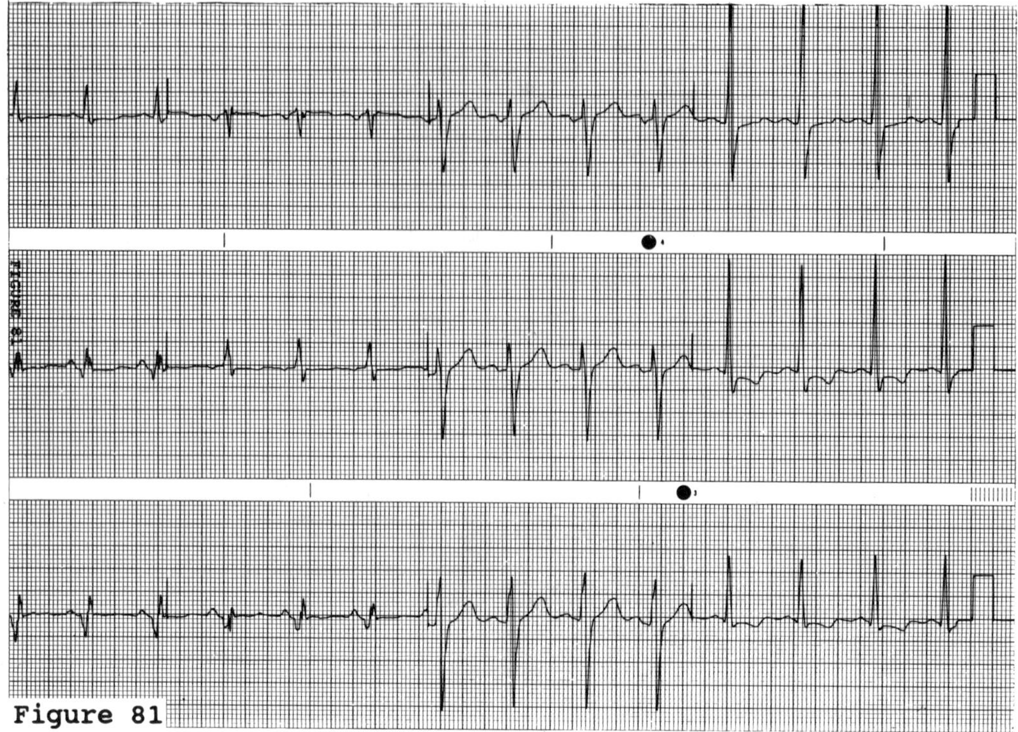

Figure 81

frontal QRS vector _back_ from the vertical position (greater than +60 degrees) it would have had from the inferior hemiblock alone, and makes it relatively _normal_ again. The QRS is slightly widened. When such patients lose their Q waves later on, they actually have lost their inferior hemiblock. Any bundle branch block or IV conduction defect may come and go from time to time, depending, presumably, on vascular supply. Having lost their Q's, their QRS usually becomes slightly narrower as well.

Because of all this, it is never quite clear _just what_ the Q waves in 2, 3, and aVF are telling us. We do _not_ know how to distinguish inferior infarction from inferior hemiblock when they coexist. It is likely, however, that if the QRS is slightly wide, the Q in 2, 3, and aVF is smooth and at least .03 sec wide, and the middle or later part of the QRS has a normal frontal axis and some notching, that we may have the combination of an inferomesial or inferobasal infarct (the notching and the normal frontal axis), plus an inferior hemiblock (the smooth wide Q's in 2, 3, and aVF). Some possible examples of this are shown in Figures 79 - 81.

Posterior Myocardial Infarction- Figures 68 and 82 - 83.

Loss of cells in this area causes an irregular anterior displacement of the QRS loop in the horizontal plane. If the lesion is near the apex, the loss occurs early in the QRS complex, and causes a taller and more prolonged early R wave in V1, V2, and V3 (over .04 seconds). If the lesion is _mesial_ or _basal_, its effects are seen later, causing an R' in these same leads in the _middle_ or the _terminal portion_ of the QRS. In any case, the ST segment is often shifted posteriorly (posterior subepicardial injury) and the T wave anteriorly (posterior ischemia), causing ST depression and tall upright T waves in V1, V2, and V3.

This record shows regular sinus rhythm, low voltage in the frontal plane, and Q waves in 2,3 aVF, V5 and V6, consistent with inferior and lateral infarction. Prominent R waves in V1 and V2 are seen, and posteroapical infarction may also be present. The frontal plane QRS axis is -90, the T axis is +60, and the P axis is +45 degrees. The horizontal plane QRS axis is difficult to plot, but has prominent anterior forces. The T axis is +70, and the P axis is 0 degrees. Suggest repeat or serial records and clinical correlation.

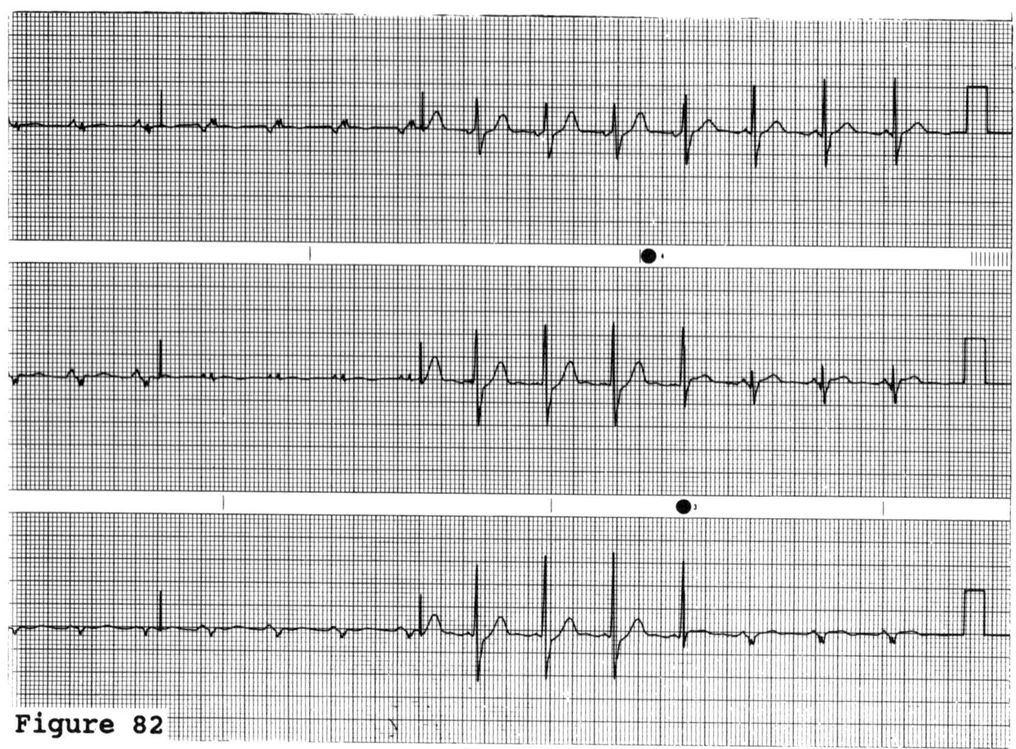

Figure 82

This record shows sinus rhythm and frequent bigeminal PVC's. The frontal plane QRS axis is +30, the T axis +40, and the P axis +45 degrees. The horizontal plane QRS axis is +5, the T axis +5, and the P axis +45 degrees. Except for the frequent bigeminal PVC's and prominent anterior forces of uncertain etiology, the record may be within normal limits. However, a posteroapical infarct cannot be completely excluded. Suggest repeat or serial records and clinical correlation. Digitalis toxicity cannot be excluded.

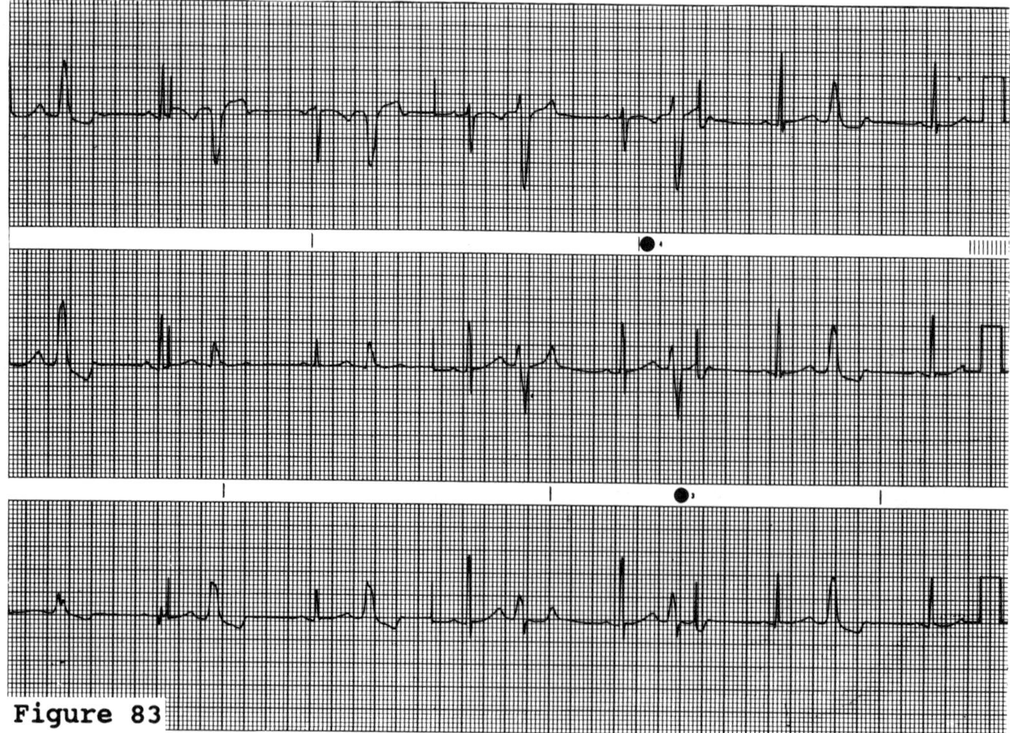

Figure 83

<u>Infarction and Bundle Branch Blocks.</u>

Most of the time the coexisting lesions are self-evident, especially when Right Bundle Branch Block is present, and septal depolarization proceeds in the usual manner, as shown in Figure 22 earlier, proceeding from left to right and anteriorly.

<u>Infarction and RBBB.</u> Figures 84 - 87.

For example, Figure 84 shows a RBBB with a combination of anteroseptal, apical, and inferior infarction, while Figures 85 and 86 show RBBB with Left Anterior Superior Hemiblock (LASHB) and anteroseptal and apical infarction. In Figure 86, the inferior forces are minimal, and the usual R in 2, 3, and aVF that one usually sees with LASHB is greatly reduced, suggesting inferior infarction as well. Figure 87 shows an especially severe example with inferior and possible apical infarction.

<u>Infarction and LBBB.</u> Figures 88 - 89.

In the normal state, the initial wave of depolarization is delivered via the left bundle to the lower left part of the interventricular septum, as shown in Figure 22. This results in the normal small to modest septal R waves one sees in V1 - V3, and often in the small narrow (less than 0.02 sec.) septal Q waves in Lead 1 and in V5 - V6.

When LBBB is present, however, the initial impulse via the left bundle is blocked. Initial depolarization now arrives via the right bundle, and septal depolarization now proceeds from right to left and posteriorly. Because of this, the initial normal septal R waves are lost or greatly diminished, as shown in Figures 44 - 46 for patients with LBBB.

Now to the EKG changes seen with LBBB and anteroseptal infarction. We generally have thought that we lose anterior forces with anterior infarc-

This record shows regular sinus rhythm, right bundle branch block, and anteroseptal, anteroapical, and inferior infarction, with T changes consistent with inferior and apical ischemia. The
frontal QRS axis is -45, the T axis is -20, and the P axis +15 degrees. The horizontal plane QRS
axis is +115, the T axis -80, and the P axis is +5 degrees. Suggest serial records.

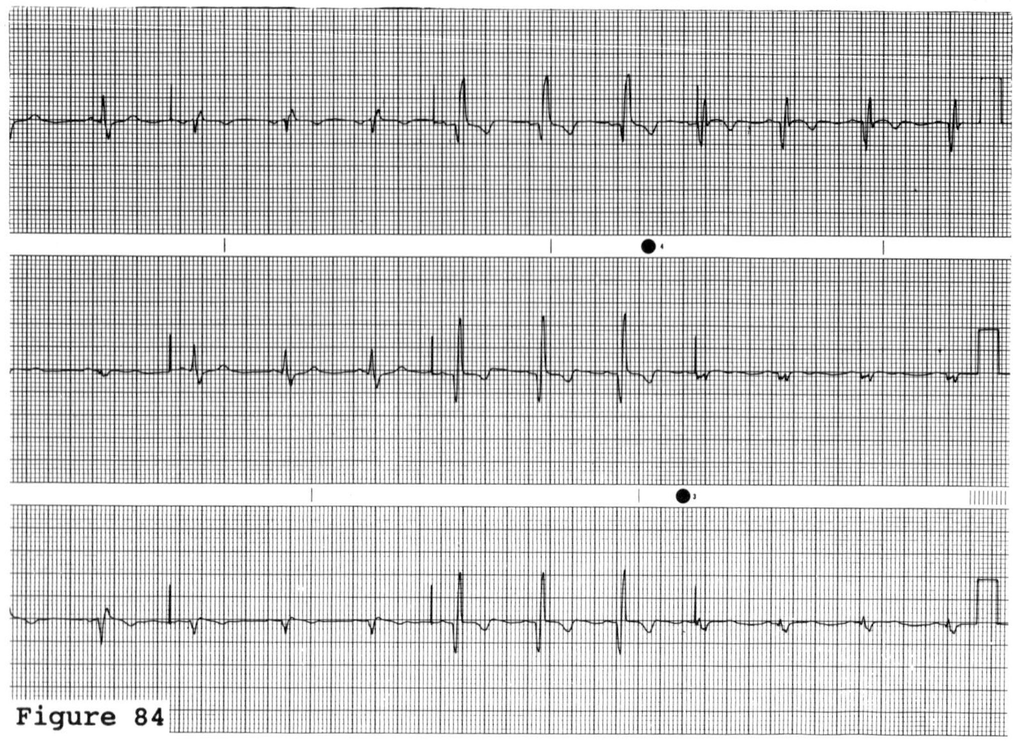

Figure 84

This record shows regular sinus rhythm, right bundle branch block, left anterior superior
hemiblock, and anteroseptal and anteroapical infarction, with T changes consistent with lateral,
posterior, and superior ischemia. Posterobasal infarction cannot be excluded. The QRS duration is
0.12 seconds. A Q is present in lead 1, which is almost .04 seconds in duration, consistent with
lateral infarction as well. The frontal plane QRS axis is -90, the T axis is +130, and the P axis
+70 degrees. The horizontal QRS axis has a double transition between V1 and V2 and between V5 and
V6. The horizontal plane T axis is +170, and the P axis is about +45 degrees. Suggest serial
records.

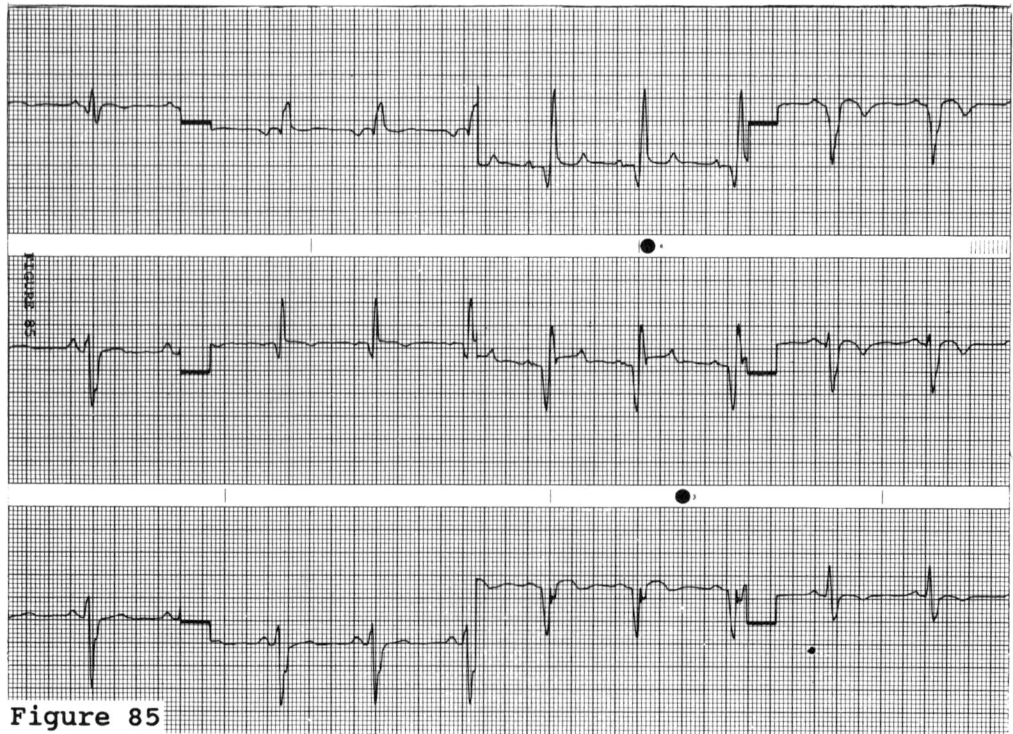

Figure 85

This record shows sinus rhythm, right bundle branch block, left anterior superior hemiblock, and anteroseptal, anteroapical, and possible inferior infarction, with possible anteroseptal sub-epicardial injury as suggested by the somewhat unusual degree of ST elevation (for RBBB) in V2 and V3. The frontal plane QRS axis is -120, the T axis is +45, the P axis is +45 degrees. The horizontal plane QRS axis is -170, the T axis is -10, and the P axis +20 degrees. The ST segment vector in the horizontal plane is perhaps +80 degrees. Suggest serial records and clinical correlation.

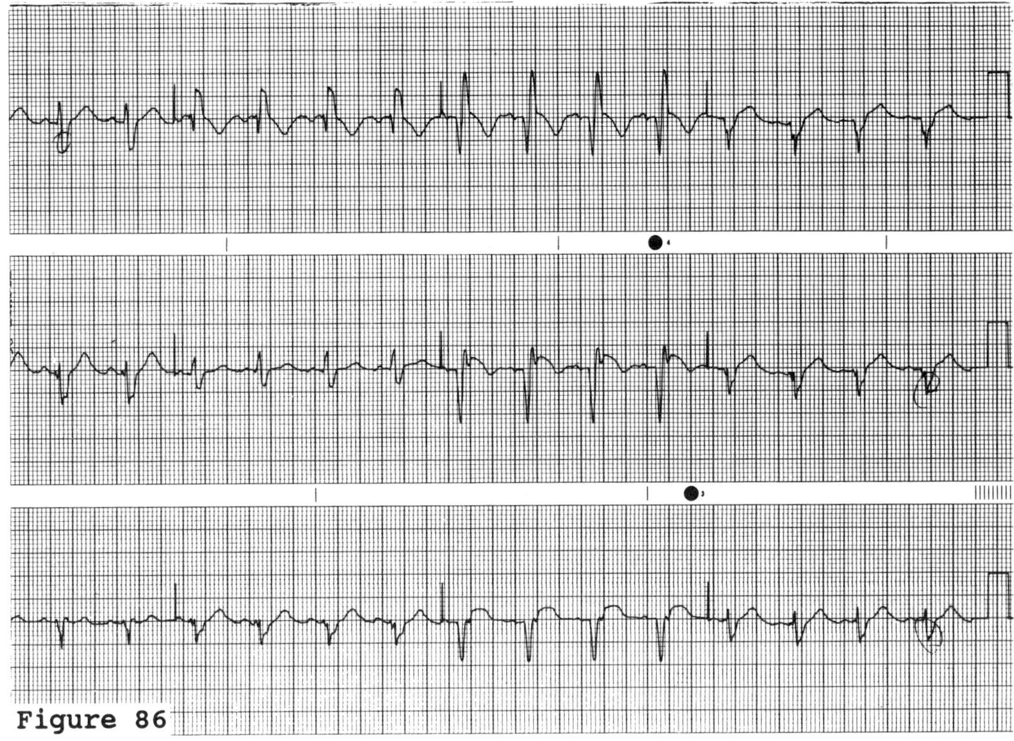

Figure 86

This record shows sinus rhythm, first degree AV block, left atrial enlargement, right bundle branch block, left anterior superior hemiblock, and probable inferior infarction, as suggested by the Q waves in 2,3, and aVF, and the lack of inferior forces. Apical and inferior ischemia and subendocardial injury cannot be excluded. The QRS duration is extremely wide at 0.18 seconds. The frontal plane QRS axis is -60, the T axis is +120, and the P axis is +40 degrees. The horizontal plane QRS axis is +90, the T axis is -70, and the P axis is 0 degrees. Suggest serial records.

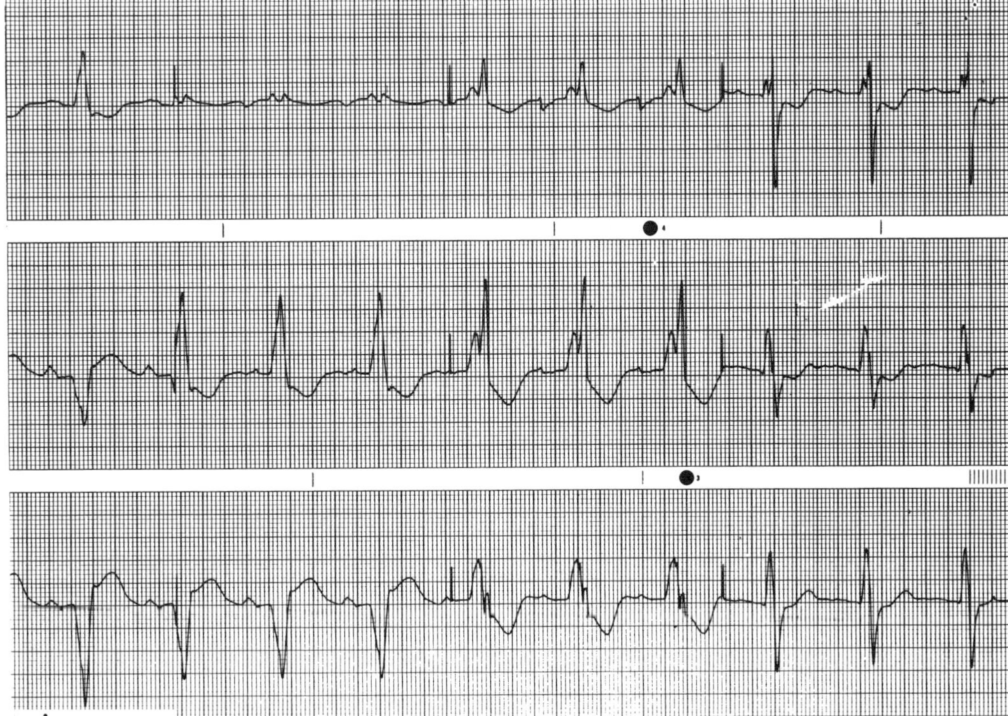

Figure 87

This record shows sinus rhythm, left atrial enlargement, left bundle branch block, and probable anteroseptal and apical infarction. A somewhat unusual amount of ST elevation is noted in V1 through V4, consistent with anterior subepicardial injury. The QRS duration is very wide (for LBBB), about 0.19 seconds, in V1. The frontal plane QRS axis is -15, the T axis is +130, and the P axis +35 degrees. The horizontal plane QRS axis is -80, the T axis is +110, and the P axis is 0 degrees. Note the unusually tall and broad R in V1 and V2 for a patient with left bundle branch block, and the abnormal R progression in V4-V6. Suggest serial records and clinical correlation.

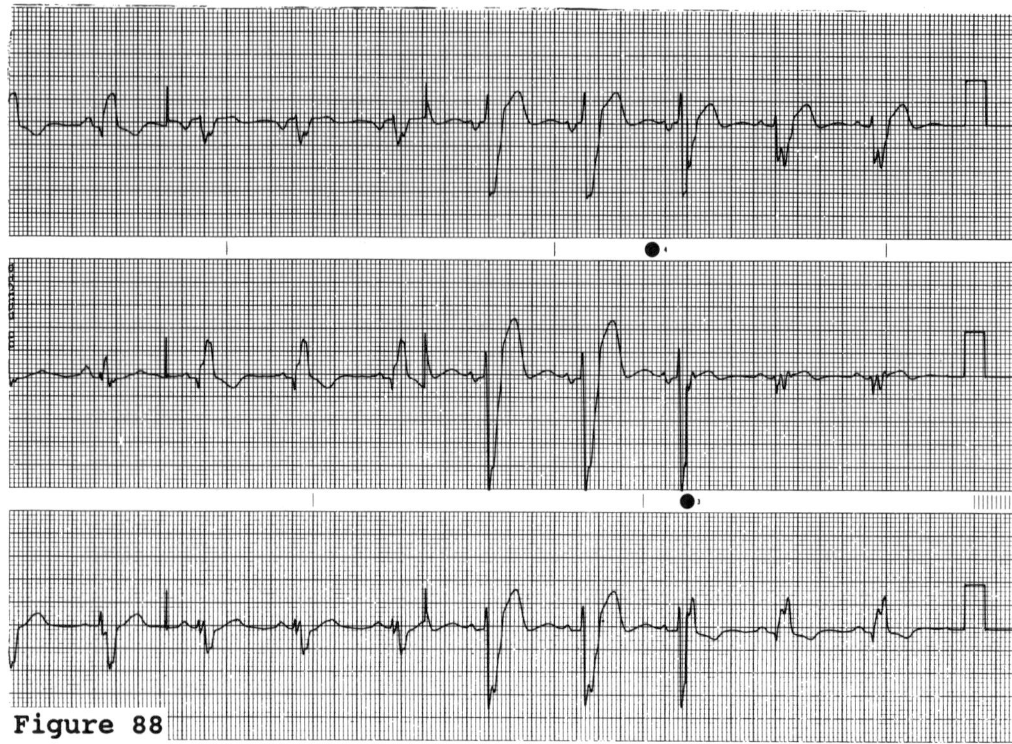

Figure 88

This record shows probable atrial fibrillation, left bundle branch block, possible left anterior superior hemiblock, and an apical infarct of undetermined age, possibly recent. The frontal plane QRS axis is -30, and the T axis is +135 degrees. The horizontal QRS axis is -75, and the T axis is +60 degrees. The tall R in V1 is consistent with anteroseptal involvement as well. Suggest serial records and clinical correlation.

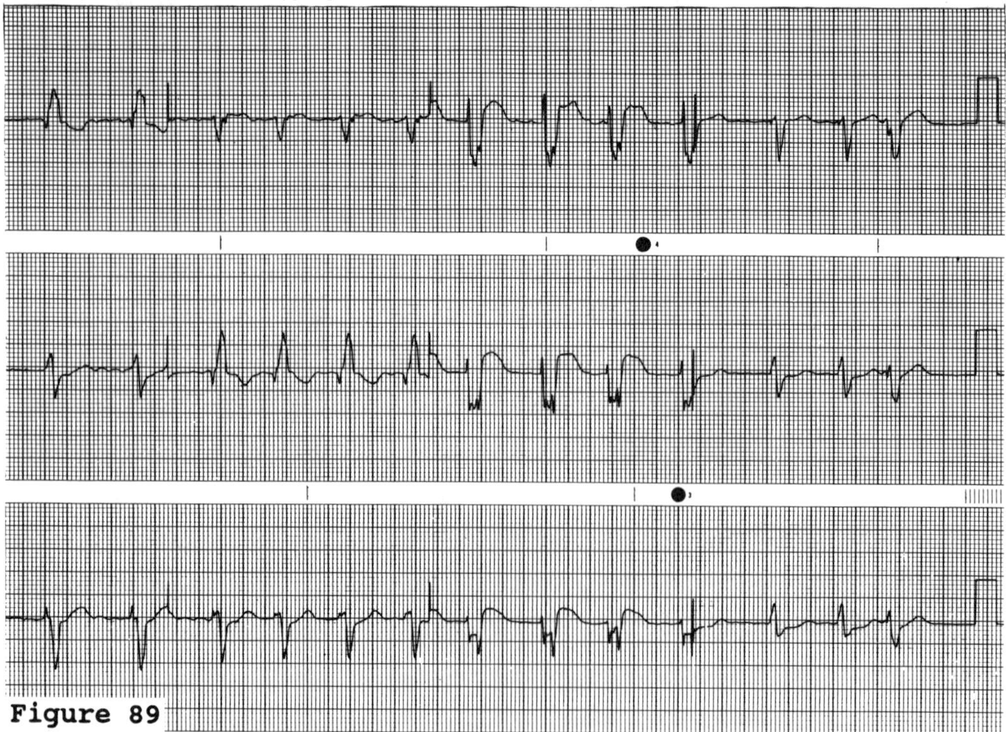

Figure 89

tion, posterior forces with posterior infarction, inferior forces with inferior infarction, and so on. This is true, but what is the real reason for this? The reason is that the wave of depolarization is usually <u>travelling</u> anteriorly in the anterior regions, inferiorly in the inferior regions, and so on. It is for <u>this</u> <u>reason</u>, and only because of this, that infarction causes the usual losses of force that we see. This is because the Purkinje system essentially delivers the impulse to the inner (endocardial) surfaces of both ventricles and to the left side of the septum, resulting in the usual pathway of ventricular depolarization shown in Figure 22. In this situation of normal intraventricular conduction, an anteroseptal infarct results in a <u>loss</u> of anterior forces in the EKG.

In LBBB, however, the septal depolarization now proceeds in the opposite direction, from right to left and posteriorly, giving us Q waves or only small and thin R waves in V1 - V3. Now exactly the same anteroseptal infarct gives us a loss of <u>posterior</u> force, since the wave of depolarization is now traveling <u>posteriorly</u> through this region, and <u>that</u> is what is now lost with the infarct. This results in a net <u>gain</u> of anterior forces in V1 - V3, with taller and broader R waves than are usually seen here with ordinary LBBB. Examples are shown in Figures 88 and 89. In addition, one may see a Q in Lead 1 and/or V6 from either a septal or a lateral infarct in the presence of LBBB.

<u>Pericarditis</u> <u>and</u> <u>Effusion</u>- Figures 90 - 91.

In pericarditis the outermost portions of the pericardium and ventricular myocardium are inflamed and develop the same K loss abnormalities of repolarization and resting potential, leading to the usual T changes and ST segment shifts.

This record shows sinus tachycardia with ST segment elevations and hyperacute T changes in many leads, consistent with pericarditis. The narrow Q in leads 1 and V6 is probably a normal septal Q. Both the frontal and horizontal plane ST segment axes are 0 degrees. Suggest serial records and clinical correlation.

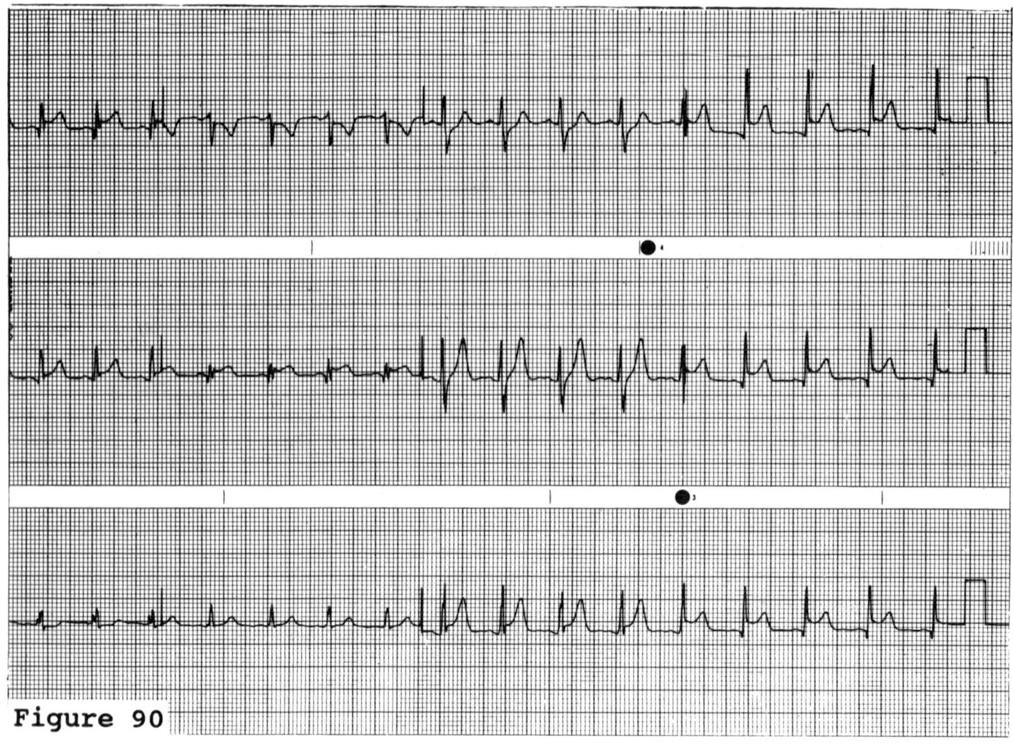

Figure 90

This record shows extremely low voltage in almost all leads, consistent with pericardial effusion. The rhythm is not clear, but examination of V1 suggests that it might be an atrial tachycardia or flutter with 2/1 AV block. The T changes are consistent with anterior and lateral pathology, pericarditis, or ischemia. The frontal plane QRS axis is biphasic in many leads and is difficult to plot. The frontal T axis also cannot be plotted. The horizontal plane QRS axis is also biphasic in many leads and difficult to plot, but it is upright in V5 and V6 and may be about +15 degrees. The frontal T axis is away from the lateral leads. Suggest serial records and clinical correlation.

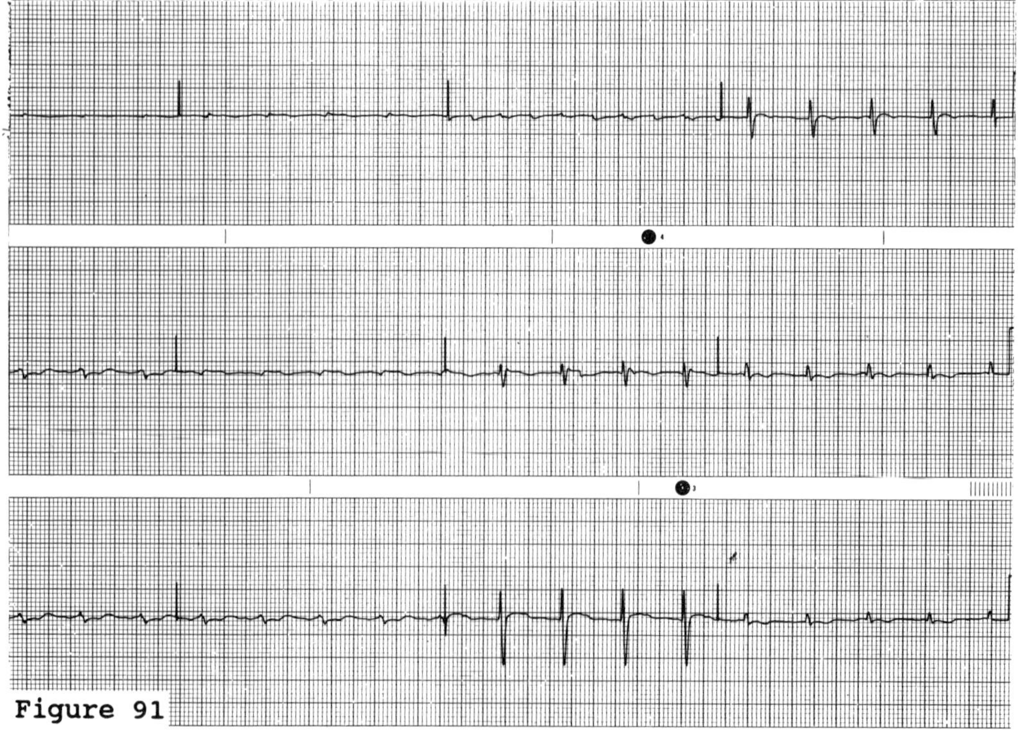

Figure 91

Since these are not localized to any one region of the myocardium but are generalized over much of its surface, pericarditis is recognized by ST elevations and T inversions (or hyperacute changes) appearing in almost all leads of the EKG, usually except aVR, usually without any localizing QRS changes to suggest an infarction. If, however, pericarditis is accompanied by significant pericardial effusion, one may see in addition a diminution in amplitude of all complexes. This appears to be caused by the interposition of the pericardial fluid between the myocardium and the electrocardiographic leads. Low voltage in general, therefore, is caused by interposed material such as an effusion, by intervening lung tissue as in emphysema, or by interposed ground substance in the myocardium, with a less vigorous spike discharge of the individual cells as in myxedema or a chronic myocardopathy.

5
Extrasystoles

<u>Normal</u> <u>Sinus</u> <u>Rhythm</u> <u>and</u> <u>Its</u> <u>Variations</u> <u>(NSR)</u>- Figure 10

The SA node usually fires spontaneously at about 70/minute. Increased vagal tone, carotid sinus pressure, and cholinergic drugs are capable of greatly slowing or transiently stopping this activity by reducing the slope of phase 4 of these cells. Sympathetic stimuli and sympathomimetic drugs will increase the rate to as high as 150-180/minute, by increasing the slope of phase 4. The P wave is followed by a normal QRS and T in .12 to .20 seconds after the beginning of the P wave. Thus the normal PR interval (from the beginning of the P wave in the earliest lead showing a P wave to the beginning of the QRS complex in the earliest lead showing a QRS) is usually within .12 to 0.20 sec. It is slightly shorter at fast rates and slightly longer at slow rates.

<u>Sinus</u> <u>Bradycardia</u>- Figure 92.

The rhythm arises from the SA node at a rate less than 60/minute. This normally occurs during sleep and in trained athletes or laborers at rest. It is produced by increased vagal tone, cholinergic drugs, digitalis, anoxia, and other causes.

<u>Sinus</u> <u>Arrhythmia</u> Figure 93.

Toward the end of inspiration, LV filling has been decreased, as pulmonary venous blood has been held in the lungs due to the decreased intrathoracic pressure, and LV output has been reduced. It is likely that baroreceptors in the aortic wall are then less stretched, and (with a slight delay) send autonomic impulses to the heart to increase its rate. Similarly,

This record shows marked sinus bradycardia at 45/minute. The frontal QRS axis is +50, the T axis is -5, and the P axis is 0 degrees. The horizontal QRS axis is -30, the T axis is +40, and the P axis is +45 degrees. While inferior ischemia cannot be completely excluded, the record may well be within normal limits. Suggest repeat or serial records and clinical correlation.

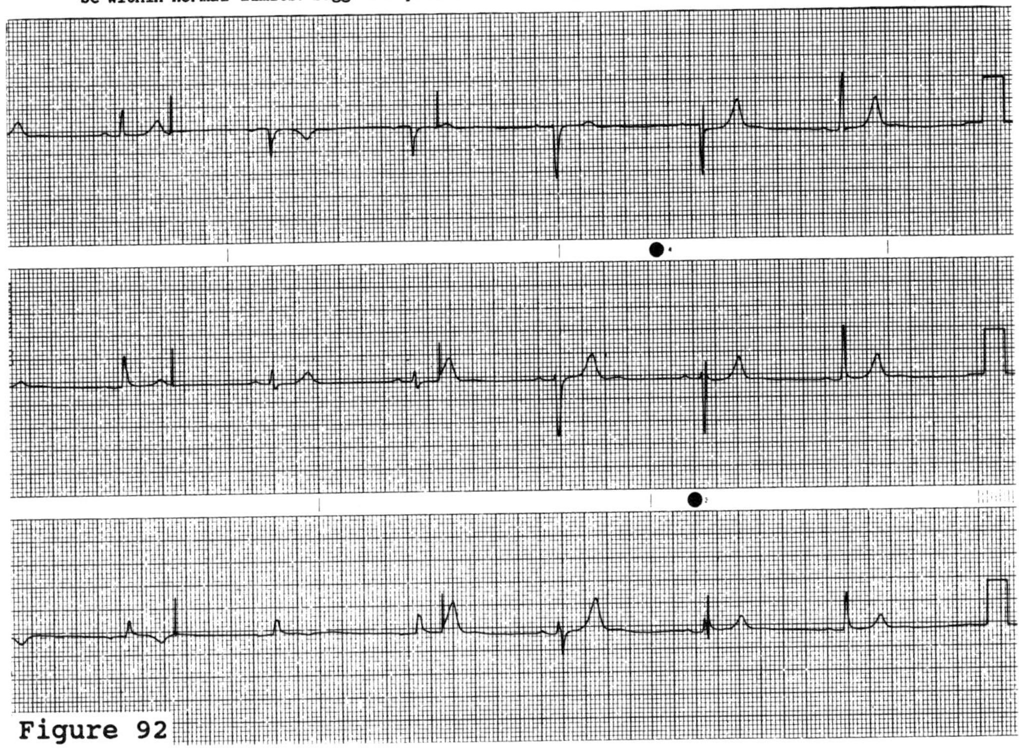

Figure 92

LV output is increased toward the end of expiration, and the aortic baroreceptors now send impulses to reduce the rate of SA nodal discharge (heart rate). Thus the cyclic changes in intrathoracic pressure which follow respiration lead to cyclic changes in cardiac output, aortic pressure, and heart rate, each of which has its own phase relationship to the respiratory cycle. Thus sinus arrhythmia is usually a sign of health, and so is the mild cyclic change in blood pressure with the respiratory cycle, which becomes accentuated, however (sometimes greatly!) with chronic obstructive lung disease or pericardial effusion. An exaggerated decrease in blood pressure with inspiration, (over 10-15 mmHg) is called a <u>paradoxical</u> <u>pulse</u>.

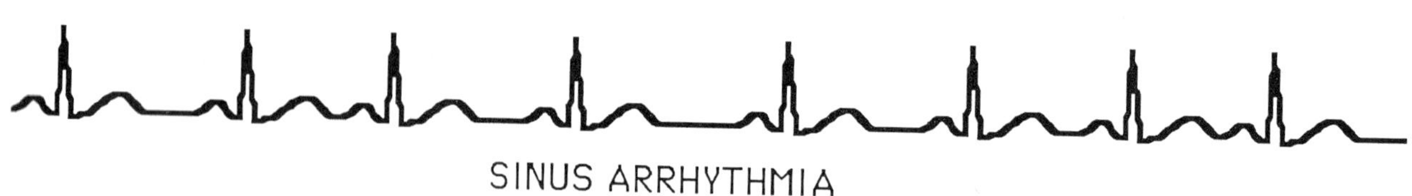

<u>Figure 93</u>

<u>The</u> <u>Paradoxical</u> <u>Pulse</u>

A <u>paradox</u>, in symbolic logic, is a set of conditions which first appear to be a logical contradiction or untruth, but which on close examination are found to be true or consistent. Now, what is paradoxical about a paradoxical pulse? Most of the time when we <u>feel</u> a change in the amplitude of the peripheral pulse, we also <u>hear</u> a change in the amplitude of the heart sounds. This relationship exists with extrasystoles, for example, and with atrial fibrillation, because of the basic length-tension relationship in muscle. Kussmaul noted that patients with pericardial effusion or tamponade

114

often had a <u>great</u> <u>diminution</u> in the amplitude of the peripheral pulse with inspiration, returning with expiration, but that there was essentially <u>no</u> <u>change</u> in the amplitude of the usually quiet heart sounds (the rhythm remaining regular). This, to Kussmaul, was the <u>paradox,</u> and this is why he named it the <u>paradoxical</u> <u>pulse</u> (large respiratory changes in pulse amplitude without corresponding changes in the amplitude of the heart sounds).

The paradoxical pulse is not reflected in the EKG, except as it may show evidence of pericardial disease. We just had to tell you about it, as the actual paradox seems generally not to be well known, and it clears up a lot of misconceptions!

<u>Wandering</u> <u>Atrial</u> <u>Pacemaker</u>

With an increase in vagal tone with respiration, and for other reasons, the atrial pacemaker may be moved from the SA node down into the specialized atrial conducting cells, and occasionally down as far as the AV node itself, as the firing of the SA nodal and other cells is suppressed by the vagal supression of phase 4 of their action potentials. There are corresponding changes in the shape of the P wave and its frontal and horizontal axes or vectors (especially the frontal, as it may move superiorly), and sometimes changes in the PR interval as well.

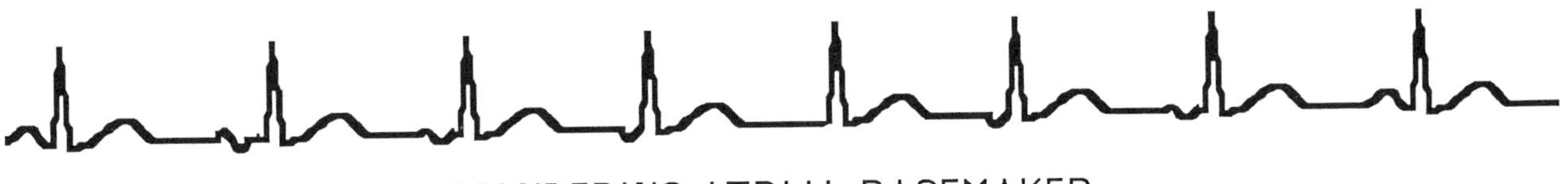

<u>Figure 94</u>

<u>Sinus</u> <u>Tachycardia</u>- Figure 95.

Usually the rhythm is called sinus tachycardia when the SA node fires at more than 100/minute. It is due to those things which increase sympathetic tone, such as fear, exercise, anger, fever, hypoxia, anemia, shock, hyperthyroidism, and cardiac failure, all of which increase the slope of phase 4 of SA nodal (and other) cells. Sympathomimetic amines, caffeine, nitrites, and tobacco may also cause sinus tachycardia.

Sinus tachycardia differs from ectopic tachycardias in its gradual onset and disappearance, and in its normal frontal and horizontal P axes or vectors. It is most helpful if the onset and disappearance can be reliably elicited by careful history-taking, or by proper vagal maneuvers, and the P axis examined.

As seen on the EKG, it will resemble a normal sinus rhythm but with a rate over 100/minute. The P wave may begin to merge with the preceding T wave. The Valsalva maneuver, carotid sinus pressure, and other vagal maneuvers transiently and gradually slow this rhythm, which gradually returns to its previous rate after the maneuver is completed.

<u>Sinus</u> <u>Standstill</u> <u>or</u> <u>SA</u> <u>Block</u>- Figures 96 - 99.

SA nodal discharge may be suppressed either by vagal tone or hyperpotassemia, and may be rendered inadequate to initiate a propagated wave of depolarization over the atria. Asystole or varying degrees of SA block may result. The AV node may fire spontaneously at its own slower rate (junctional or nodal escape) if the period of asystole is long enough. Treatment consists of atropine, correction of electrolyte imbalance, or, if the arrhythmia leads to frequent disabling syncopal episodes, a pacemaker. An idealized example is shown in Figure 96, and two possible records and one probable clinical example are shown in Figures 97 - 99.

116

This record shows sinus tachycardia at 143/minute, and ST elevations in many leads consistent with pericarditis and/or anteroseptal, anteroapical, inferior, and lateral subepicardial injury with hyperacute T changes. No definite evidence of infarction can be seen, although the R progression between V1 and V4 is minimal, and a small Q may be present in V4. The frontal plane QRS axis is +60, the T axis is +60, and the P axis +60 degrees. The horizontal plane QRS axis is -20, the T axis is +45, and the P axis 0 degrees. The frontal plane ST segment vector is +60 degrees. The horizontal plane ST segment vector is about +70 degrees. Suggest serial records and clinical correlation.

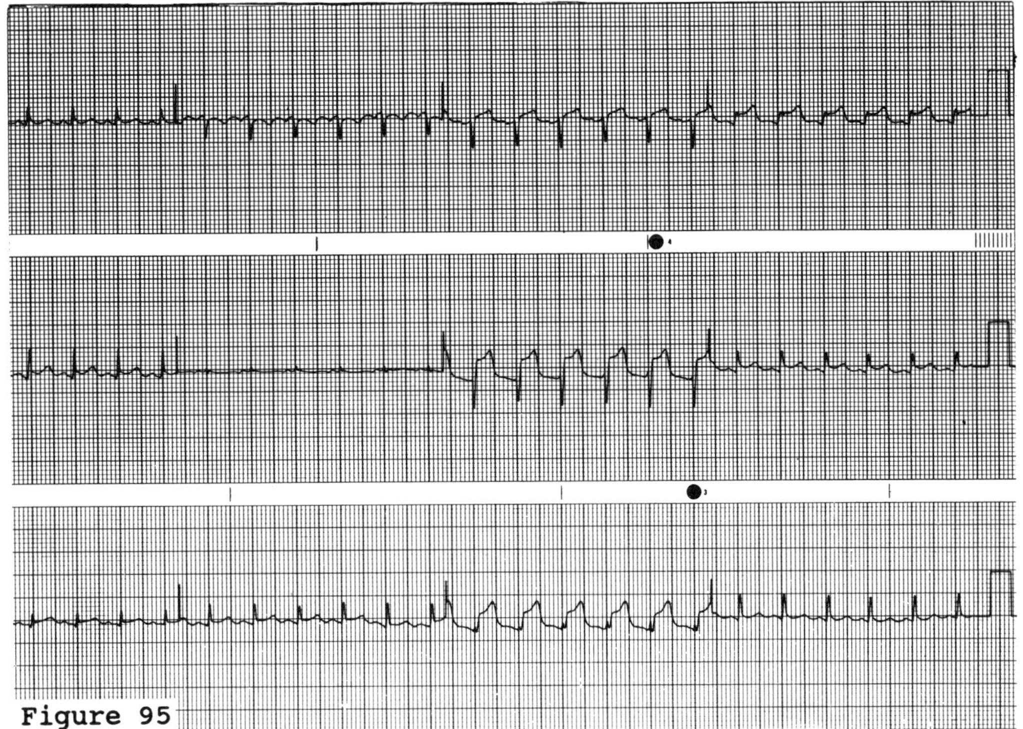

Figure 95

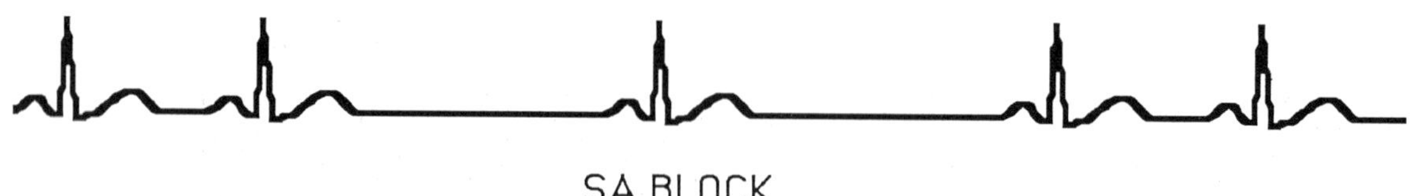

FIGURE <u>96</u>

<u>Extrasystoles:</u> <u>General</u> <u>Aspects.</u>

As we have already seen, the capacity for spontaneous firing exists in the SA node (about 70/minute), the AV node (about 50/minute), and in the Purkinje cells of the Bundle of His and its ramifications (about 30-40/minute).

Anoxia, ischemia, sympathomimetic amines, digitalis, and cardiac enlargement (stretching the sarcomeres) can increase the rate of slow diastolic depolarization of the above cells (phase 4), and therefore can greatly increase their rate of spontaneous discharge.

Single spontaneous discharges of atrial, AV nodal, or Purkinje tissue are called extrasystoles. These often occur in perfectly normal hearts under the influence of excitement (sympathomimetic amines). In people with normal hearts they usually disappear or become less frequent with exercise (overdriven by the sinus tachycardia), while extrasystoles due to organic heart disease usually become more frequent with exercise (probably because of increasing ischemia, with an increasing slope of phase 4).

118

This record shows regular sinus rhythm with two episodes of possible SA block. However, these
pauses may actually be due to nonconducted atrial extrasystoles which may be present just behind the
last QRS complex in leads aVR, aVL, and aVF, and just behind the last QRS complex in V1-V3. The QRS
duration is .14 seconds. First degree AV block and probable left atrial enlargement are present. An
intraventricular conduction defect, possibly left bundle branch block with a lateral infarct of
undetermined age, is present. The frontal plane QRS axis has almost no net deflection in any lead,
and may be straight posterior. The T axis is +60 degrees. There is an M-shaped P wave in lead 2,
and the P axis is about +30 degrees. The horizontal plane QRS axis is about -130, the T axis +40,
and the P axis about 0 degrees. Suggest serial records and clinical correlation.

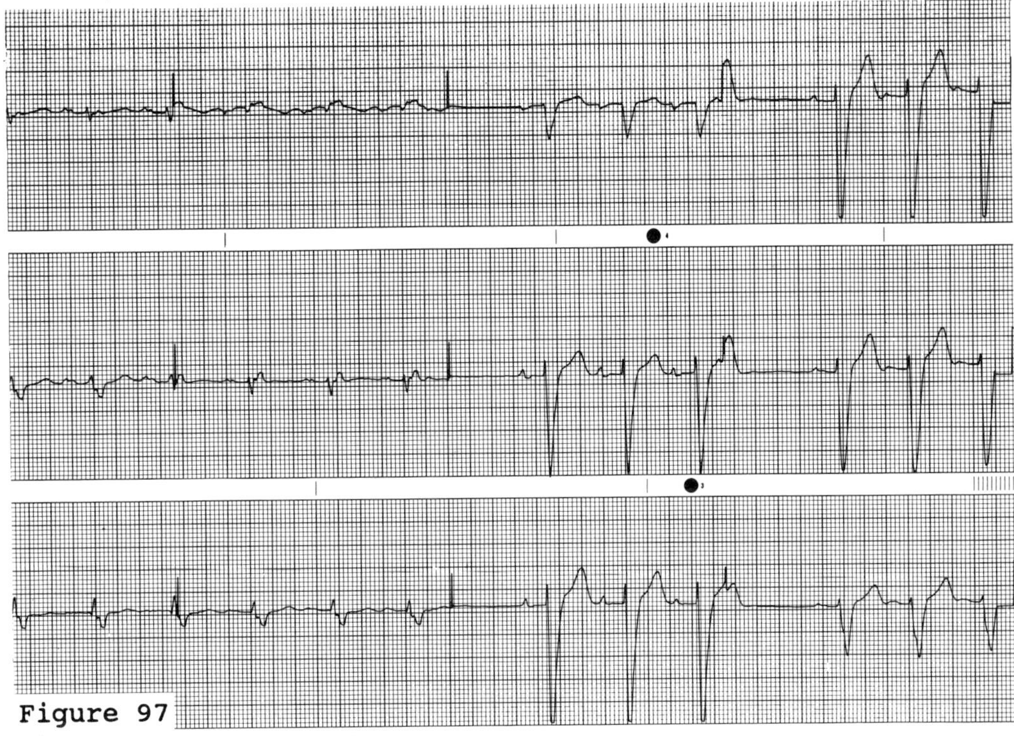

Figure 97

This record shows sinus bradycardia, first and second degree AV block with probable ventricular
escape, and right bundle branch block with left superior branch hemiblock in the few conducted beats
seen. SA arrest cannot be clearly seen in this record, as the escape beat comes just before the next
P wave is due to fire. Suggest repeat or serial records and clinical correlation.

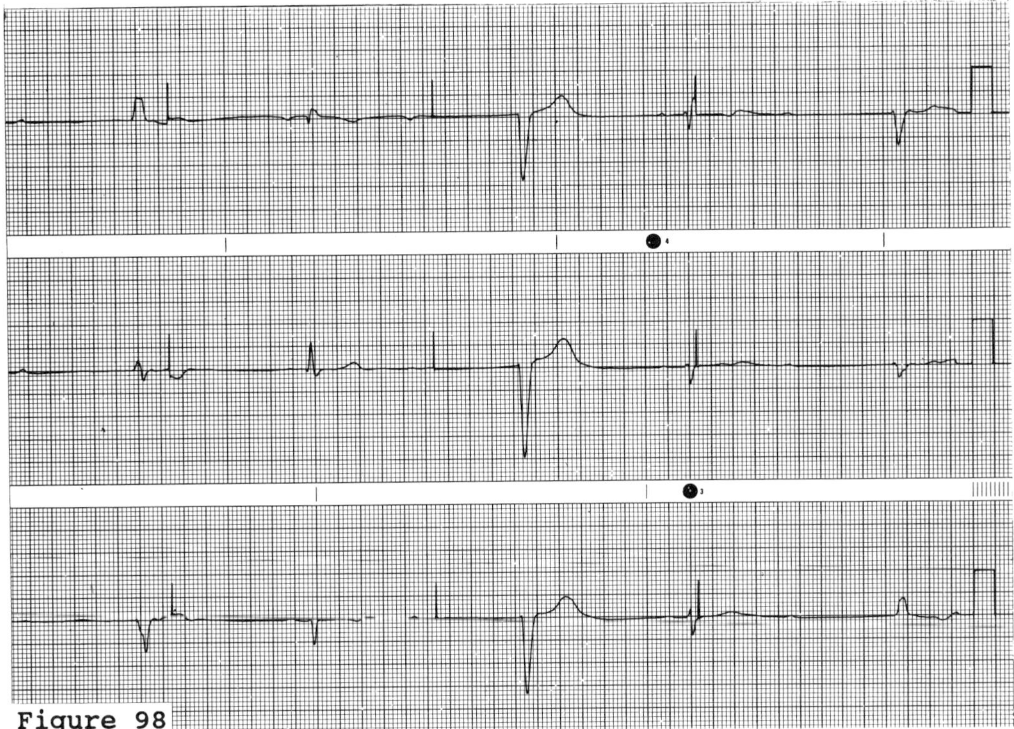

Figure 98

This record shows sinus rhythm and evidence of probable Mobitz Type 2 SA block or sinus arrest. Since it occurs periodically after every 3 conducted beats but is not accompanied by a change in shape of the P waves or a shortening of the P-P interval, the record may well represent Mobitz Type 2 second degree SA block. The T waves are somewhat peaked, and hyperkalemia cannot be excluded. Suggest repeat or serial records and clinical correlation.

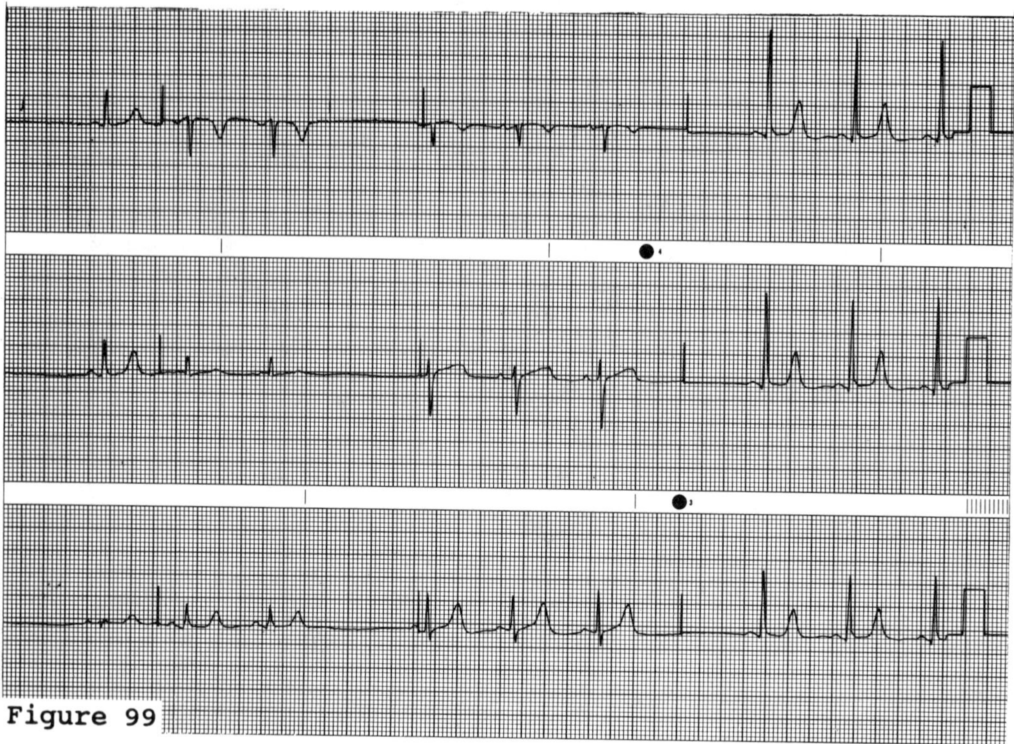

Figure 99

Clinically, infrequent extrasystoles occurring in people with normal hearts usually do not warrant treatment. If they are frequent or bothersome, however, a proper workup should be done and treatment considered.

<u>Atrial Extrasystoles</u>- Figure 100 - 103.

Atrial extrasystoles (premature atrial contractions, PAC's) may occur in normal people, or in patients with diseases leading to atrial enlargement or involvement of atrial tissue, such as mitral stenosis, acute cor pulmonale (pulmonary embolism), hyperthyroidism, or myocardial infarction involving the atria (usually the left). EKG recognition is based on a P wave of unusual shape and axis, followed in .12 seconds or more by a normal QRS complex and T wave. However, atrial extrasystoles may also fail to be conducted, or may be propagated with aberrant intraventricular conduction. Other examples are shown in Figures 101 - 103.

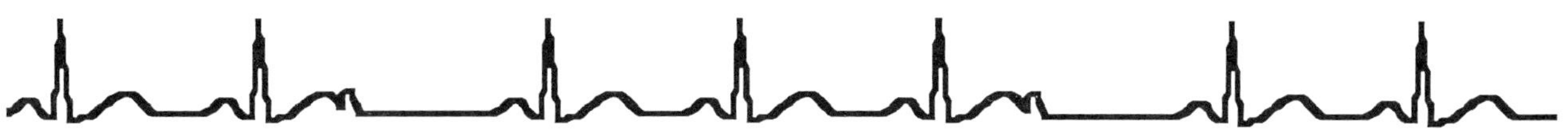

ATRIAL EXTRASYSTOLES (NONCONDUCTED)

<u>FIGURE 100</u>

This record shows regular sinus rhythm, frequent nonconducted atrial extrasystoles, and T changes consistent with left ventricular strain and/or lateral ischemia. The frontal plane QRS axis is -40, the frontal plane T axis about 180, and the P axis is +40 degrees. The horizontal plane QRS axis is -20, the T axis is +120, and the P axis is +5 degrees. Suggest serial records.

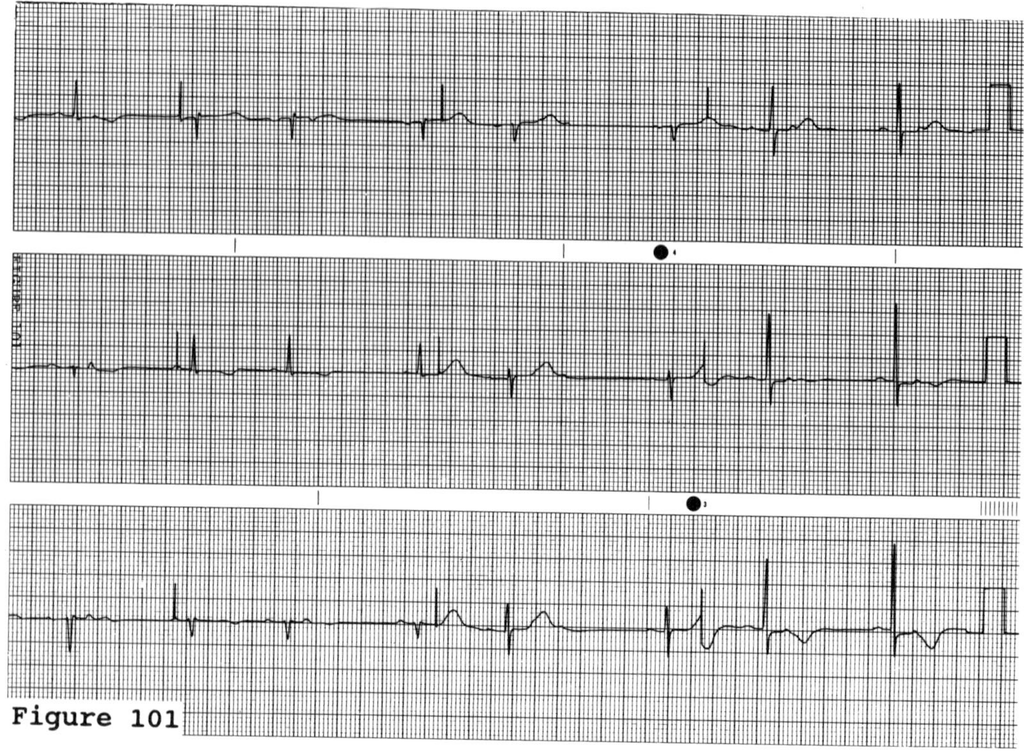

Figure 101

This record shows sinus rhythm and frequent atrial extrasystoles, often in bigeminy. The frontal plane QRS axis is -10, the T axis is +135, and the P axis is +70 degrees. The frontal plane P axis of the atrial extrasystoles is about -90 degrees. The horizontal plane QRS axis is -40, the T axis is +140, and the P axis is +5 degrees. The record shows sinus rhythm, frequent atrial extrasystoles, possible left ventricular enlargement, and T changes consistent with left ventricular strain and/or lateral ischemia. Suggest repeat or serial records and clinical correlation.

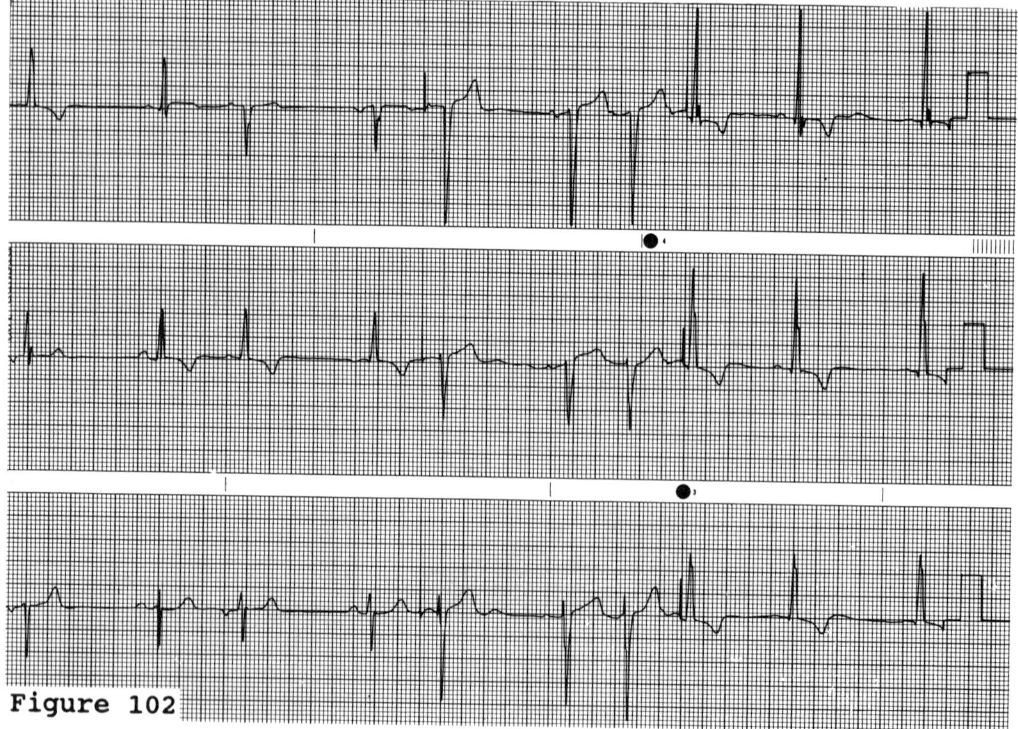

Figure 102

This record shows sinus rhythm and occasional atrial extrasystoles. The frontal plane QRS axis
is 0, the T axis is 180, and the P axis is +35 degrees. The horizontal plane QRS axis is -40, the T
axis -90, and the P axis is +5 degrees. The record shows sinus rhythm, frequent atrial extrasystoles, and T changes consistent with anterior and apical ischemia. Suggest serial records.

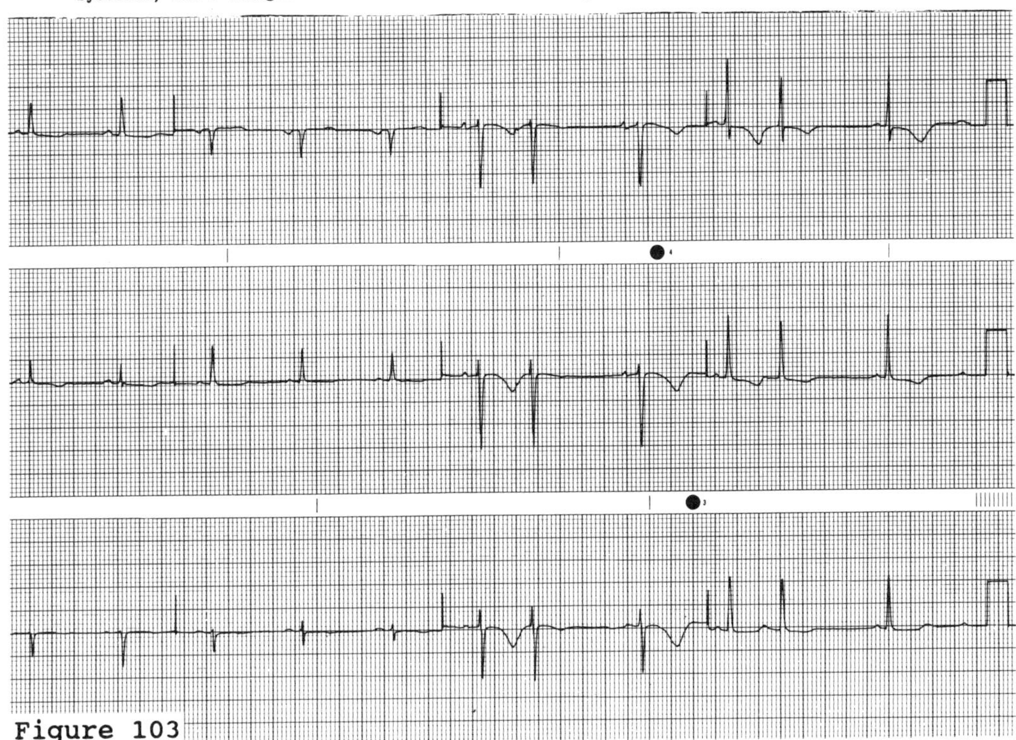

Figure 103

Here conduction proceeds over the atria in a retrograde direction so that the P wave is inverted in most leads but is usually upright in aVR. Thus the frontal P vector is usually directed superiorly. The focus is closer to the His bundle, thus slightly delaying the P wave and <u>shortening</u> the PR interval to less than 0.12 second. The QRS and T waves are usually normal. Junctional extrasystoles have been classified as described below, though this may not be as accurate as once was thought.

<u>Upper</u> <u>Junctional</u> <u>or</u> <u>Nodal</u> <u>Extrasystoles</u> give rise to the least P wave delay. The usually inverted P wave has a <u>short</u> <u>PR</u> <u>interval</u> of less than 0.12 seconds, as shown in Figure 104. Figure 105 also shows an example of either a low atrial or upper junctional extrasystole.

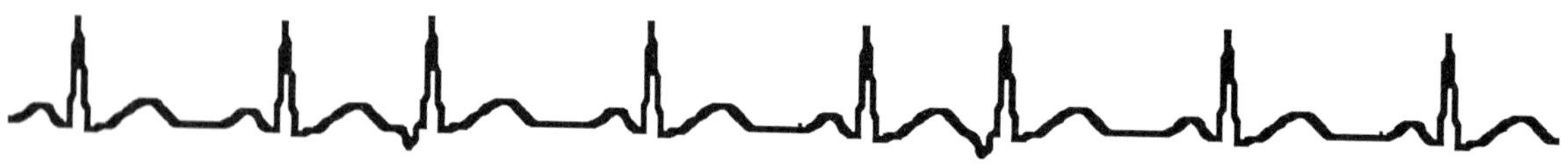

<u>Figure 104</u>

124

This record shows sinus rhythm and a low atrial or upper junctional extrasystole (the last
event - the retrograde P wave - in leads 1,2, and 3). The frontal plane QRS axis is +45, the T axis
+60, and the P axis is +60 degrees. The horizontal plane QRS axis is -30 degrees. The T axis is
+135, and is consistent with possible apical and lateral ischemia. An abnormal precordial R
progression is noted, reflecting anterior infarction, possibly acute. The horizontal plane ST segment vector is +60 degrees. This record shows sinus rhythm, occasional low atrial or upper
junctional extrasystoles, and anteroseptal infarction with anterior subepicardial injury and apical
ischemia. Suggest serial records.

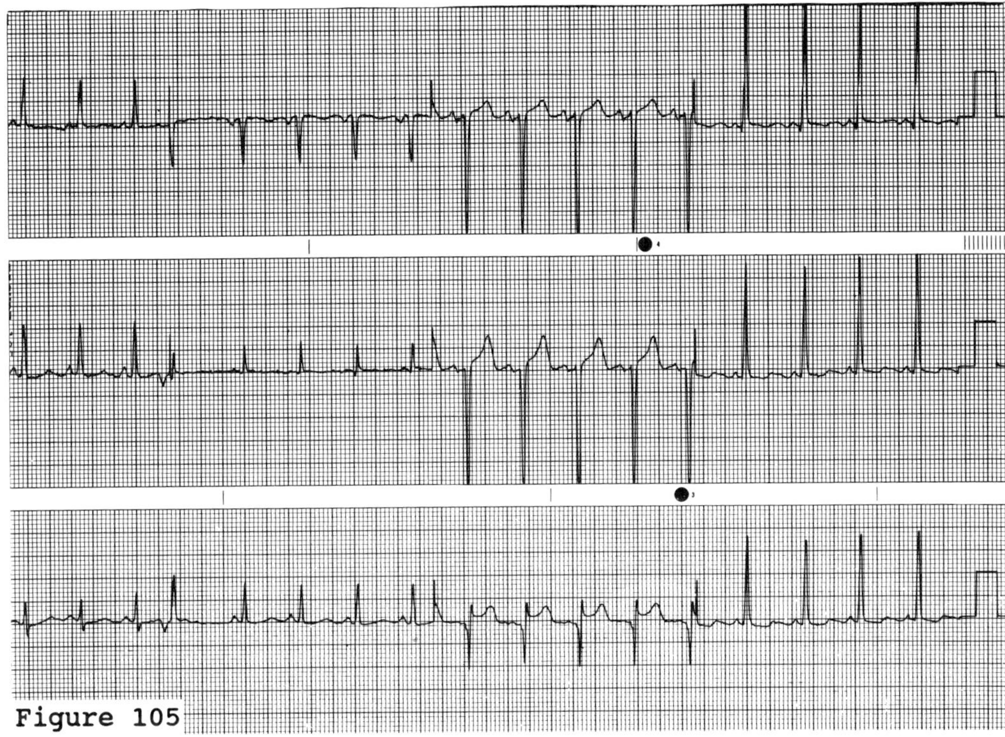

Figure 105

<u>Mid-Junctional</u> <u>or</u> <u>Mid-Nodal</u> <u>Extrasystoles</u> cause more delay to the P wave. As a result, there is no PR interval, and the P wave is buried and lost <u>in</u> the QRS complex, often distorting it slightly, as in Figure 106. A clinical example is shown in Figure 108, in the second unpaced QRS complex in Leads aVR, aVL, and aVF. This extrasystole is then followed by a normal (not a retrograde) P wave, which, however, fails to be conducted.

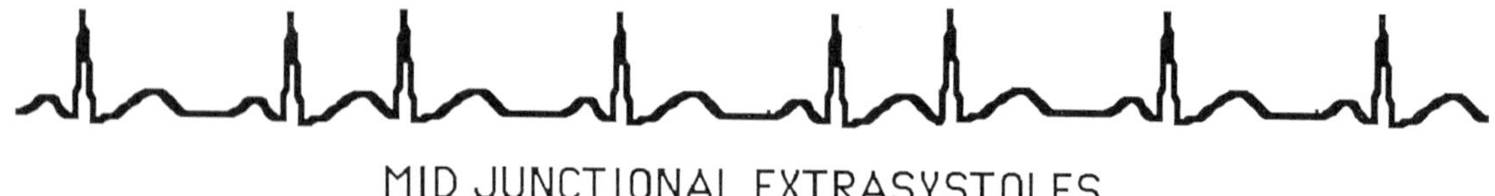

<u>Figure</u> <u>106</u>

<u>Lower</u> <u>Junctional</u> <u>or</u> <u>Lower</u> <u>Nodal</u> <u>Extrasystoles</u> cause still further delay in the retrograde atrial depolarization, causing the inverted P wave now to appear <u>behind</u> the QRS complex, in the ST segment, as in Figure 107.

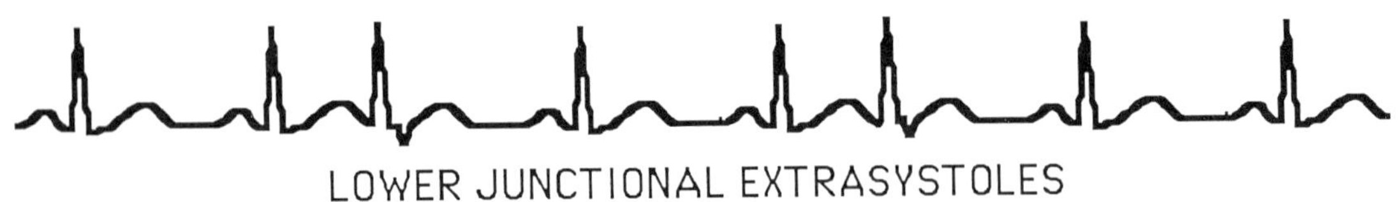

<u>FIGURE</u> <u>107</u>

This record shows a pacemaker functioning possibly in the fixed-rate mode, but possibly in the QRS inhibited mode (see the last QRS complex in V4-V6). It appears not to sense many QRS complexes and it often fails to capture the ventricle to produce a QRS complex. Random variation in the apparent pacemaker spike height is seen. Second degree AV block and occasional junctional escape (V1-V3 and V4-V6) is seen. T changes suggest inferior and apical ischemia. The frontal QRS axis is +50, the T axis is -45, the P axis +30 degrees. The horizontal QRS axis is -40, the T axis +165, (although a second transition between V5 and V6 is seen), and the P axis is difficult to plot. This record shows second degree AV block and a probable nonsensing, noncapturing (possibly fixed-rate) pacemaker. T changes suggesting inferior and apical ischemia are noted. Suggest serial records and evaluation of the pacemaker.

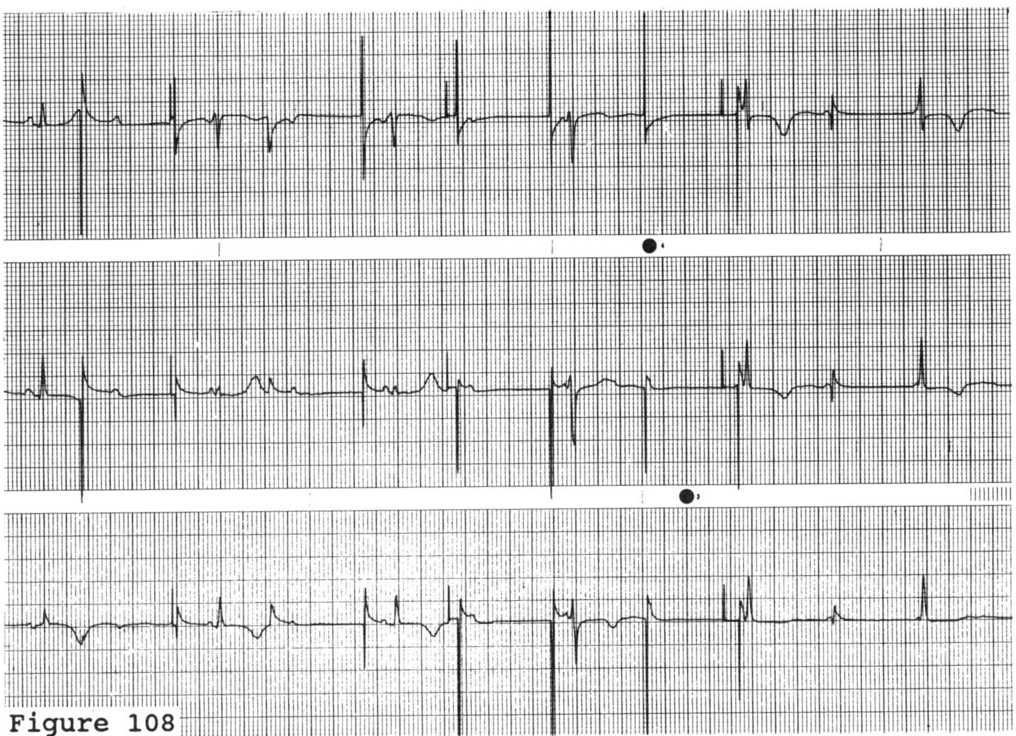

Figure 108

<u>Ventricular (Purkinje Cell) Extrasystoles</u>

Ventricular extrasystoles (premature ventricular contractions, PVC's) may arise from any portion of the bundle of His or its branches. They may be either unifocal or multifocal in origin.

PVC's cause a wide, bizarre QRS complex, usually more than .12 seconds in duration, as the pathway of ventricular depolarization does not proceed normally. The ST segment may be displaced, and the T wave vector is usually in the opposite direction from the QRS vector, as is Figures 109 - 112.

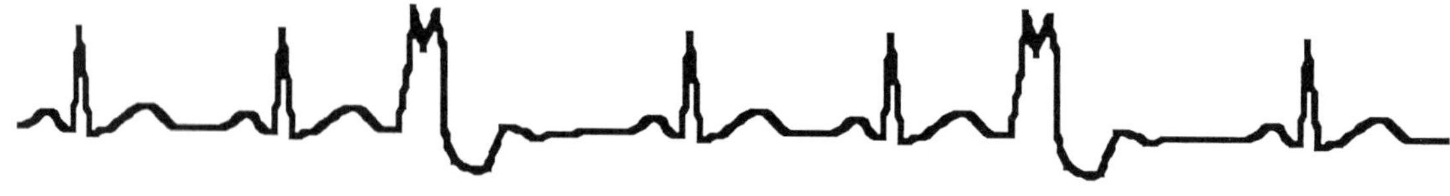

<u>FIGURE 109</u>

Extrasystoles arising from the Purkinje system of the left ventricle usually have a QRS complex resembling that of right bundle branch block, and those arising in the right ventricle will usually have a QRS resembling that of left bundle branch block.

Ventricular extrasystoles are not preceded by a P wave. In some cases retrograde atrial conduction may occur and a delayed retrograde P wave may be seen. The frequently seen pause following a ventricular extrasystole (the so-called "compensatory pause") is a very bad misnomer. Nothing is being

This record shows sinus rhythm and multifocal ventricular extrasystoles. The frontal plane QRS
axis is +160, the T axis is +90, and the P axis is +60 degrees. The horizontal plane QRS axis shows
a double transition between and V1 and V2 and almost at V6. The horizontal T axis is about +5, and
the P axis is +5 degrees. A possible junctional extrasystole or wandering atrial pacemaker is
present in V4-V6, with the QRS firing very shortly after a normally timed P wave. Left atrial
enlargement is present. The record is consistent with left atrial enlargement, pulmonary disease,
and possible right ventricular enlargement. The T changes noted appear non-specific. They do not
suggest right ventricular strain. Suggest repeat record and clinical correlation.

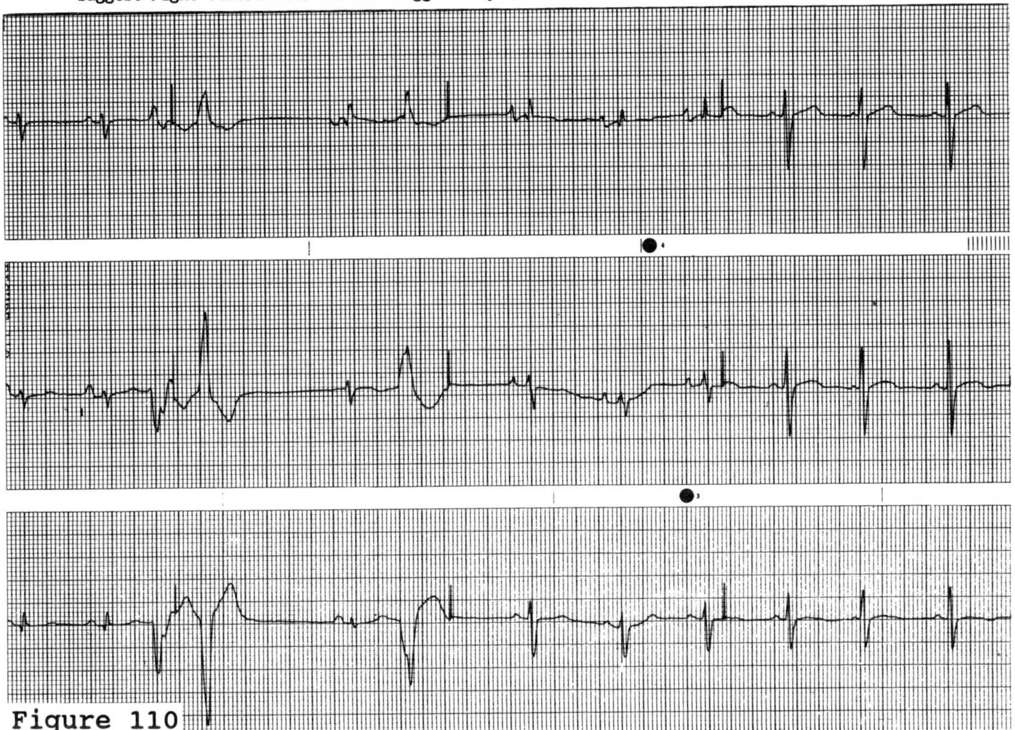

Figure 110

This record shows regular sinus rhythm with repetitive and multifocal ventricular extrasystoles. The frontal plane QRS axis is -100, the T axis +75, and the P axis +40 degrees. The
horizontal plane QRS axis is 180 degrees. The T axis has a double transition between V1 and V2 and
possibly between V4 and V5. It is away from V5 and V6. The P axis is +5 degrees. The record shows
sinus rhythm, several ventricular extrasystoles (some of which are multifocal), a probable
junctional extrasystole in aVR, aVL, and aVF, right bundle branch block, left anterior superior
branch hemiblock, an anterior infarct of undetermined age, possibly recent, and T changes consistent
with lateral ischemia and/or left ventricular strain. Suggest serial records.

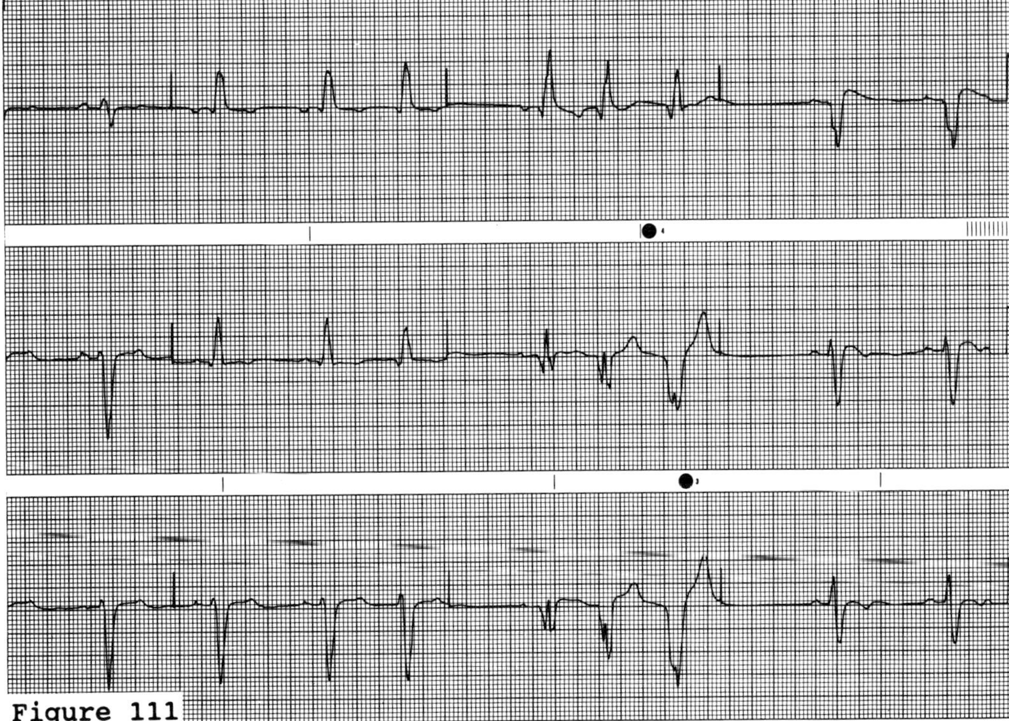

Figure 111

   This record shows sinus rhythm and frequent ventricular extrasystoles, often in trigeminy.
Digitalis toxicity may be present. The frontal plane QRS axis is +90, the T axis is +40, and the P
axis is +45 degrees. The horizontal QRS axis is -40, the T axis is +45, and the P axis is +45
degrees. Except for the PVC's, the record may well be within normal limits. Suggest repeat record
and clinical correlation.

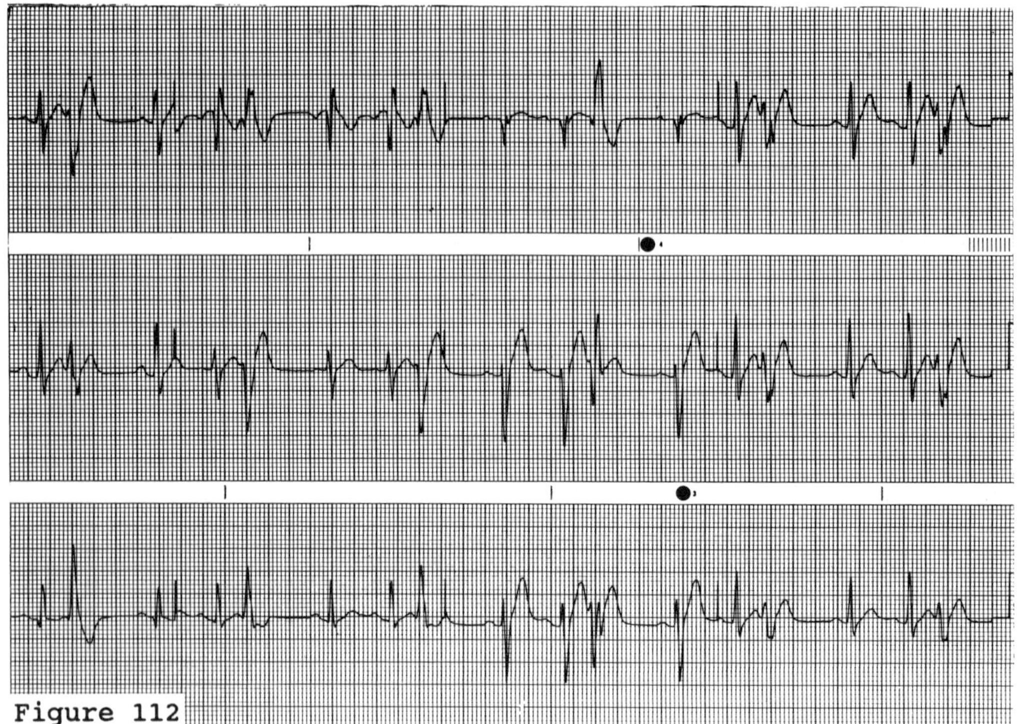

Figure 112

compensated for. The PVC merely blocks the next normal P wave, and everything usually waits for the <u>next</u> P wave to come along. Because of this, the P - P interval seen across such a PVC is often that of the interval between two normal P waves. PVC's may also be <u>interpolated</u> between 2 normal P waves, without any such pause.

Treatment of Extrasystoles

Every patient with extrasystoles requires a complete medical evaluation, an EKG or VCG, and appropriate laboratory studies. He may feel the extrasystoles, may be greatly disturbed by them, and may possibly develop a cardiac neurosis. He will require calm reassurance during the diagnostic studies. However, if he is unaware of them or if they are of no consequence, no treatment may be required.

On the other hand, if the extrasystoles appear to be forerunners of a more serious arrhythmia (as in a myocardopathy or a myocardial infarct, for example), drug therapy may be indicated. If PVC's are due to cardiac failure (elevated atrial pressures, increased sarcomere length, increased slope of phase 4), they may subside after digitalis, diuretics, salt restriction, and perhaps afterload reduction. Digitalis must, however, be used with caution here in the presence of ventricular premature beats. They must be watched carefully to see if they improve or not as the patient's failure improves.

VENTRICULAR EXTRASYSTOLES DUE TO AUTOMATICITY OR RE-ENTRY

Parasystole and Variably-Coupled PVC's

Automatic regular spontaneous discharge of Purkinje cells usually will lead to PVC's with regular intervals between them, unless ventricular tissue is made refractory by another depolarizing event just prior to one of the automatic discharges. In this situation, the R - R interval of the PVC's

will be a multiple of some basic R - R interval of discharge, and the
interval between a preceding normally conducted QRS complex and a subsequent
PVC will usually be a varying one. Such automatic, regular PVC's have been
called <u>parasystolic,</u> and the rhythm disturbance has been called <u>Parasystole.</u>

<u>Re-entry</u> <u>and</u> <u>Fixed-Coupled</u> <u>PVC's</u>

On the other hand, conduction may proceed through an ischemic area of
ventricular myocardium extremely slowly, and by very complicated pathways
(5) as shown in Figure 113.

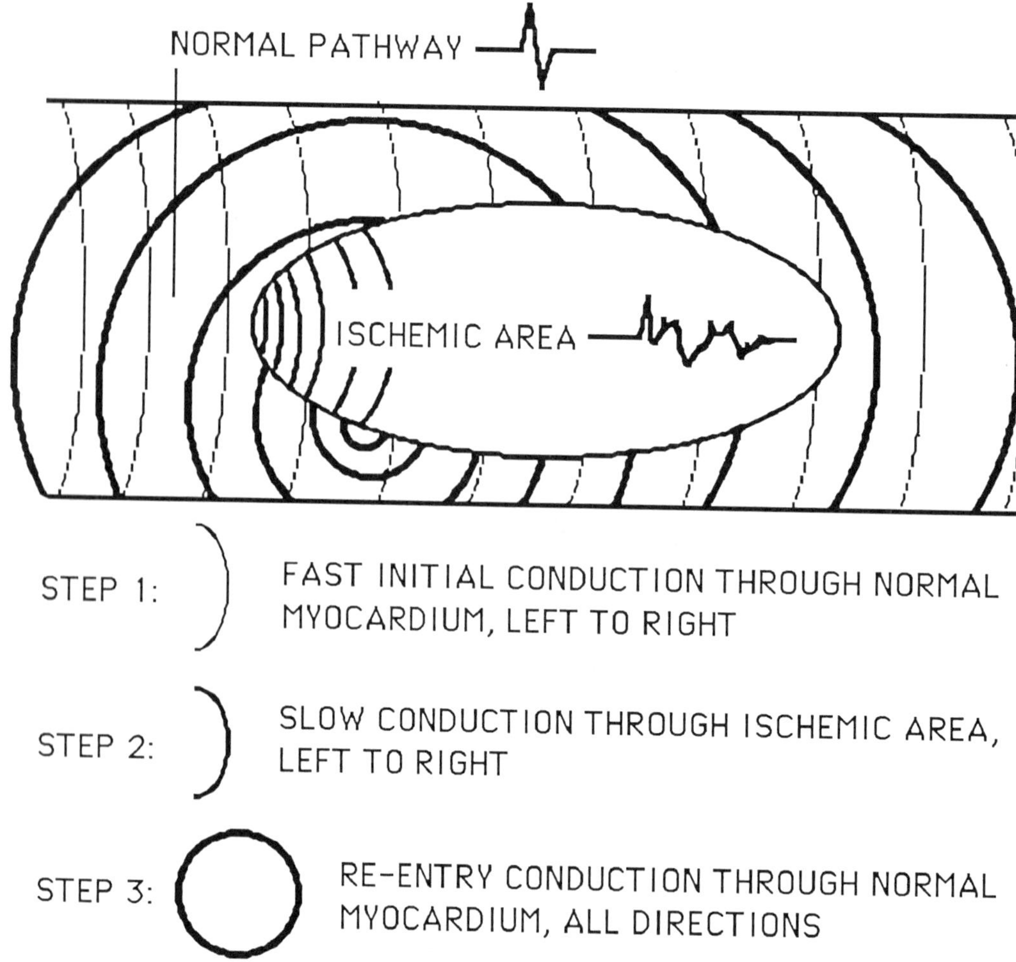

<u>FIGURE 113</u>

Conduction through such slow and labyrinthine pathways can take well over .25 sec or more. It is not surprising, therefore, that such a slowly moving wave front should sooner or later encounter, at its borders, some nonischemic cells which have recovered and are ready to respond to another stimulus. Here they then receive such a stimulus, and the result is a re-entry PVC, usually with a fixed time interval from the preceding QRS. In general, then, PVC's showing fixed coupling are probably due to re-entry, while those showing variable coupling and some sort of basic underlying regularity are more likely to be due to automatic firing of Purkinje cells.

In general, automatic extrasystoles are treated with those drugs that decrease or abolish the slow diastolic depolarization which leads to spontaneous discharge. This can usually be accomplished without significant alteration of the normal spontaneous discharge of normal SA nodal, AV nodal, or Purkinje tissue. Quinidine, pronestyl, and potassium have such an effect. If unsuccessful, other drugs such as norpace, bretylium, magnesium sulfate, or atropine have been used.

For fixed-coupled PVC's, as illustrated in Figure 114, that labyrinthine communication pathway is often like a fragile house of cards, and almost anything that can alter the conduction in any way may be effective against them. Drugs that shorten the refractory period, such as lidocaine, may stop them, as well as those that slow phase 4 depolarization and bring the cell to threshold later, and also those that slow intraventricular conduction. Many different types of drugs have been useful here, and have made significant reductions in the incidence of PVC's. On the other hand, few have been completely successful. Many patients with refractory PVC's and other arrhythmias) are extremely tense people, and difficult to treat.

This record shows sinus rhythm and frequent ventricular extrasystoles appearing in bigeminy. The frontal plane QRS axis is +10, the T axis is +30, and the P axis is +40 degrees. The horizontal plane QRS axis is 0, the T axis +5, and the P axis is +45 degrees. Digitalis toxicity may be present. Except for the frequent bigeminy, the record otherwise appears within normal limits. Suggest repeat record.

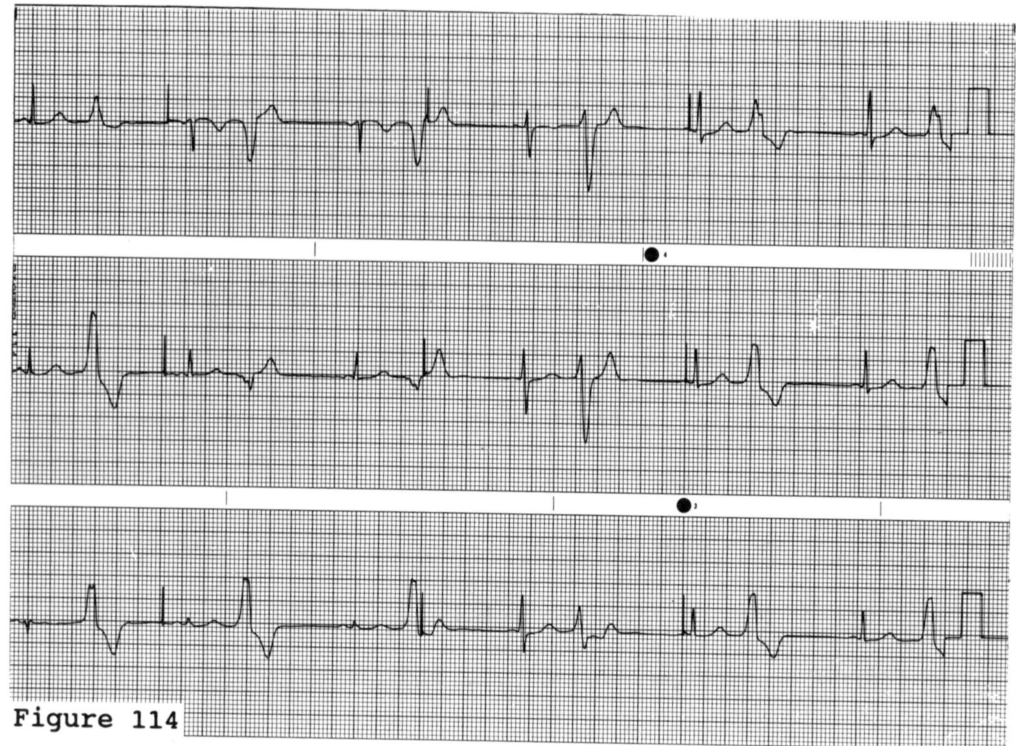

Figure 114

6
The Ectopic Arrhythmias

<u>Analysis</u> <u>of</u> <u>Ectopic</u> <u>Tachycardias</u>

Physical examination is often informative, but never conclusive.

1. One may find a rapid, regular heart rate with absolutely no change in the quality of the heart sounds, suggesting or consistent with some sort of a supraventricular tachycardia.

2. One may find an almost completely regular heart rate, but with slight changes in the timing and quality of the heart sounds from time to time, suggesting or consistent with a ventricular tachycardia, and the varying relationship between P and QRS that can affect the first sound.

3. One may find a grossly irregular rate suggesting atrial fibrillation or multiple extrasystoles, or

4. A rate which is irregular, but which makes sudden jumps which are multiples of a basic rate, suggesting atrial tachycardia or flutter with varying degrees of ventricular response.

5. A pulse deficit may be present due to poor ventricular ejection.

6. An imperceptible heart beat.

7. Mechanical pulsus alternans. This must be differentiated from bigeminy. Its regularity helps.

<u>Vagal</u> <u>Maneuvers</u>

Vagal maneuvers such as the Valsava, eyeball pressure, or carotid sinus pressure will gradually slow a sinus tachycardia, will minimally slow (but often abruptly abolish) an atrial tachycardia, but will not affect a ventricular tachycardia, since Purkinje fibers and the ventricular myocardium clinically are uninfluenced by acetylcholine or its congeners. In helping us to recognize and understand an arrhythmia, vagal maneuvers are often helpful by increasing the amount of AV block and slowing the ventricular rate if it responds. Even if the rate or AV block is not greatly altered, this may allow one to take a good look at the P waves to see what is going on in the atria. In atrial flutter, vagal maneuvers often reduce the ventricular rate to sub-multiples of the original rate.

Carotid sinus pressure involves massage of the carotid sinus under the angle of the jaw when the patient is in the supine position, and is best done with hard-copy electrocardiographic monitoring. It should begin gently, and the degree of pressure should be increased as required by the response of the arrhythmia. Pressure should be maintained for only 10-15 seconds at most, as elderly patients with carotid arterial disease may sometimes have reversible symptoms of carotid vascular insufficiency, and occasionally a frank cerebral thrombosis may be precipitated by this maneuver. Bilateral carotid sinus pressure is absolutely contraindicated. Massage over the right carotid sinus may be more likely to affect the SA node, since the right vagus supplies mainly that area. Massage over the left carotid sinus may be more likely to affect the degree of AV block produced, since the left vagus supplies mainly the AV node. The carotid sinus maneuver may be reinforced by breath holding, by the Valsava, or by eyeball pressure. One may, however, produce a detached retina by injudicious eyeball pressure.

All too often, arrhythmias are approached by a routine EKG. The value of vagal maneuvers done under direct EKG monitoring is then completely lost. When doing any vagal maneuvers, always make sure you do them with a <u>hard copy</u> printed record. Do not be wondering what it was that just went off the scope on the monitor. Always have a secure record that you can put a ruler

This record shows an atrial tachycardia with 2/1 AV block, best shown in V1. An anteroseptal infarct, possibly recent, is also present, with ST changes consistent with anterior subepicardical injury, and T changes suggesting possible apical and lateral ischemia and/or left ventricular strain. Low voltage in the frontal plane is also seen. The frontal QRS axis is -15 degrees. The T axis is difficult to plot. The horizontal plane QRS axis is -60, the ST segment vector is +130, and the T axis is difficult to plot. Each QRS complex may well be fired not by the immediately preceding P wave but by the P wave buried in the T wave in front of it. Pulmonary disease cannot be excluded. Suggest serial records.

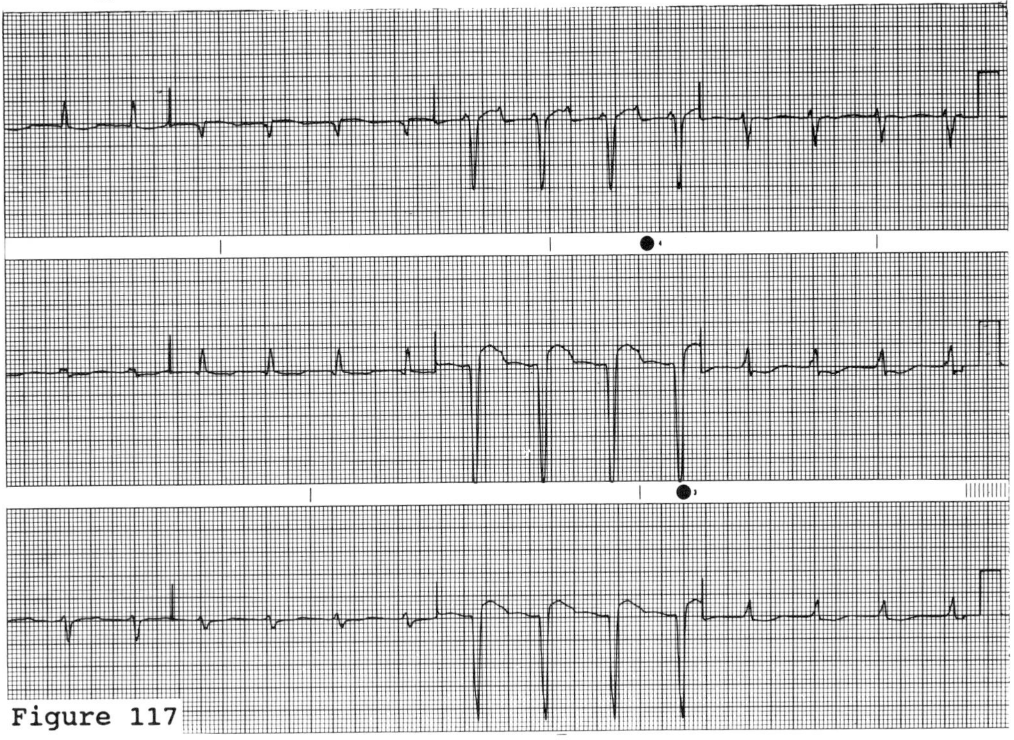

Figure 117

This record shows a rapid atrial tachycardia (almost an atrial flutter), and varying AV block. The frontal plane QRS axis is +105 degrees. The T axis is difficult to plot. The horizontal plane QRS axis is -35, and the T axis is also -35 degrees. Pulmonary disease may be present. Anterior T inversions consistent with anterior ischemia and/or right ventricular strain are present. Suggest serial records and clinical correlation.

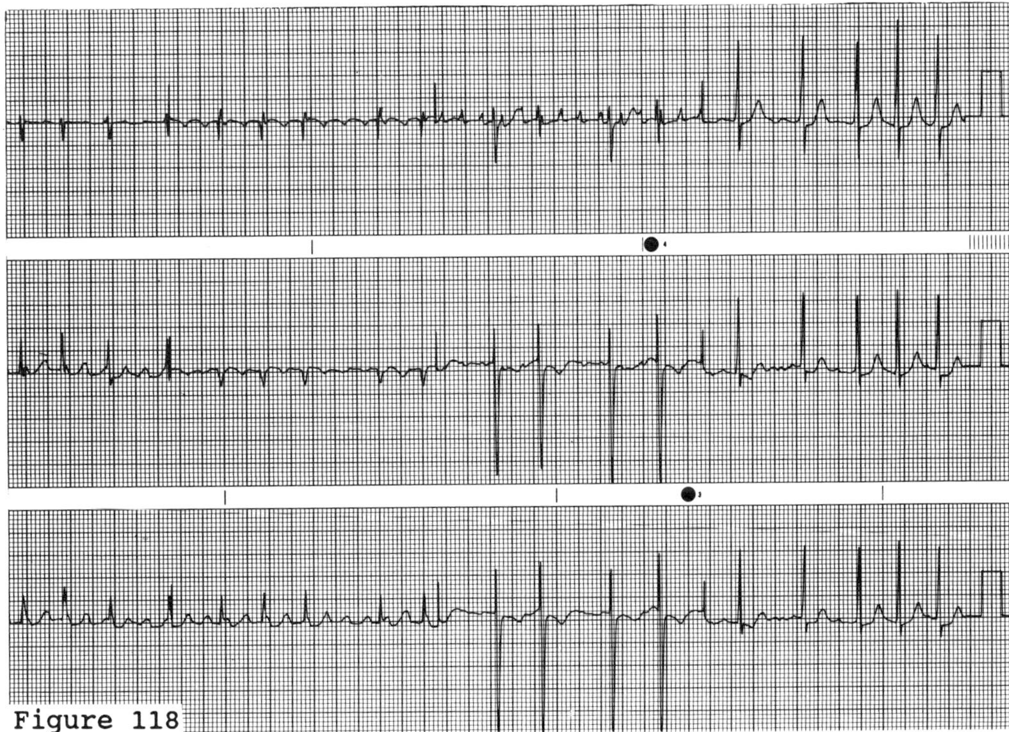

Figure 118

    This record shows an atrial tachycardia with 2/1 AV block. Low frontal plane QRS voltage is
present. The frontal plane QRS axis is +30, and the T axis 180 degrees. The horizontal plane QRS
axis is -35, and the T axis is +135 degrees. The record shows an atrial tachycardia with 2/1 AV
block, possible pulmonary disease, and lateral T changes consistent with apical and lateral
ischemia. Suggest serial records.

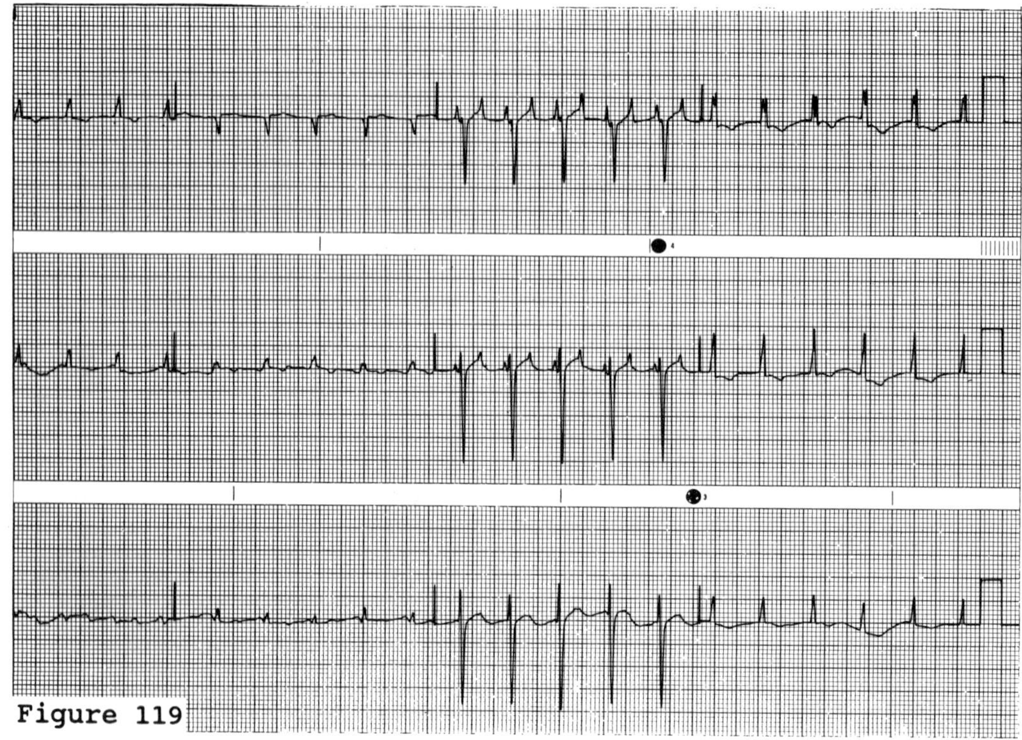

Figure 119

<u>Junctional</u> <u>Rhythm</u> <u>or</u> <u>Tachycardia</u>

Here the EKG looks like a string of junctional extrasystoles. Figures 120 - 125 show various examples. Treatment is usually the same as that of an atrial tachycardia. Junctional tachycardias can also be produced by digitalis toxicity.

<u>Atrial</u> <u>Flutter</u>- Figures 126 - 130.

Atrial flutter commonly consists of sawtooth P waves occurring in many leads with a basic rate of about 300/minute, followed by 2:1 or 3:1 AV block with a resultant ventricular rate of about 150 or 100/minute. Vagal maneuvers often suddenly slow the ventricular rate to lower sub-multiples and allow better inspection of the flutter waves. This arrhythmia may well represent an atrial tachycardia running as fast as it can, whose basic rate is about 300/minute, and 1 to 1 AV conduction may occasionally occur, as in a possible example in Figure 130. There is no sharp differentiation between atrial tachycardia and atrial flutter. As the basic atrial rate is increased over 200/minute, the P waves become more and more saw-tooth in their appearance, and resemble more and more those seen with atrial flutter. Similarly, as the atrial rate increases over 160-200/minute, varying degrees of AV block usually occur. For the mechanism of varying degrees of AV block, see the Wenckebach phenomenon later on. Digitalis is used in the treatment of atrial flutter to increase the degree of AV block and thus protect the ventricles from the disastrous possibility of 1:1 AV conduction. When this has been accomplished, digitalis may be withdrawn and while a person is excreting his digitalis, the atrial arrhythmia may be attacked with cardioversion, quinidine or procainamide. Sometimes digitalis will degrade a flutter to atrial fibrillation, which then often converts to sinus rhythm

This record shows an ectopic low atrial or upper junctional rhythm. The frontal plane QRS axis is +45, the T axis is 0, and the P axis is -30 degrees. The horizontal plane QRS axis is -60, the T axis is -100, and the P axis is +5 degrees. The record shows a low atrial or upper junctional tachycardia, probable acute anteroseptal infarction, with ST segment changes consistent with anterior supepicardial injury and T changes consistent with anterior and apical ischemia. Suggest serial records.

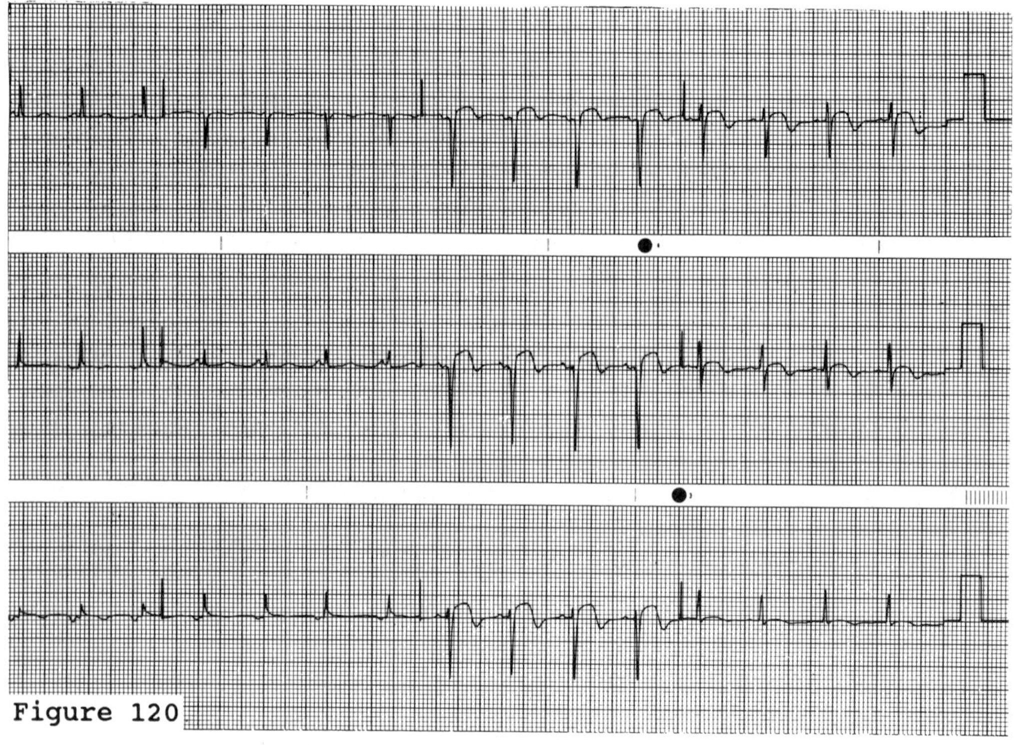

Figure 120

This record shows a junctional rhythm at about 70 per minute. No P waves can be seen. The frontal plane QRS axis is +85, and the T axis is -105 degrees. The horizontal plane QRS axis is -45, and the T axis is +140 degrees. The record shows a junctional rhythm, T changes consistent with lateral ischemia and/or left ventricular strain, and a non-specific intra-ventricular conduction defect. The rhythm may even arise from a focus in the bundle of His close to the branches, with failure of retrograde V-A conduction to the atrium. Suggest serial records and clinical correlation.

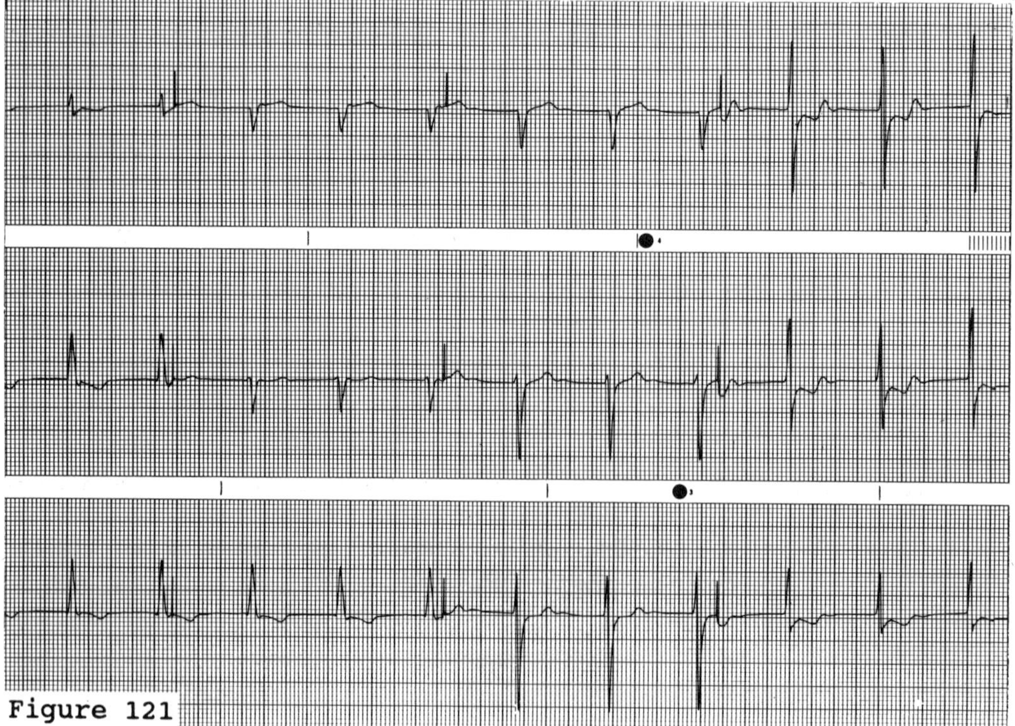

Figure 121

This record shows a probable low junctional rhythm, with retrograde V-A conduction, best seen in leads 3 and aVF. The frontal plane QRS axis is +120, and the T axis is -70 degrees. The horizontal plane QRS axis is -90, and the T axis is +50 degrees. The record shows a low junctional rhythm and T changes consistent with inferior ischemia. Small narrow Q waves are present in 2, 3, and aVF, but are not necessarily indicative yet of inferior infarction. Suggest serial records.

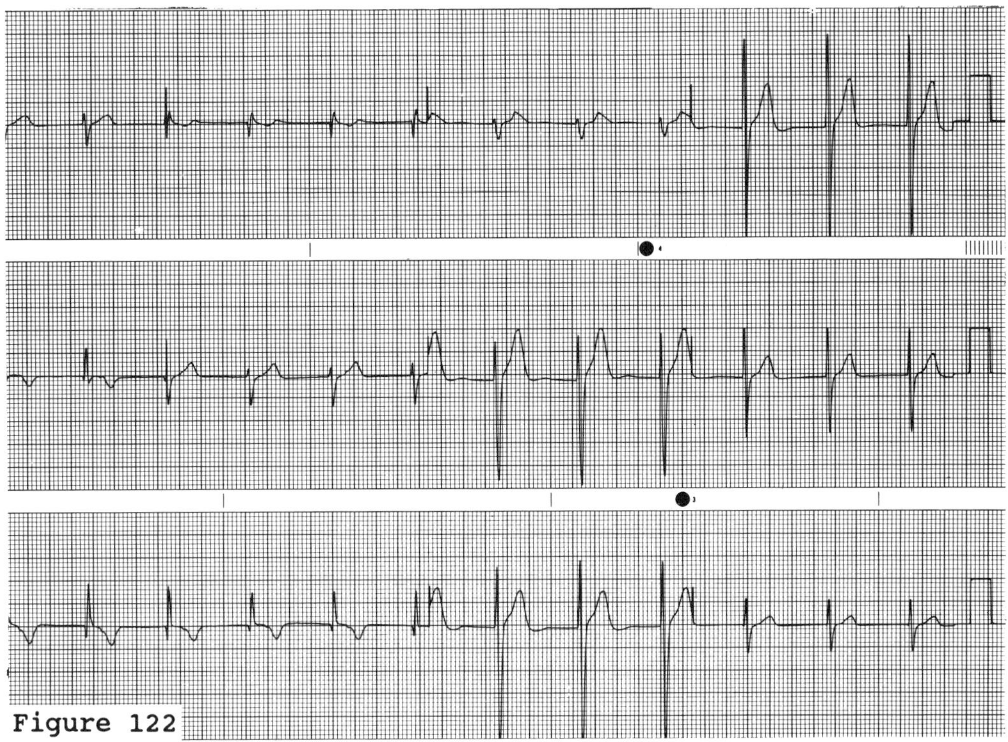

Figure 122

This record shows a probable low junctional tachycardia with retrograde P waves appearing behind the QRS, best seen in V1 and V2. The frontal QRS axis is +5, and the frontal T axis is difficult to plot. The retrograde P waves have a frontal axis of about -90 degrees. The horizontal plane QRS axis is -30 degrees. The T axis is difficult to plot, but the T waves are flat in V6. The horizontal plane ST segment vector is about -135 degrees. The record shows a low junctional tachycardia with ST changes consistent with apical subendocardial injury and ischemia. Suggest serial records.

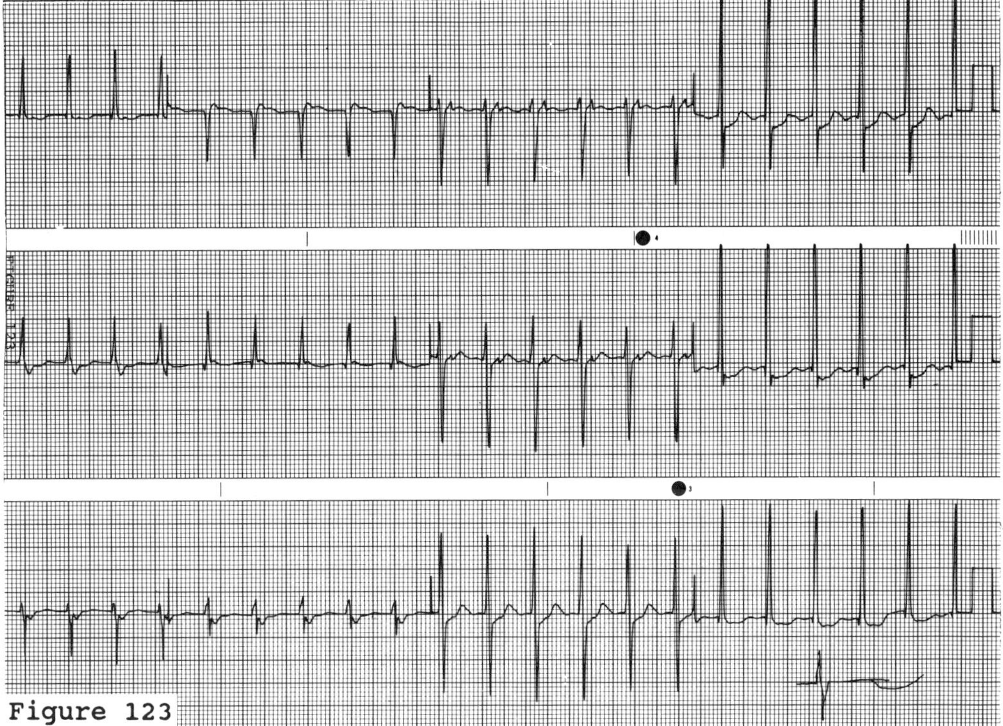

Figure 123

This record shows a low junctional brachycardia. Retrograde P waves appear behind the QRS, with occasional first degree V - A block. The frontal plane QRS axis is 0, the T axis is +15, and the retrograde P axis is about -90 degrees. The horizontal plane QRS axis is 0, the T axis is +5, and the retrograde P axis about +135 degrees. Except for the low junctional rhythm, the record may otherwise be within normal limits. Suggest repeat record.

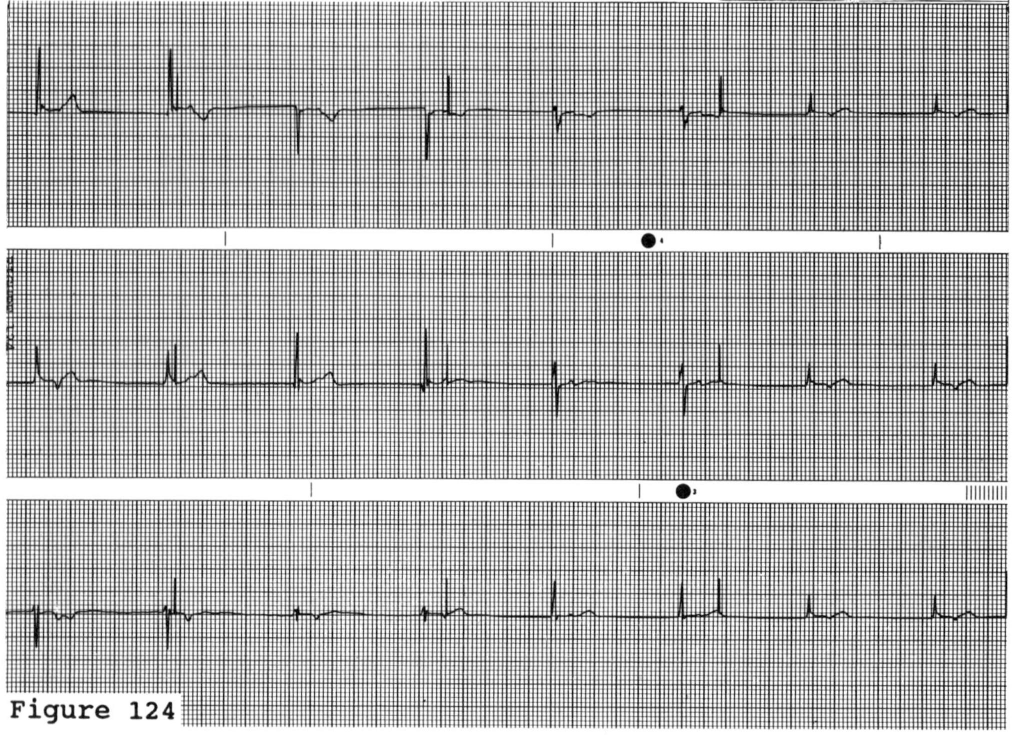

Figure 124

This record shows a probable low junctional rhythm, though an ectopic atrial rhythm with a long PR interval and severe first degree AV block cannot be excluded. Low voltage is noted, especially in the frontal plane, but also in the precordial leads. The frontal QRS axis is +60. The T axis is difficult to plot. No P waves can clearly be seen in the frontal plane. The horizontal QRS axis is -40, and the T axis is -170 degrees. The retrograde P axis is anterior, perhaps about +90 degrees. The record shows a probable low junctional rhythm and possible pulmonary disease or pericardial effusion. An anteroseptal infarct cannot be completely ruled out from the marginal R progression in V1 through V3. T changes consistent with anterior and lateral ischemia are present. Suggest serial records and clinical correlation.

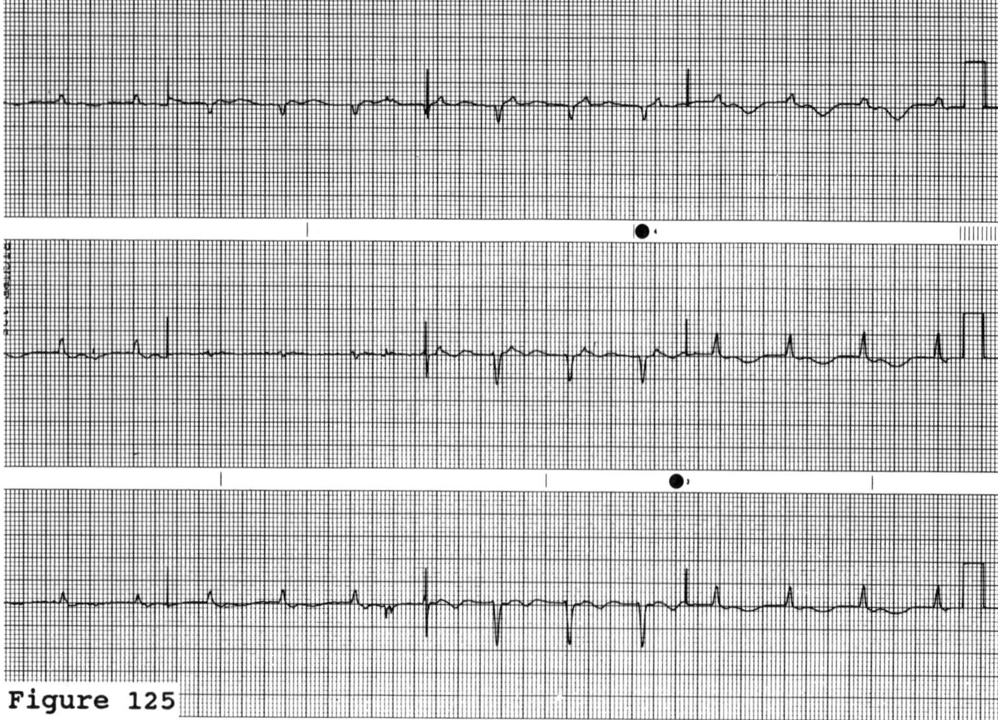

Figure 125

This record shows atrial flutter with 2/1 AV block and T changes consistent with apical, lateral, and possible inferior ischemia. The frontal plane QRS axis is -60 degrees. The frontal plane QRS duration is not wide enough to call a left anterior superior hemiblock. The frontal plane T axis cannot be plotted. The horizontal plane QRS axis is -30, and the T axis is +170 degrees. Suggest serial records.

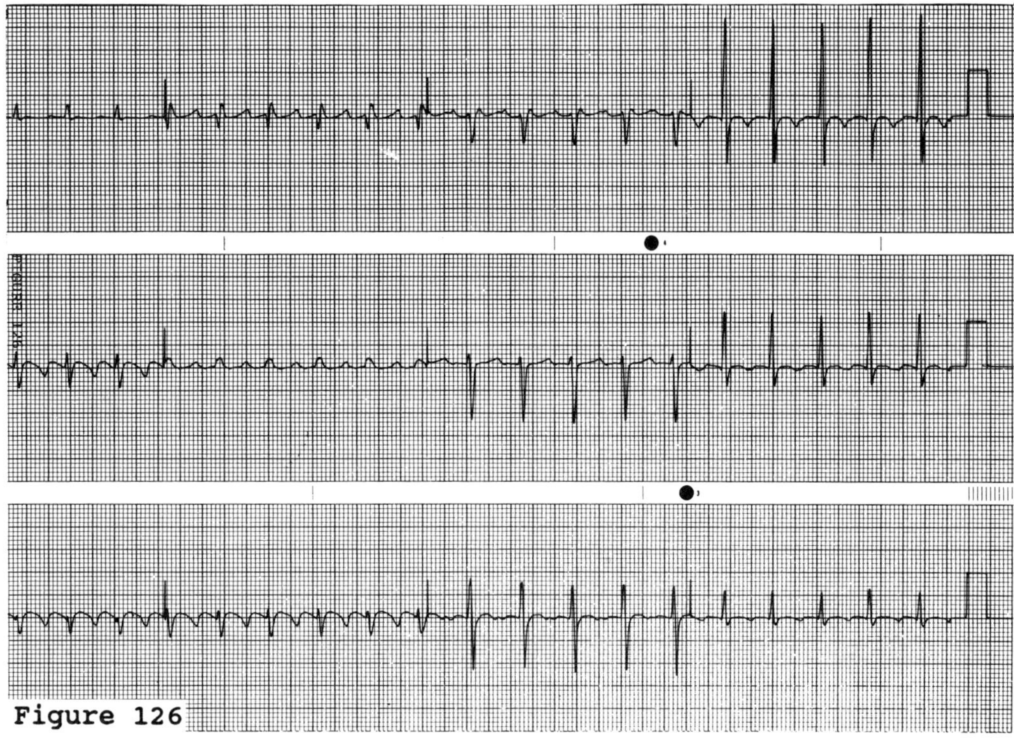

Figure 126

This record shows atrial flutter with 2/1 AV block and non-specific ST-T changes. The frontal plane QRS axis is 95 degrees. The T axis cannot be plotted. The horizontal plane QRS axis is -45 degrees. The T axis cannot be plotted. Suggest repeat record.

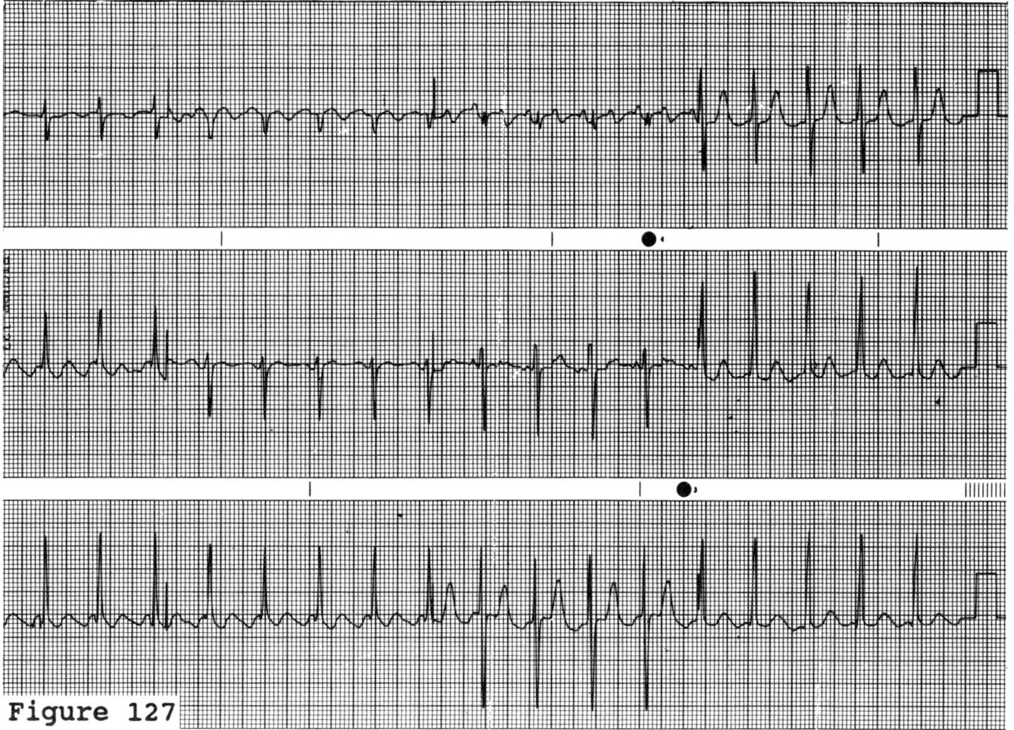

Figure 127

This record shows a probable atrial flutter with 2/1 AV block and non-specific ST-T changes.
The frontal plane QRS axis is +60 degrees. Low voltage is noted in the frontal plane. The horizontal plane QRS axis is -40 degrees. Pulmonary disease cannot be excluded. Suggest repeat record.

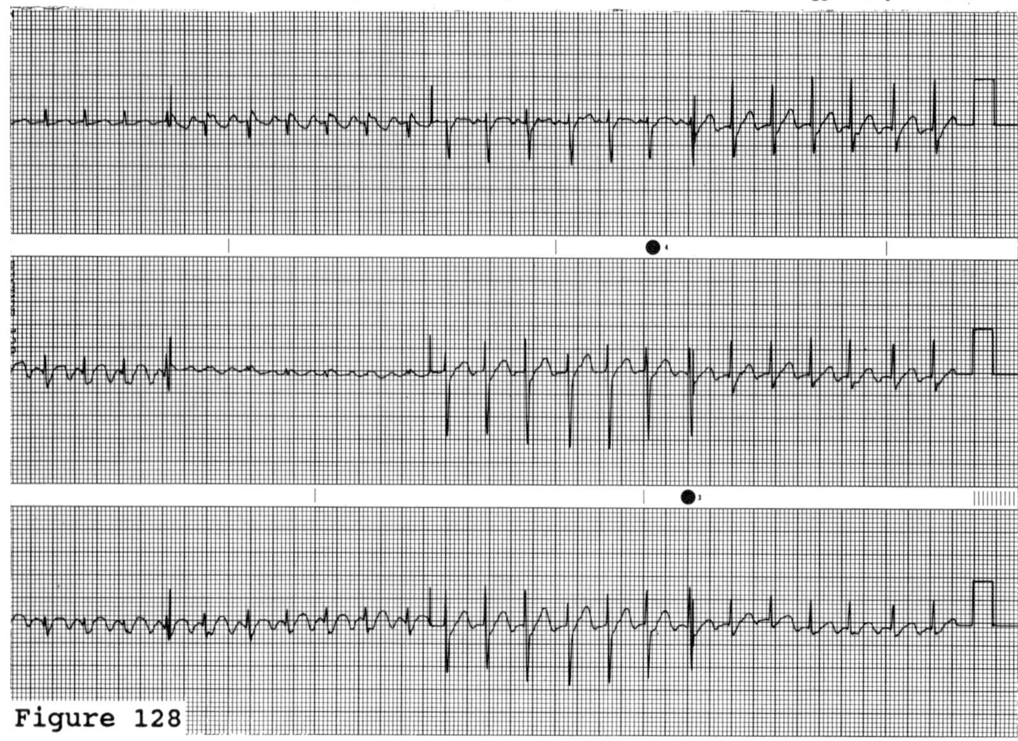

Figure 128

This record shows an atrial flutter with variable AV block. The frontal plane QRS axis is +100
degrees. The T axis cannot be plotted. The horizontal plane QRS axis is -40 degrees. The T axis is
difficult to plot, but inverted T waves are present in V5 and V6, consistent with lateral ischemia
and/or left ventricular strain. A slightly wide QRS complex is present. Left ventricular enlargement may be present. This, combined with the vertical frontal plane axis, also suggests that
combined right and left ventricular hypertrophy cannot be excluded. Suggest repeat or serial records
and clinical correlation.

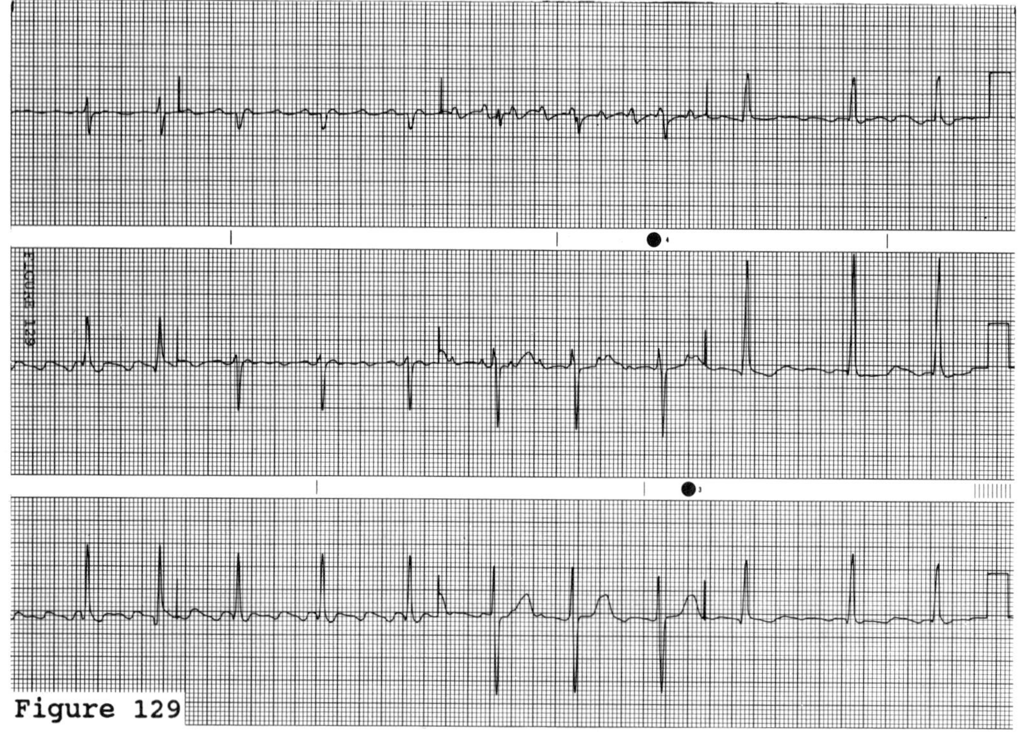

Figure 129

146

This record shows an extremely rapid arrhythmia, probably of supraventricular origin, possibly atrial tachycardia or flutter with 1/1 AV conduction. A ventricular tachycardia, however, cannot be completely excluded. The rate is about 240/minute. An intraventricular conduction defect, possibly right bundle branch block and left anterior superior hemiblock, may be present. An inferior infarct cannot be excluded. Suggest serial records.

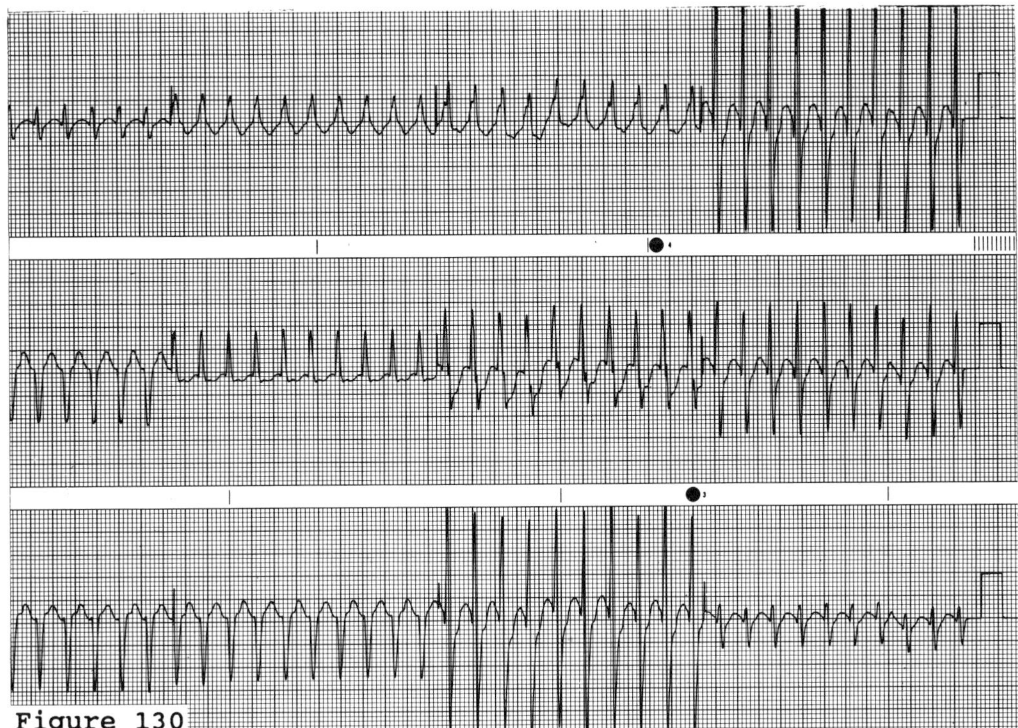

Figure 130

upon withdrawal of digitalis. Cardioversion by itself is most useful for flutter. Flutter may also occur as a manifestation of digitalis toxicity.

<u>Atrial</u> <u>Fibrillation</u>- Figures 131 - 136.

This consists of disorganized, random atrial fibrillatory waves in the EKG, plus normal QRS complexes occurring usually at a completely random and irregularly irregular rate. Atrial depolarization proceeds in a disorganized, random fashion. The AV node becomes stimulated in a random fashion. Atrial fibrillation occurs in conditions characterized by atrial enlargement or fibrosis, such as mitral stenosis, and hypertensive and/or arteriosclerotic cardiovascular disease. It also occurs in occult hyperthyroidism. Physical examination reveals an irregularly irregular pulse. Cardiac failure may be precipitated, due primarily to the resulting rapid ventricular rate and poor diastolic filling, but also to the loss of atrial function and its atrial kick, which usually reduces cardiac output about 25 percent, unless other mechanisms can compensate for this. In patients with significant aortic stenosis, atrial fibrillation may be a preterminal event unless emergency valve surgery is done, as such patients have usually exhausted their other compensatory mechanisms, and unless successfully cardioverted, do extremely poorly without their atrial kick. Cardiac output may drop by 50, not just 25, percent, and they may deteriorate rapidly.

<u>Treatment</u> <u>of</u> <u>Atrial</u> <u>Fibrillation</u>

If the episodes are infrequent, no therapy may be necessary. Some people have paroxysmal atrial fibrillation when they smoke or drink, and these factors should be avoided.

The drug of choice for control of the ventricular rate is digitalis. While or after the ventricular rate is being or has been controlled, one must also decide whether or not to convert the fibrillating atria. Other

This record shows coarse atrial fibrillation. Low frontal plane voltage is present, and prominent tall and wide R waves are seen in V2. The frontal plane QRS axis is +15 degrees. The T axis cannot be plotted. The horizontal plane QRS axis has a double transition, and excess anterior forces are present. The T axis may be about +45 degrees. The record shows atrial fibrillation and a possible posteroapical infarction of undetermined age. Non-specific T wave changes are seen. Pulmonary disease cannot be excluded. Suggest serial records and clinical correlation.

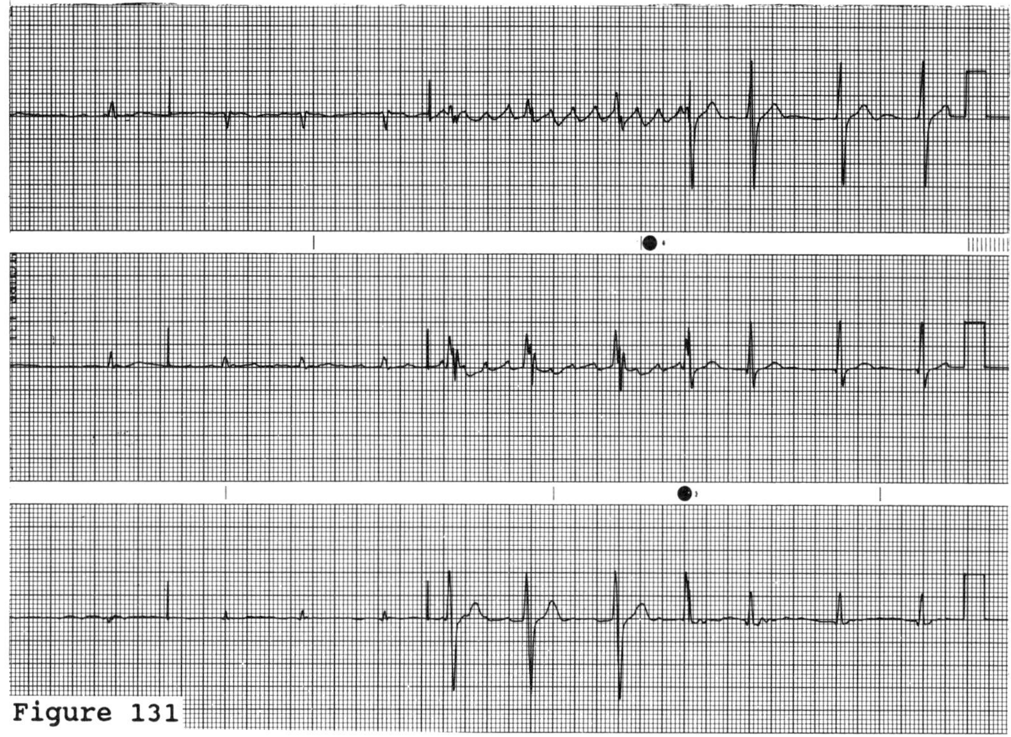

Figure 131

This record shows coarse atrial fibrillation and T wave changes consistent with left ventricular strain and/or lateral ischemia. The frontal plane QRS axis is +70 degrees. The T axis cannot be plotted. The horizontal plane QRS axis is -40, and the T axis is +120 degrees. Suggest repeat or serial records and clinical correlation.

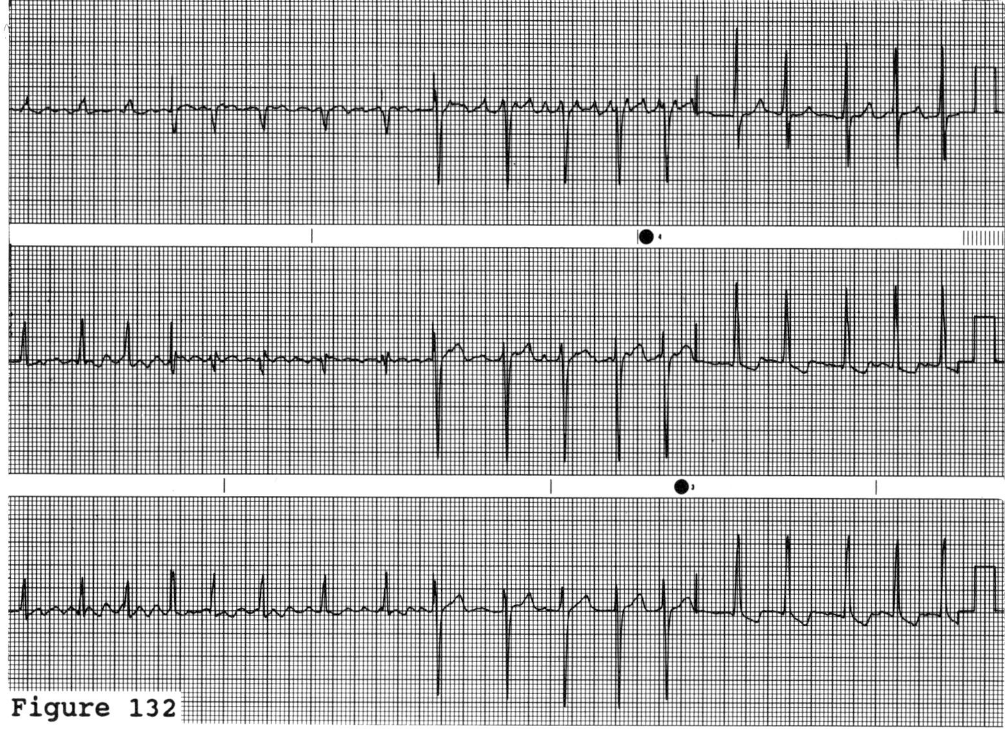

Figure 132

This record shows atrial fibrillation and nonspecific ST-T changes. The frontal plane QRS axis is +70 degrees. The T axis cannot be plotted. The horizontal plane QRS axis is -10, and the horizontal T axis is +10 degrees.

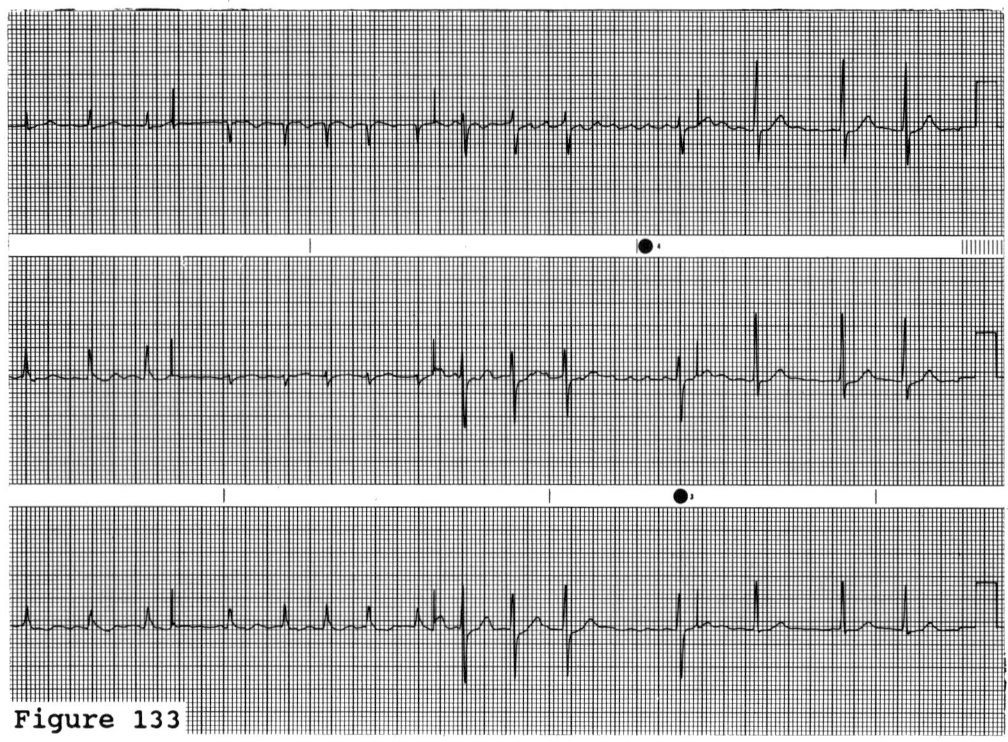

Figure 133

This record shows atrial fibrillation and prominent U waves in V2 and V3, although terminal T inversion consistent with possible anterior ischemia cannot be excluded. The frontal plane QRS axis is +45, and the T axis +60 degrees. The horizontal plane QRS axis is -30 degrees. The T axis is difficult to plot. It depends on what one thinks is a T, a terminally inverted T, or a U wave. Anterior ischemia cannot be excluded. Suggest repeat or serial records and clinical correlation.

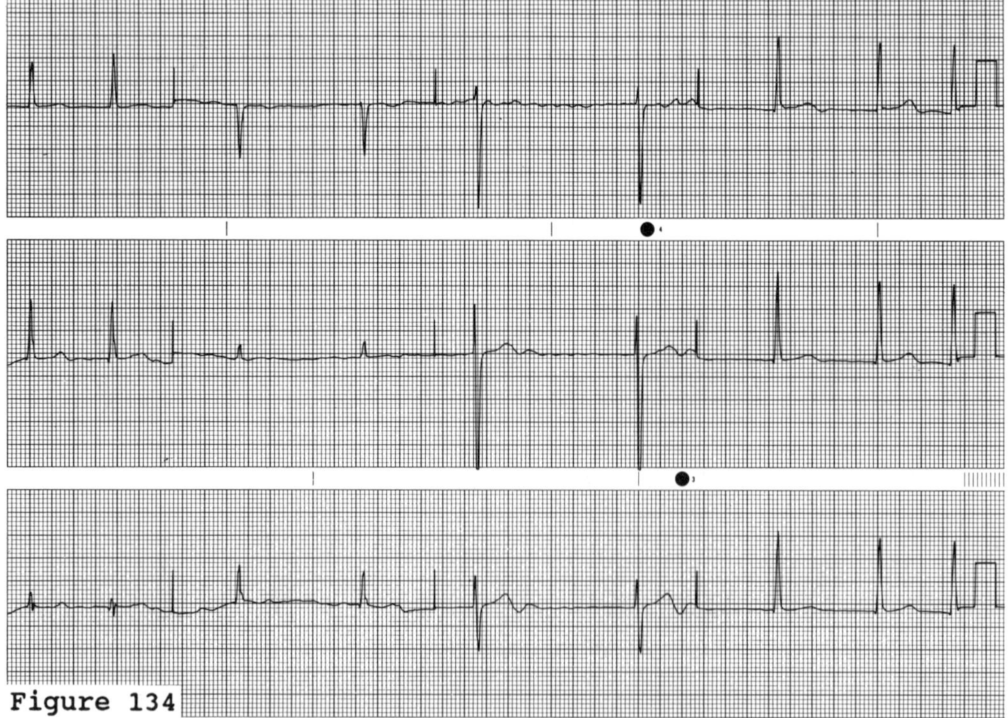

Figure 134

This record shows an atrial tachycardia with 2/1 AV block, best shown in V1. An anteroseptal infarct, possibly recent, is also present, with ST changes consistent with anterior subepicardical injury, and T changes suggesting possible apical and lateral ischemia and/or left ventricular strain. Low voltage in the frontal plane is also seen. The frontal QRS axis is -15 degrees. The T axis is difficult to plot. The horizontal plane QRS axis is -60, the ST segment vector is +130, and the T axis is difficult to plot. Each QRS complex may well be fired not by the immediately preceding P wave but by the P wave buried in the T wave in front of it. Pulmonary disease cannot be excluded. Suggest serial records.

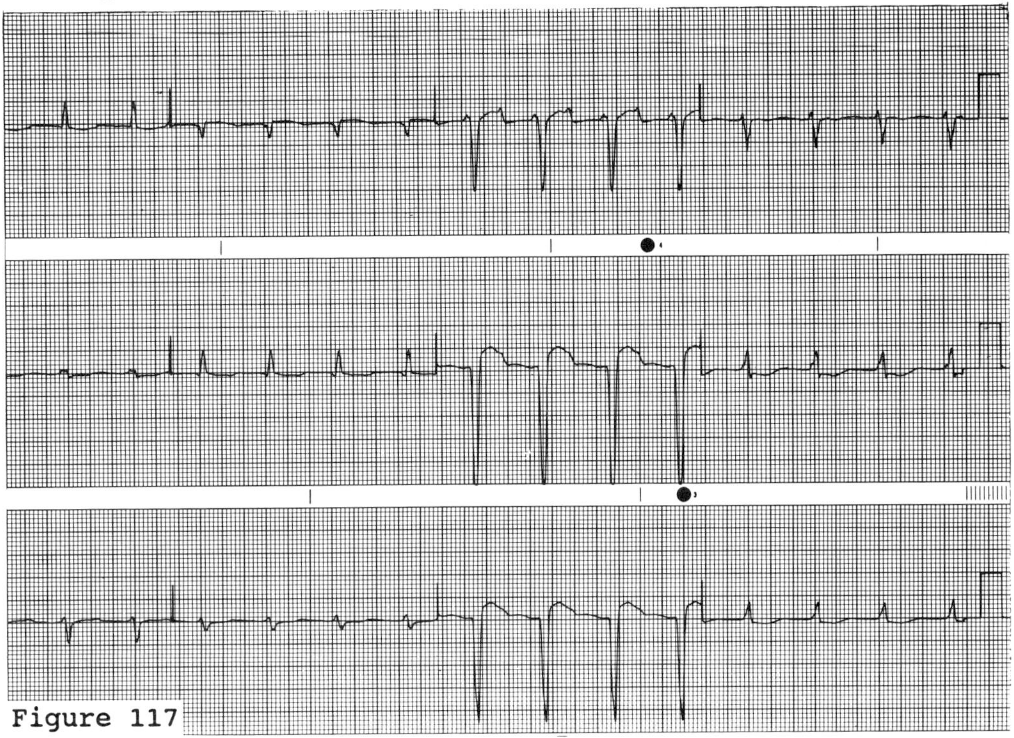

Figure 117

This record shows a rapid atrial tachycardia (almost an atrial flutter), and varying AV block. The frontal plane QRS axis is +105 degrees. The T axis is difficult to plot. The horizontal plane QRS axis is -35, and the T axis is also -35 degrees. Pulmonary disease may be present. Anterior T inversions consistent with anterior ischemia and/or right ventricular strain are present. Suggest serial records and clinical correlation.

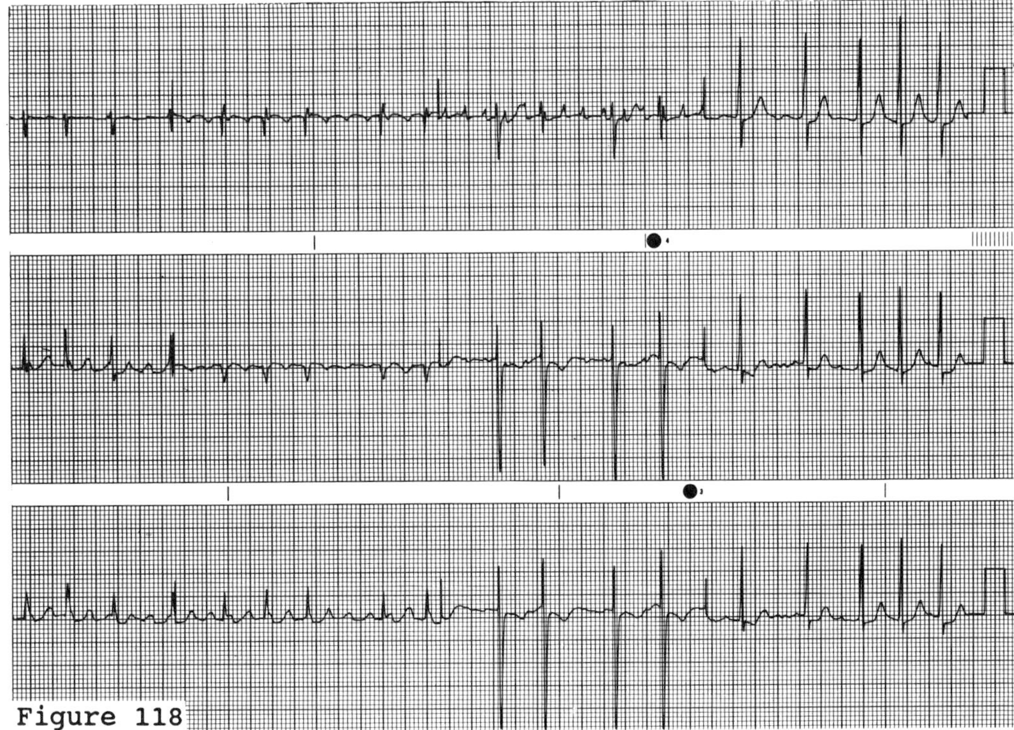

Figure 118

This record shows an atrial tachycardia with 2/1 AV block. Low frontal plane QRS voltage is present. The frontal plane QRS axis is +30, and the T axis 180 degrees. The horizontal plane QRS axis is -35, and the T axis is +135 degrees. The record shows an atrial tachycardia with 2/1 AV block, possible pulmonary disease, and lateral T changes consistent with apical and lateral ischemia. Suggest serial records.

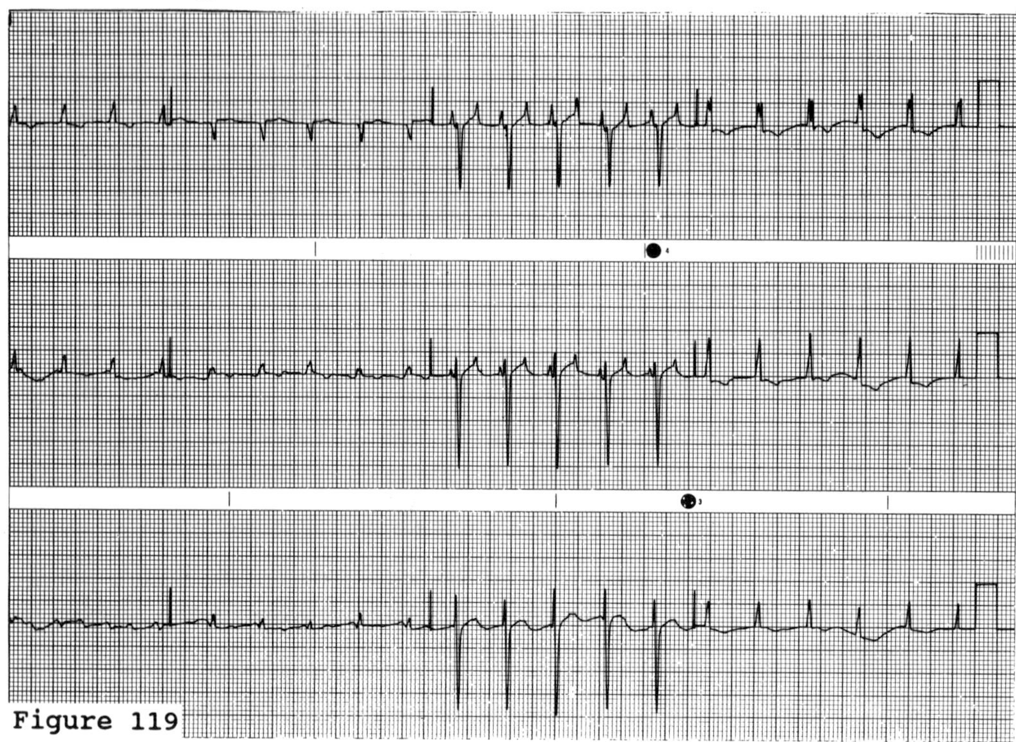

Figure 119

This record shows atrial fibrillation and typical scooped ST-T changes with a short QT interval, consistent with digitalis effect. The frontal plane QRS axis is +70 degrees. The T axis is difficult to plot. The horizontal plane QRS axis is -10, and the T axis is approximately +10 degrees.

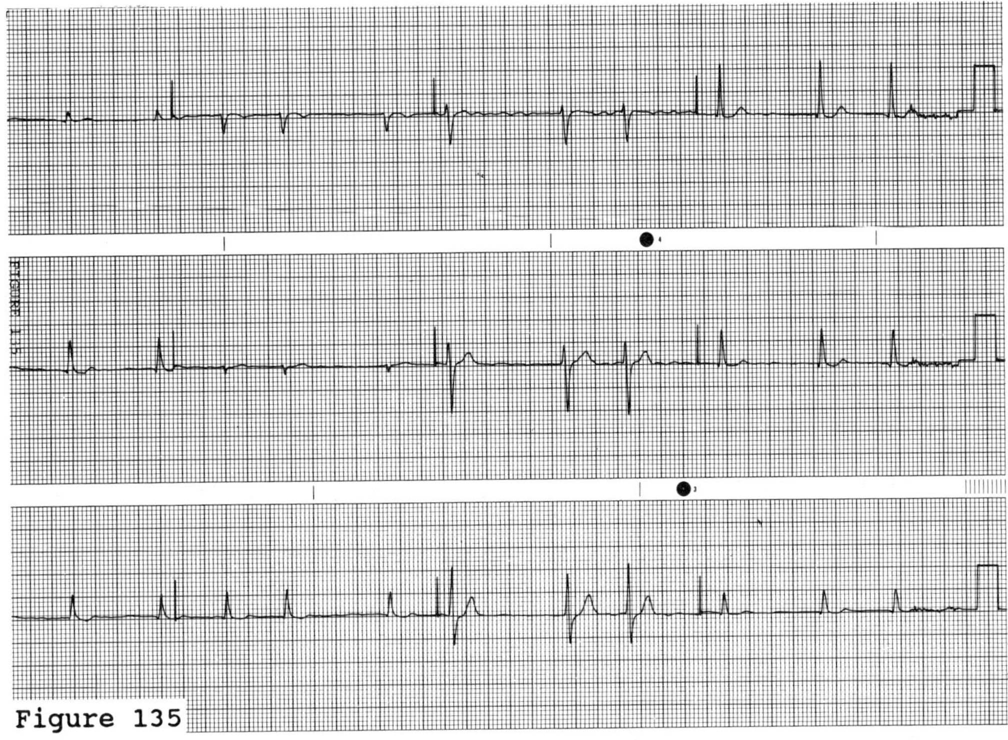

Figure 135

This record shows an irregularly irregular ventricular rate and very fine occasional baseline wiggles, as noted in leads 2, V1, and V2, which are consistent with atrial fibrillation. ST-T changes consistent with combined digitalis effect and left ventricular strain and/or lateral ischemia are present. The frontal plane QRS axis is +30 degrees. The T axis cannot be plotted. The horizontal plane QRS axis is -10 degrees. The T axis is away from V5 and V6. The record shows probable atrial fibrillation and ST-T changes consistent with a combination of digitalis effect and left ventricular strain and/or lateral ischemia. Suggest repeat or serial records if clinically indicated.

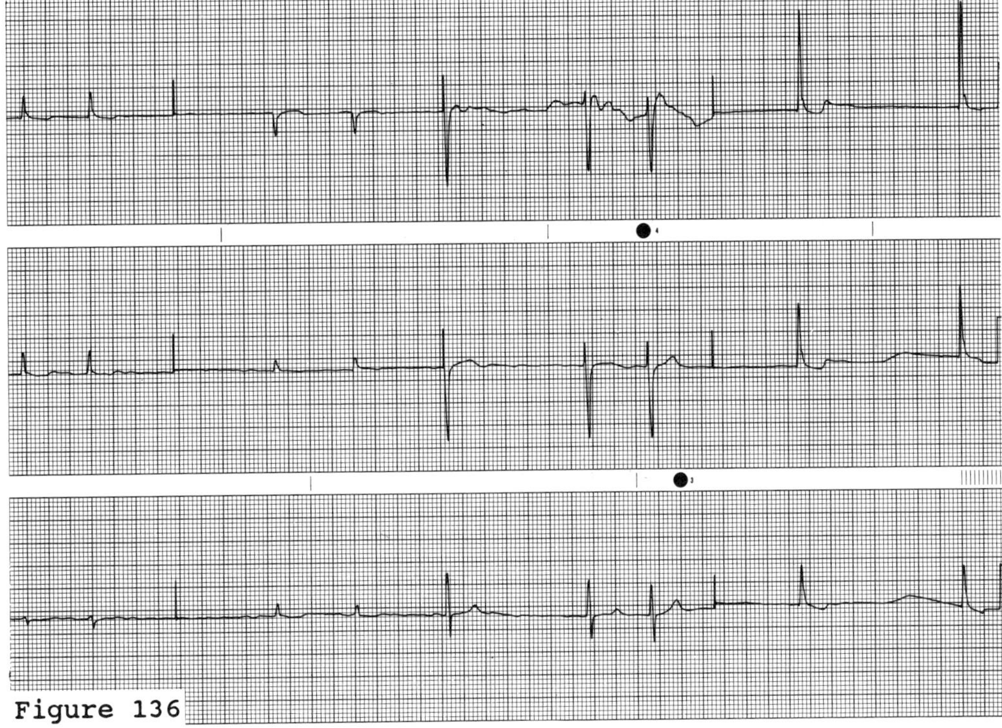

Figure 136

things being equal, conversion to sinus rhythm adds a potential 25% or greater increase in cardiac output at any given venous pressure. Conversely, a normal cardiac output can be obtained at a lower venous pressure. The incidence of arterial thrombosis and thromboembolic phenomena, especially strokes, is significant with atrial fibrillation and is much less with normal sinus rhythm. If fibrillation has been of more than a few days duration, conversion (usually with oral quinidine plus elective electrical cardioversion) must proceed with caution following an adequate period (2-3 weeks) of anticoagulant therapy in order to avoid suddenly dislodging an embolus as the atria begin to contract in unison again. Conversion may also be accomplished by correction of the underlying disease which in many cases involves cardiac surgery. In summary, patients with atrial fibrillation usually should be given digitalis to control the ventricular rate, and/or to achieve conversion to sinus rhythm. The advantages of restoring sinus rhythm must be balanced against the dangers inherent in conversion and the likelihood of maintaining successful conversion. Calcium channel blockers may also be used to slow or convert atrial fibrillation, but they have a varying negative inotropic effect.

AV Dissociation by Interference (Accelerated Idioventricular Rhythm)

Figures 137 - 138.

In this arrhythmia, as shown in Figure 137, there are two foci, one in the atrium and one in the AV node or the Purkinje system. The one in the AV node or Purkinje system fires at a faster rate than the atrial one. Usually the atrial impulse falls on refractory junctional or Purkinje tissue, but every now and then it gets through in the normal fashion, and a normal QRS complex following a P wave (ventricular capture) will be seen, usually

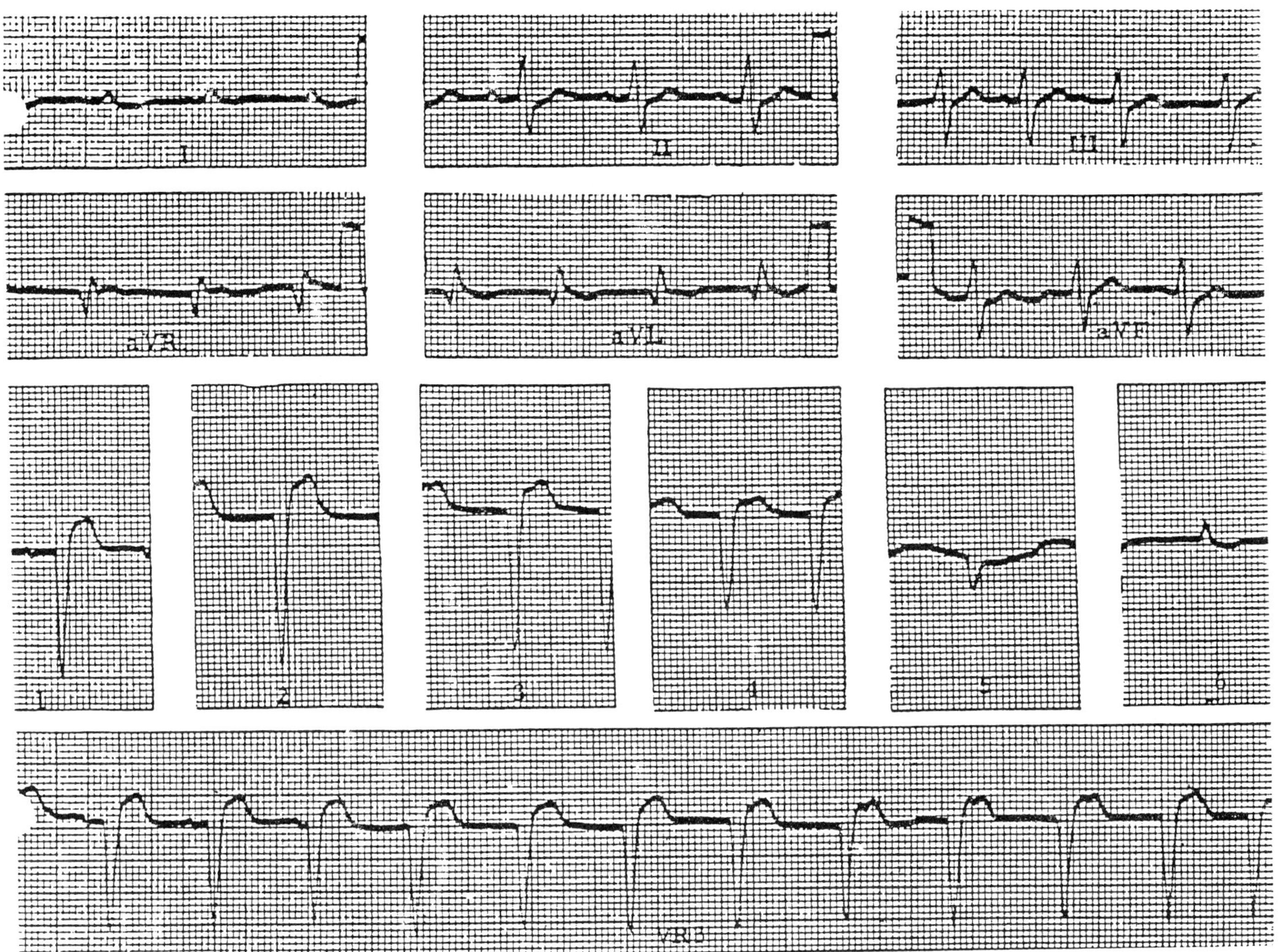

This record shows evidence of sinus rhythm complicated by a lower focus discharging at a slightly faster rate. Because of this, the lower focus represents either an accelerated idioventricular rhythm or a junctional rhythm with somewhat aberrant intraventricular conduction. The QRS complex is not wide enough to qualify as a completely idioventricular rhythm. One must then consider the significance of the Q waves in V1 through V5. The frontal plane QRS axis is diphasic in many leads and probably has a mean direction of 0. The frontal plane T axis is about + 85 degrees. The horizontal plane QRS axis has a transition between V5 and V6, and is about minus 85 degrees. The horizontal plane T axis has a transition in the opposite direction at V5. It is, therefore, about + 100 degrees. The horizontal plane ST segment vector is displaced almost straight at lead V2 at a direction of about + 90 degrees.

This record shows an accelerated junctional or idioventricular rhythm. An anteroseptal and anteroapicial infarct may well be present, with evidence of possible anterior subepicardial injury. Digitalis toxicity may well be present. Suggest serial records and clinical correlation.

FIGURE 137

153

        This record shows atrial fibrillation and a regular ventricular rhythm. It may represent either
an accellerated idioventricular rhythm or a junctional rhythm with left bundle branch block,
possible left anterior superior hemiblock, and a possible inferior, apical, and lateral infarct of
undetermined age. The QRS duration is about .14 seconds. The frontal plane QRS axis is -30, and
the T axis is +150 degrees. The horizontal plane QRS axis is about -135, and the T axis is +45
degrees. Digitalis toxicity may be present. Suggest serial records and clinical correlation.

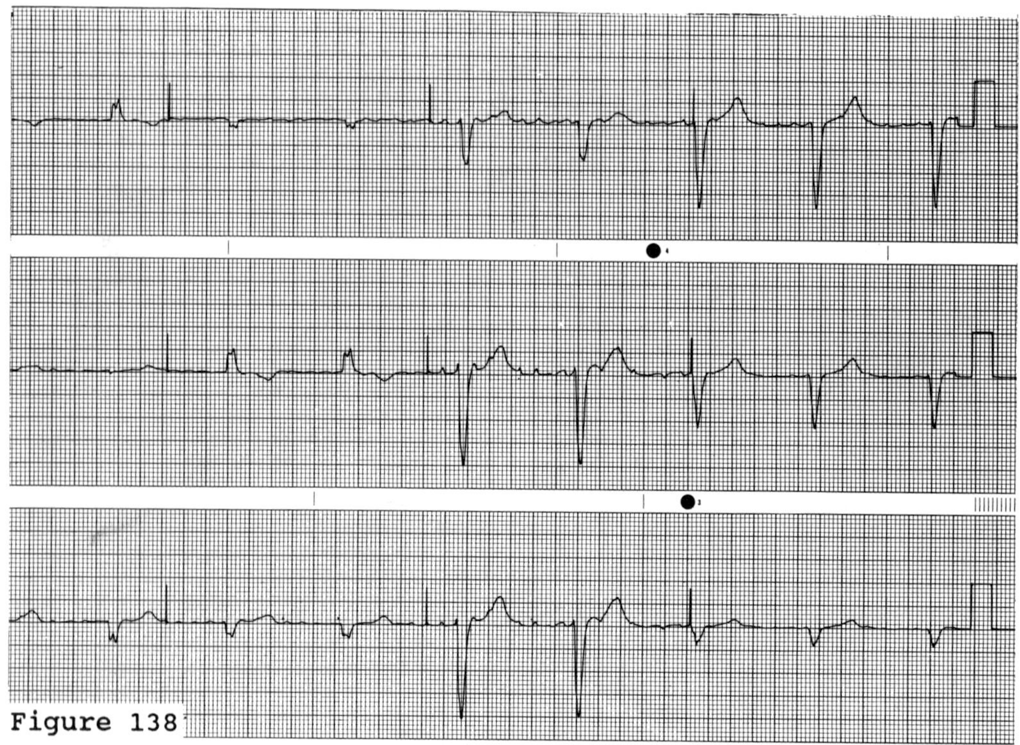

Figure 138

154

occurring earlier than the regular R-R interval. This arrhythmia is recognized by regular P waves and by regular QRS complexes, but the QRS complexes occur at a slightly faster rate than the P waves. Often the P waves seem to "march through" the QRS complexes with successive beats. Occasionally a P wave followed by a normal PR interval and a normal QRS and T wave will be seen as ventricular capture occurs. Clinically, this arrhythmia is commonly caused by digitalis toxicity, ischemia, or anoxia. It is often successfully abolished by atropine or atrial pacing, thus increasing the atrial rate but not really treating the underlying problem, or by treatment of digitalis toxicity or other causes of ectopic firing in cells. Figure 138 shows another variety of this in a patient with atrial fibrillation, who has developed complete AV block, and who may have an idioventricular rhythm accellerated to 53/minute. This figure probably also represents significant digitalis toxicity.

<u>Ventricular</u> <u>Tachycardia</u>- Figures 139 - 140.

This is always serious, and is usually associated with serious organic heart disease, commonly with acute myocardial infarction. It may however, be a direct or indirect result of these diseases plus digitalis toxicity. It may also be seen following high levels of quinidine, pronestyl, or lidocaine, sensitivity to tobacco or coffee, hyperthyroidism, during cardiac catheterization, or as a result of hyperpotassemia.

Symptoms occurring with ventricular tachycardia are often more serious and devastating than those with supraventricular tachycardias, usually because of the more serious underlying heart disease and physiology. Angina, hypotension, shock and congestive failure often occur. Clinically, one can suspect ventricular tachycardia when one listens to a rapid, almost, but not quite, regular rate, and hears slight variations in the strength of the

This record shows a probable ventricular tachycardia in a 67 year old patient who was receiving digitalis.

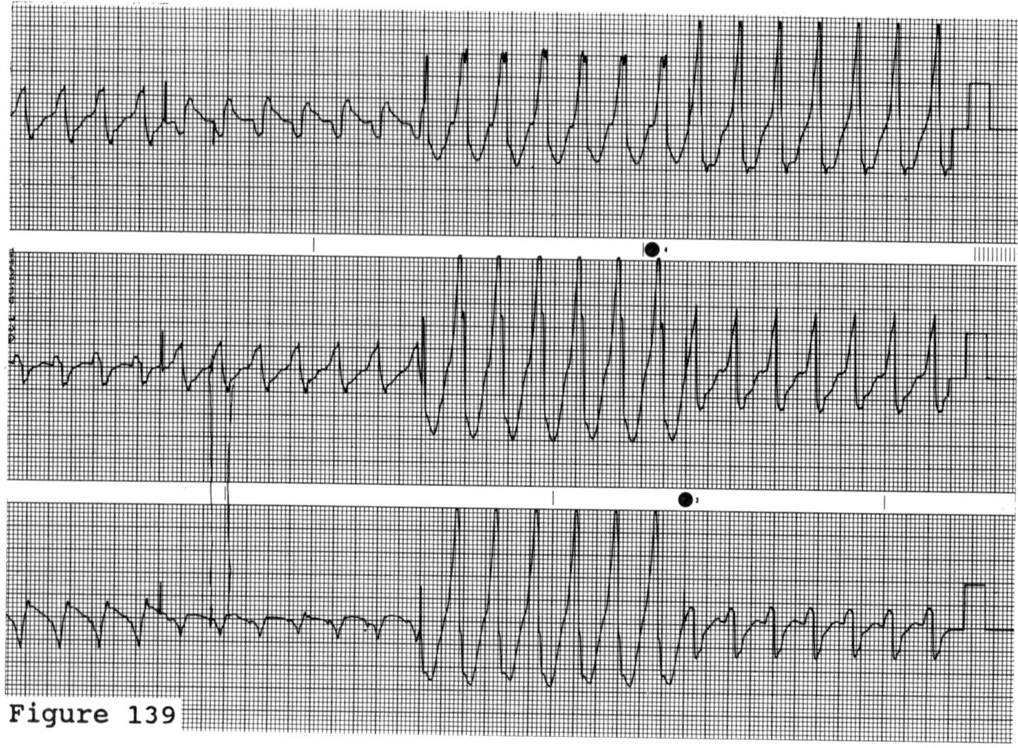

Figure 139

This record shows a probable ventricular tachycardia.

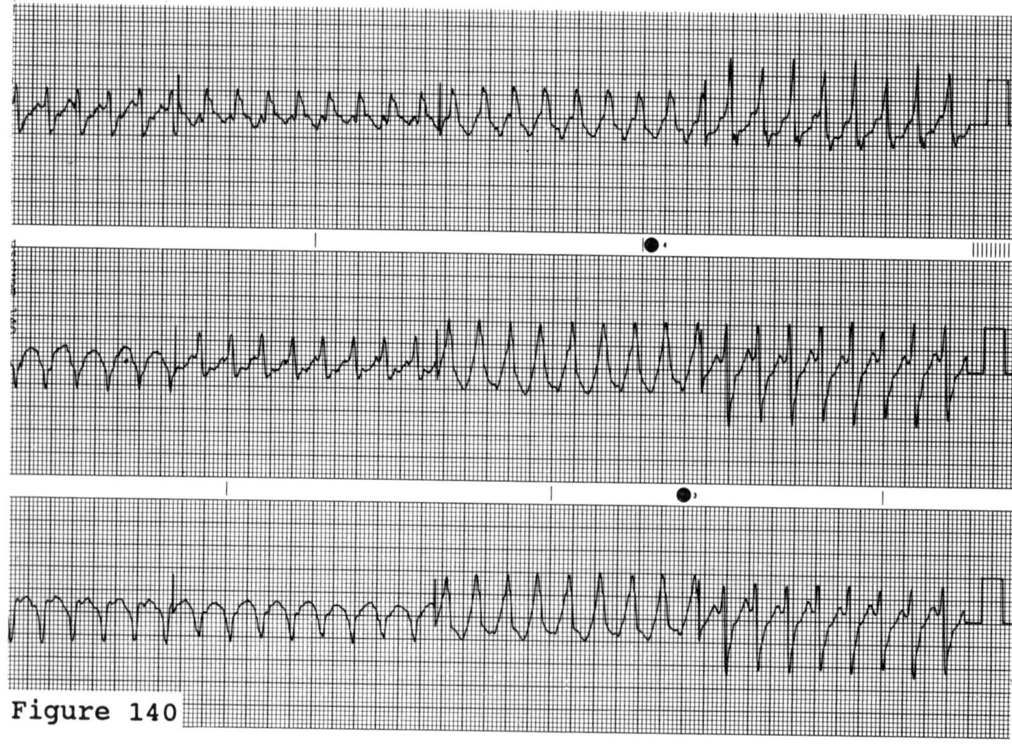

Figure 140

heart sounds or an occasional atrial sound interspersed. Vagal maneuvers are without effect. Exact diagnosis is established by the electrocardiogram, especially if an esophageal lead can also be used, and by the lack of response to vagal maneuvers while under direct EKG monitoring. Ventricular tachycardia is recognized electrocardiographically by bizarre QRS complexes which may vary somewhat in shape from beat to beat, and which may not be precisely regular. Occasional P waves may be seen, and it will be clear that the atrial rhythm is <u>unrelated</u> to the ventricular rhythm. It is this fact, plus the lack of response to carotid sinus pressure, that differentiates this arrhythmia from a supraventricular tachycardia with bundle branch block, or atrial fibrillation in a patient with WPW.

<u>Treatment</u> <u>of</u> <u>Ventricular</u> <u>Tachycardia</u>

The urgency of treatment of most arrhythmias depends upon the magnitude of hemodynamic trouble caused by the arrhythmia and by the likelihood of ventricular fibrillation. Intravenous therapy under continuous monitoring is usually required. There are three main approaches:

1. <u>Cardioversion</u>.

The urgency of treatment depends upon the patient's ability to tolerate the arrhythmia. If shock is present and mental status is confused, cardioversion is usually the procedure of choice, accompanied by some sort of drug treatment directed against the suspected etiologies of his arrhythmia. Cardioversion is also best for someone with WPW and fast atrial fibrillation, whose EKG may suggest VT and whose ventricular rate may be accelerated by lidocaine, which shortens the refractory period as it also reduces the slope of phase 4 in nonischemic Purkinje cells.

2. <u>Lidocaine</u>

Short of cardioversion, lidocaine is usually the drug of choice for VT.
This might well be given, under continuous EKG monitoring, as a pharmacokinetically designed regimen consisting of

1. A loading infusion (not a rapid bolus!) over 3-5 min to achieve a
target serum level (2.0 or 3.0 ug/ml at first), followed by

2. One or more tapering infusion steps during the distribution phase
of the drug (about 2-4 hours), followed by

3. A final maintenance infusion.

For a 70kg patient, whose cardiac output is 70% of normal for his age,
one might consider the following regimen to get one started until a more
precise regimen (6) can be utilized. Patients of different body weight
should receive appropriately adjusted regimens.

	Age under 60	Age over 60
Loading infusion (given over 5 min)	65 mg	65 mg
Then a Distribution infusion (give over 30 min)	2.5 mg/min	2.5 mg/min
Then a Maintenance infusion (thereafter)	0.8 mg/min	0.6 mg/min

If the loading infusion does not result in control of the arrhythmia,
it might be repeated twice more (if needed), giving each new loading
infusion over 5 minutes as before. If control is achieved after the 2nd
loading infusion, the subsequent 30 minute distribution and final
maintenance infusions to consider giving might be twice the values shown
above. If the 3rd loading infusion is needed, the distribution and
maintenance infusions might be 3 times those shown above. All such
lidocaine regimens are only a guide. Therapy should be followed up with a

serum level obtained out of the opposite arm at the end of the initial
loading infusion which achieves a response (not more than 3 such loading
infusions), a subsequent level 1 1/2 hours later, and a level as needed
thereafter. The regimens shown here are derived from a computer program for
developing pharmacokinetically designed lidocaine infusion regimens (6). A
rationale for the serum level monitoring strategy is also available (7,8).

3. <u>Procainamide</u>

With continuous EKG monitoring, procainamide might be given intra-
venously as a loading infusion at a rate not to exceed 25mg/min, above which
hypotension may occur from vasodilation and negative inotropic effects
resulting from excessive serum levels during this phase of therapy. The
following regimens, adjusted to body weight, might be considered

	Creatinine Clearance			
(For a 70 kg patient)	75	50	25	0
Loading Infusion (1 hour)	700mg	700	675	650
Maintenance infusion (thereafter)	130mg/hr	100	80	60

If the patient responds at the very end of the 1 hour loading infusion,
his serum level should usually be about 6ug/ml, in the upper therapeutic
range. If he responds in some fraction of that hour, his probable serum
level is probably that same fraction of 6, and his maintenance infusion rate
should be that same fraction of the infusion rate shown above. For example,
if the arrhythmia should respond in 20 minutes (1/3 hour), his estimated
serum level is 1/3 of 6, or 2, and the optimal maintenance rate should be
implemented then (<u>do not continue the loading infusion beyond the time at</u>

which the patient responds), at 1/3 of the maintenance infusion rates shown above. These approximate regimens are guides to initiate therapy. They have also been developed from pharmacokinetic models and computer software designed for this (8). Serum levels should be drawn at the end of the loading infusion (opposite arm) or when the patient's arrhythmia responds (when the loading infusion should also stop), and 6 hours later, or as needed. Serum creatinine should also be drawn and creatinine clearance estimated (8).

Other Approaches:

4. <u>Quinidine</u>

Intravenous quinidine under careful direct writing EKG control has been used in the past. One might put 0.8 grams of quinidine into 500 cc. of 5% dextrose in water and run it in a slow intravenous drip, carefully monitoring its effects by EKG. This has become less fashionable in recent years, however.

5. <u>Potassium</u>

Since ventricular tachycardia may also be produced by digitalis toxicity, intravenous potassium may well be indicated (8).It may be useful to aim for a serum potassium of about 6mEq/L, to help get digitalis off the receptor sites on the cell membranes. Sixty mEq. of potassium chloride might be put in 500 cc. of 5% dextrose in water and dripped slowly, under careful continuous EKG monitoring.

This deadly arrhythmia, which arises from multiple Purkinje fiber discharges in a disorganized manner and/or (more probably) disorganized pathways of ventricular depolarization, causes a total loss of ventricular function and consequent circulatory arrest. It can only be abolished by external counter shock, supplemented by cardiac massage and assisted respiration. It may commonly occur from a ventricular tachycardia, with Stokes-Adams attacks, or with an acute myocardial infarct.

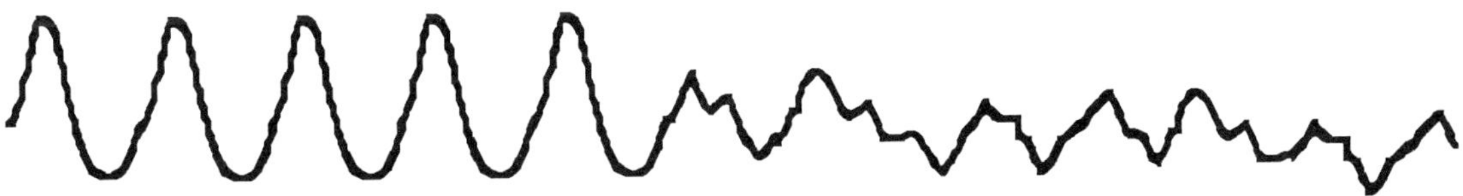

Figure 141

161

7
Conduction Disturbances

<u>DISTURBANCES OF AV CONDUCTION</u>

Figure 142 shows how factors depressing AV nodal response to stimuli cause first a delay in impulse conduction and finally failure of nodal transmission. Following a nonpropagated impulse, however, enough time has often elapsed for nodal recovery and for normal impulse conduction to occur once again. This is the cause of the Wenckebach phenomenon, of variable AV conduction, and (when these events stimulating the AV node happen in a rapid and random sequence), of the irregularly irregular rate in patients with atrial fibrillation.

<u>First Degree AV Block</u>- Figures 143 - 146.

Here the P-R interval is prolonged beyond .20 seconds, sometimes as long as .60 seconds, due to delay in the AV nodal response to atrial stimuli, but every atrial impulse is still conducted down to the ventricles. The properly synchronized "atrial kick" sets the ventricular sarcomeres at their proper end-diastolic length prior to systole. This is diminished or lost when the PR interval exceeds approximately .25 sec, and cardiac output is reduced, just as if atrial fibrillation had occurred.

<u>Second Degree AV block and the Wenckebach Phenomenon</u>- Figures 147 - 152.

The presence of any dropped beats due to failure of AV nodal transmission constitutes second degree AV block. If the atrial rate is too fast (above about 150/minute) or if the AV node is diseased or under the influence of vagal tone, cholinergic drugs or digitalis, the nodal delay prior to the firing of an adequate propagated impulse may progessively increase. Finally, the node may fail to fire, just as shown in Figure 142. This

A

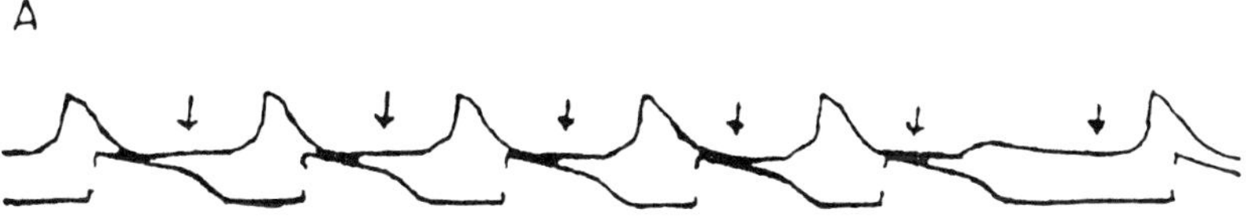

B

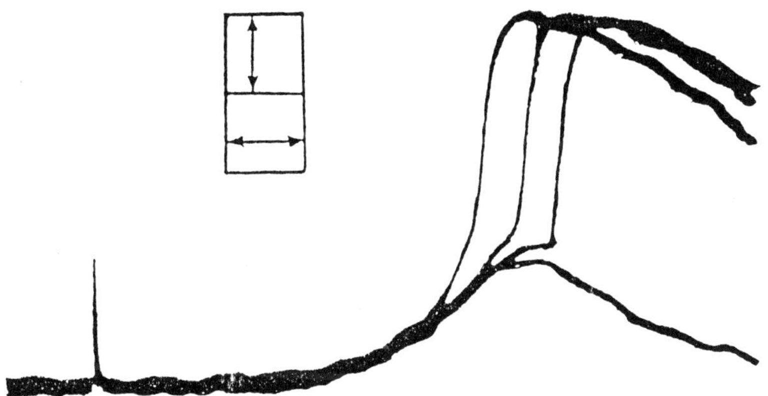

(A) Transmembrane potentials recorded from atrio-
ventricular node (upper trace) and His bundle of
rabbit heart showing the changes in nodal activity
associated with the development of Wenckebach
periodicity. Note progressive increase in duration
of the initial step of the nodal response, progressive
increase in time interval between stimulation of the
atrium (arrow) and the response of the bundle of His,
and the shortening of this interval after failure of
nodal transmission. (B) Unpublished record obtained
by A. Paes de Carvalho showing clearly the changes
in activity of a single nodal fiber in rabbit heart
during one Wenckebach period. Calibrations represent 15 mv and 25 msec.

ELECTROPHYSIOLOGY OF THE HEART, B.F. Hoffman
and P.F. Cranefield, McGraw-Hill Book Company, Inc.,
New York, 1960, p. 173

This record shows sinus bradycardia and first degree AV block. The P-R interval is approxi-
mately .30 seconds. The frontal plane QRS and T axis are both +75,and the P axis is +60 degrees.
The horizontal QRS axis is -30, and the horizontal T axis is +5, and the P axis is +10 degrees.
Suggest repeat record.

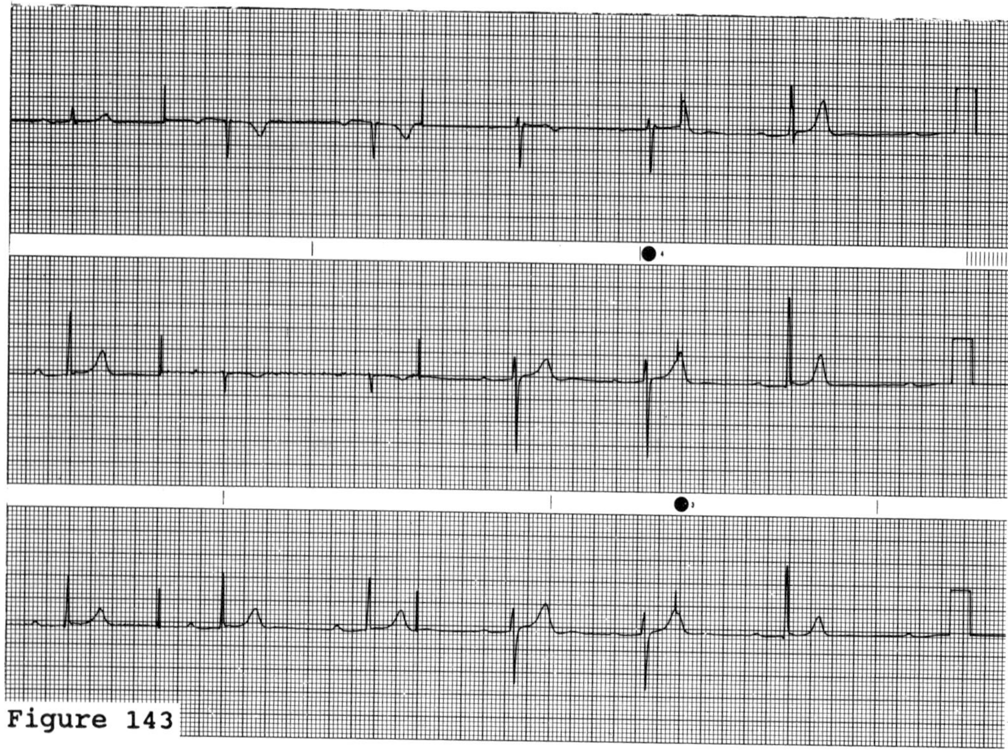

Figure 143

This record shows sinus rhythm and first degree AV block. The P-R interval is about .33
seconds. The frontal plane QRS axis is -30, the T axis -15, and the P axis is +30 degrees. The
horizontal plane QRS axis is -90, the T axis is -100, and the P axis is +5 degrees. The record
shows sinus rhythm with first degree AV block, abnormal left axis deviation, and T changes consistent with anterior and apical ischemia. Suggest serial records.

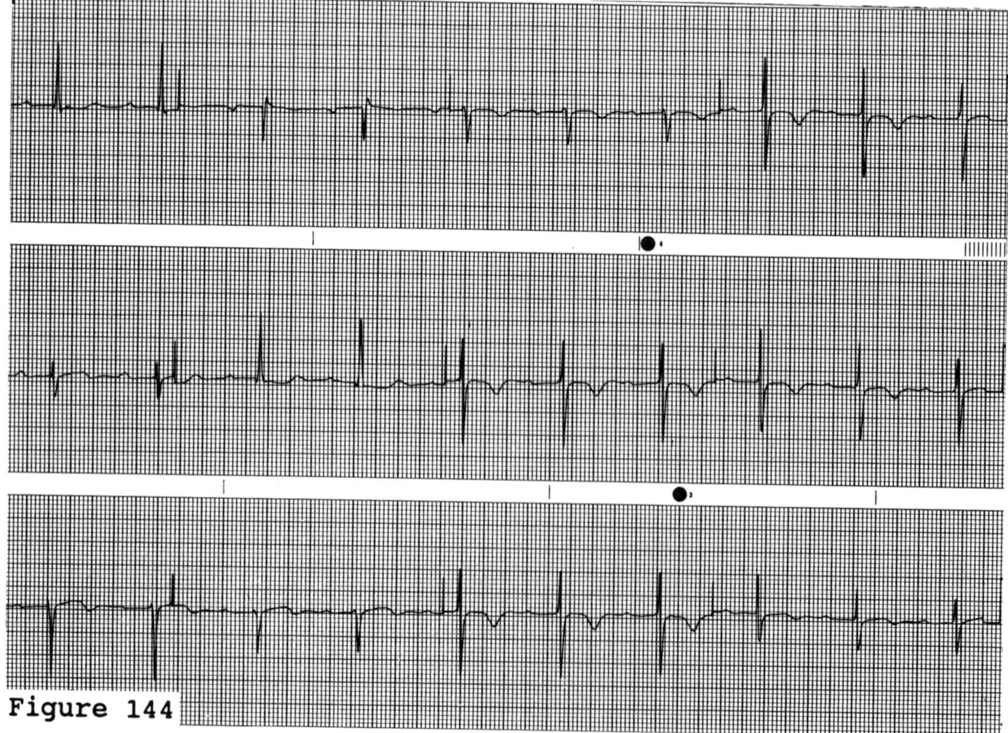

Figure 144

This record shows sinus tachycardia and first degree AV block. The PR interval is about .26 seconds. The frontal plane QRS axis is +30, the T axis -120, and the P axis approximately +60 degrees. The horizontal plane QRS axis is -20, the T axis is +135 degrees, and the P axis is difficult to plot. The record shows sinus tachycardia, first degree AV block, and T changes consistent with inferior and lateral ischemia. Minimal Q waves are present in V2 and V3. Suggest serial records and clinical correlation.

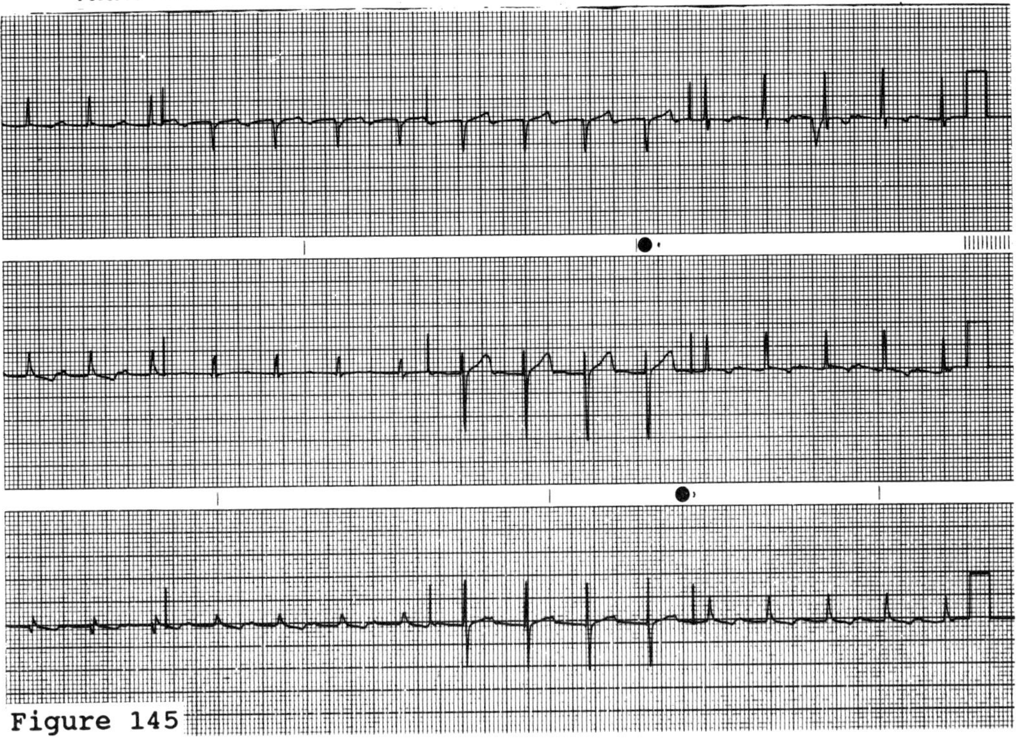

Figure 145

This record shows sinus rhythm with first degree AV block. The PR interval is about .28 seconds. The frontal plane QRS axis is +40, the T axis is +70, and the P axis is +60 degrees. The QT interval is also quite prolonged. The horizontal plane QRS axis is -50, the T axis is +110, and the P axis is +80 degrees. The QRS duration is .13 seconds. LBBB or severe left ventricular hypertrophy may be present, with T changes consistent with left ventricular strain and/or lateral ischemia. The notched R in V6 following the smooth tall R in V5 suggests that apical or lateral infarction cannot be excluded. Suggest serial records and clinical correlation.

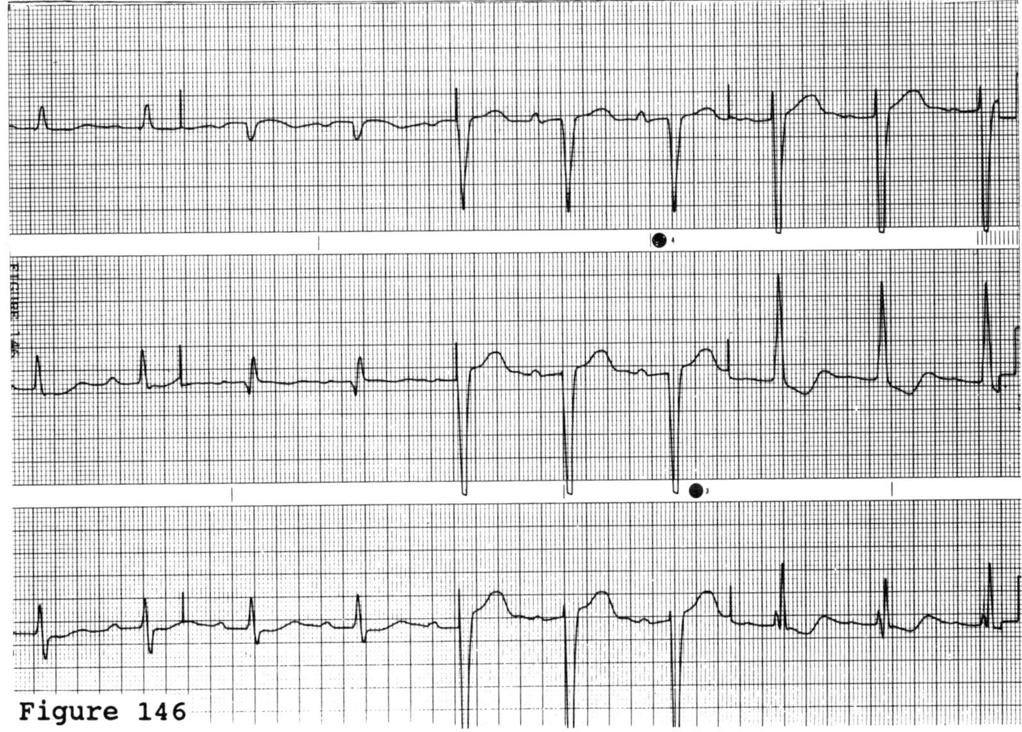

Figure 146

This record shows Mobitz type 1 second degree AV block, the Wenckebach phenomenon. It is best seen in the center of the record in the complexes which go from leads aVR, aVL, and aVF to V1, V2, and V3, where the PR initially is .24 seconds and then becomes .27 and .32 seconds before conduction fails. The frontal plane QRS axis is +50, the T axis +45, and the P axis +60 degrees. The horizontal plane QRS axis is -10, the T axis +5, and the P axis +45 degrees. Suggest repeat record.

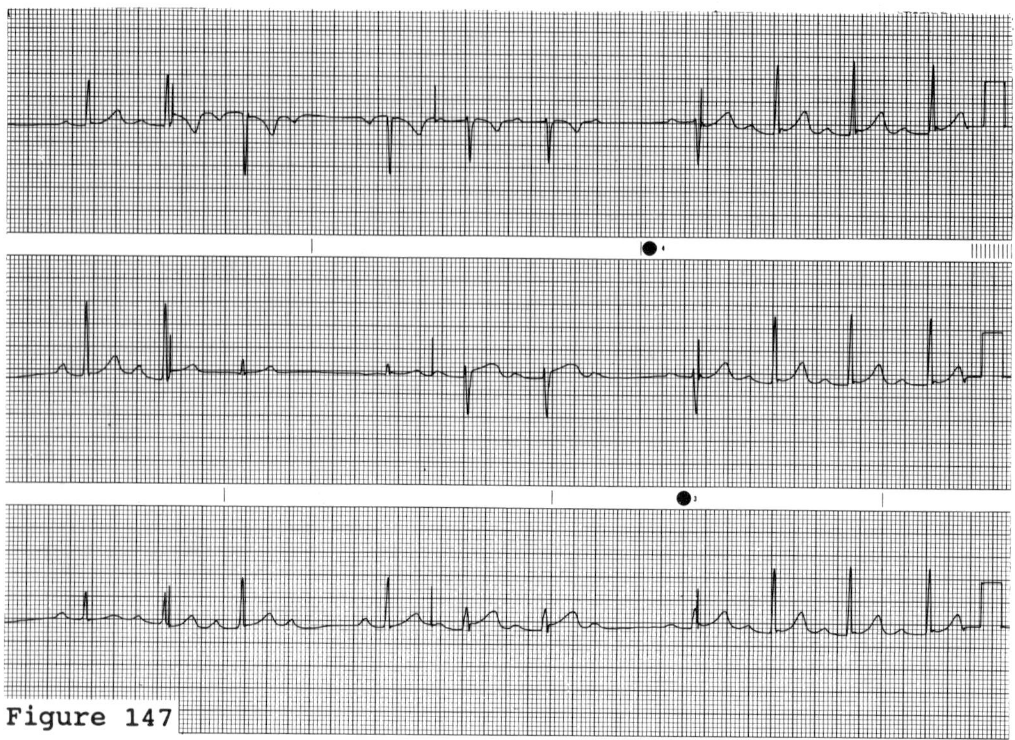

Figure 147

This technically poor record in the limb leads shows 2/1 AV block, with an occasional junctional or ventricular escape as noted in the second QRS complex of leads V1, V2, and V3. The frontal QRS axis is 0, the T axis perhaps +45 degrees. The P axis cannot be plotted due to technical artifact. The horizontal plane QRS axis is -5, the T axis +10, the P axis +10 degrees. Suggest repeat record.

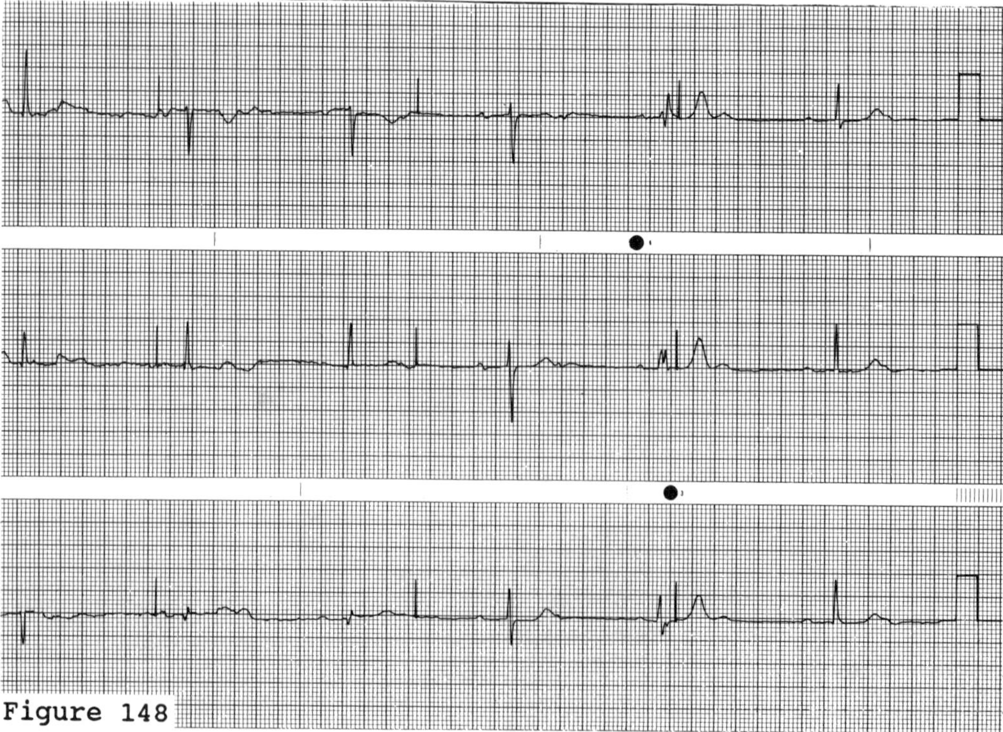

Figure 148

This record shows first degree AV block and 2/1 second degree AV block. The frontal plane QRS
axis is 0, the T axis is +60, and the P axis +45 degrees. The horizontal plane QRS axis is -10, the
T axis +45, and the P axis +45 degrees. Suggest repeat record.

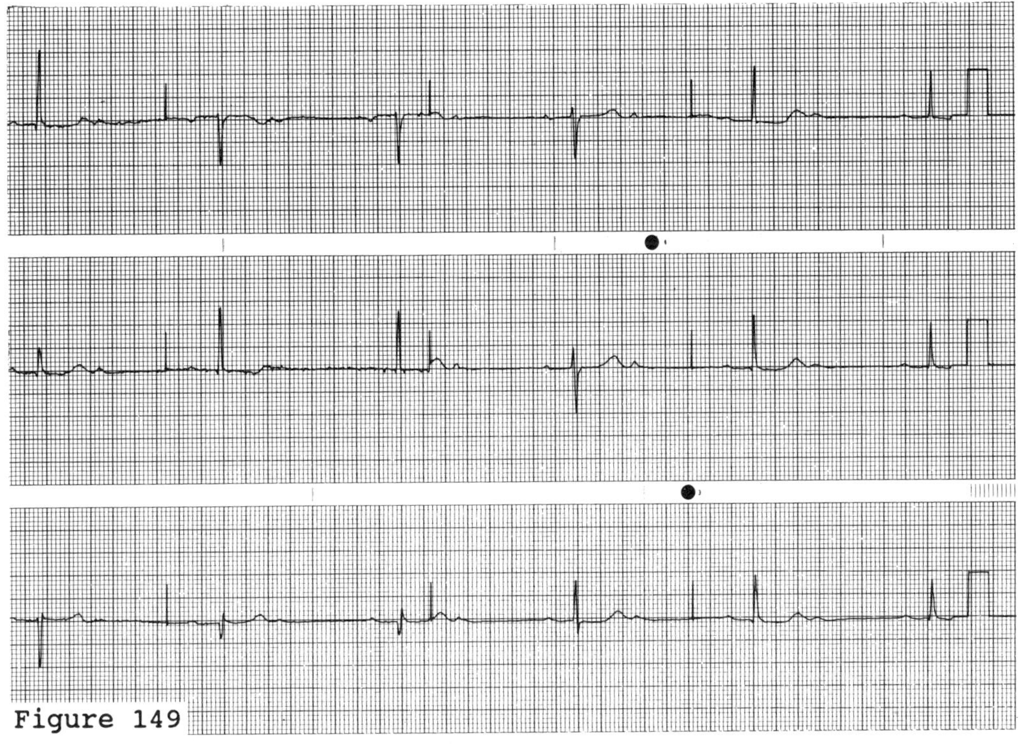

Figure 149

This record shows first degree AV block and probable Mobitz type 2 second degree AV block, as
shown in leads 1, 2, and 3 through aVR, aVL, and aVF. No definite P waves can be seen any place in
V4 through V6. The frontal plane QRS axis is +45, the T axis +45, the P axis +90 degrees. The
horizontal plane QRS axis is -35, the T axis is +5, and the P axis +90 degrees. Suggest repeat
record.

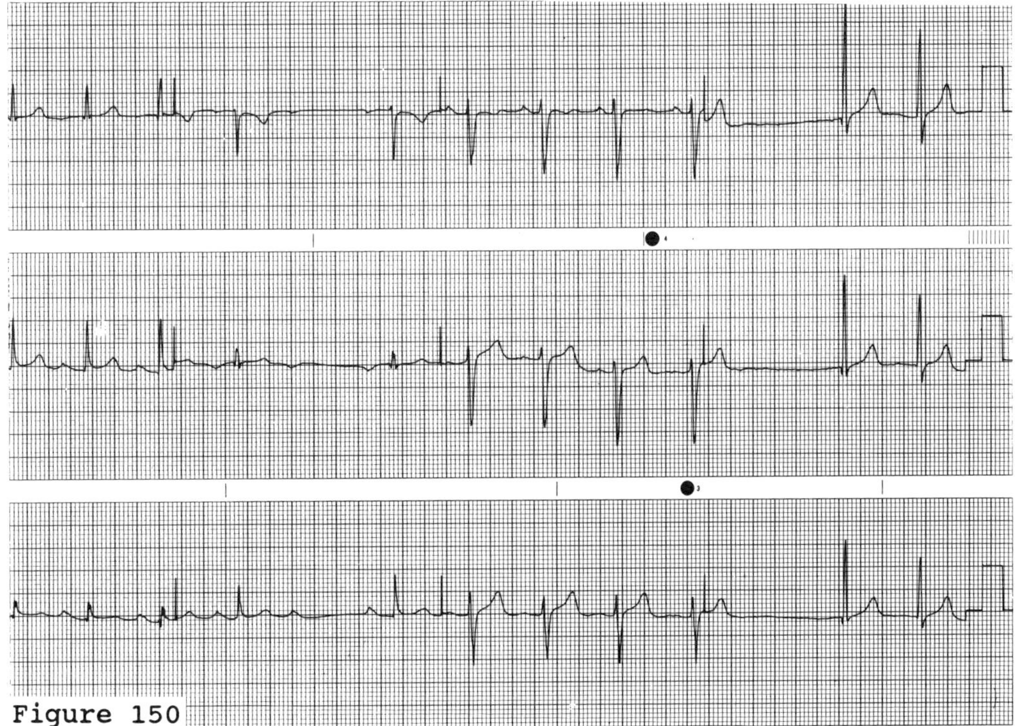

Figure 150

    This record shows sinus rhythm with second degree AV block, often 2/1, with the Wenckebach
phenomenon, and occasional junctional escape beats. The frontal plane QRS axis is biphasic in many
leads, and somewhat low voltage is present. The T axis is +60, and the P axis is +75 degrees. The
horizontal plane QRS axis is -45, the T axis is +45, and the P axis is +45 degrees. The record
shows a relatively high degree of second degree AV block, with varying P-R intervals, the Wenckebach
phenomenon, and some probable junctional escape beats.

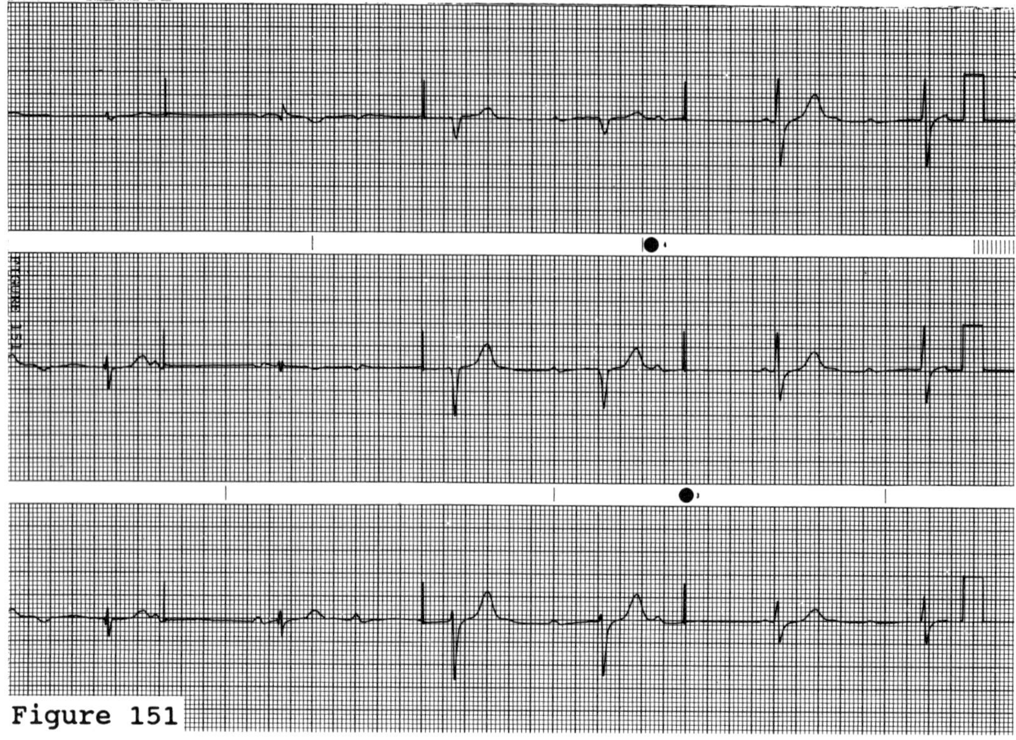

Figure 151

    This record shows atrial flutter and high grade second degree AV block. It almost resembles
third degree AV block but the R-R intervals are not quite regular. Digitalis toxicity may be present, as the ventricular rate is only 38/minute. The QRS duration is .11 seconds. The frontal plane
QRS axis is +40 degrees. The T axis is difficult to plot. The horizontal plane QRS axis is -55, the
T axis is +135 degrees. Left ventricular hypertrophy may well be present, with T changes consistent
with left ventricular strain and/or lateral ischemia. Suggest repeat or serial records and clinical
correlation.

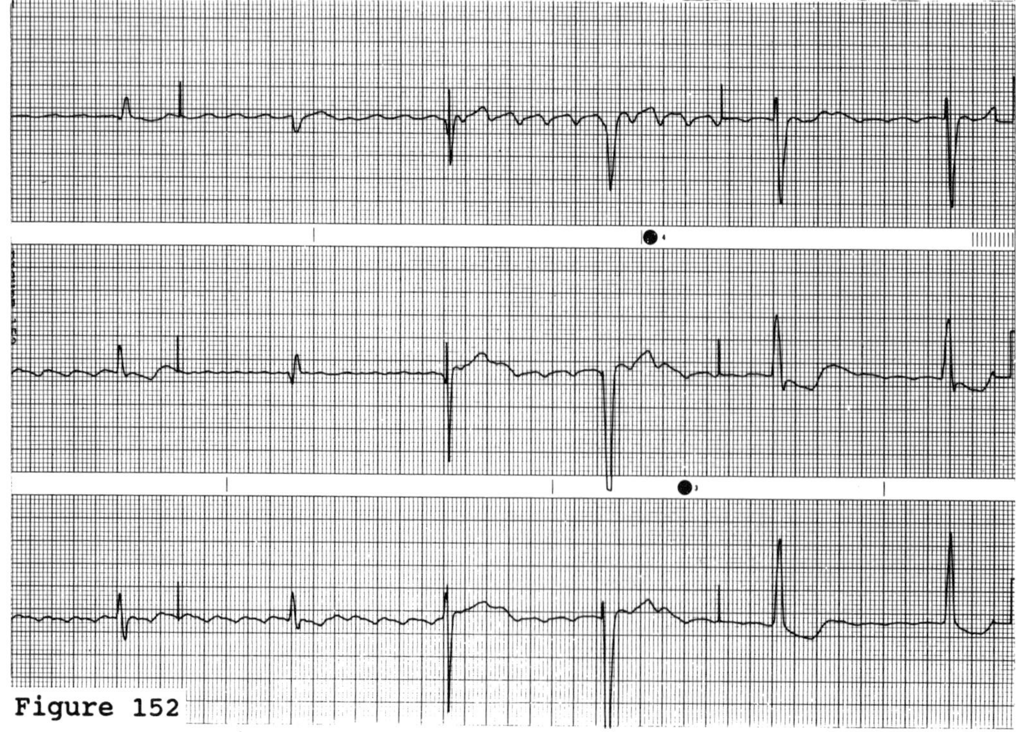

Figure 152

results in a dropped beat following a series of beats which show a progressively increasing P-R interval. This is the Wenckebach phenomenon. The node then has time to recover and the cycle repeats itself. If infrequent beats are dropped one may see, for example, a 6:5 AV block, but if the atrial rate is faster or the AV node more sluggish, more beats will be dropped, resulting in 2:1, 3:1, or even 6:1 AV block, or greater.

Mobitz Type 1 and Type 2 Second Degree AV Block

The Wenckebach phenomenon has also been called Mobitz Type 1 AV Block. The lengthening PR interval shows its presence, and it therefore gives warning of the impending tendency to drop beats. As we have seen, it is associated with malfunction of AV nodal or junctional cells, especially those of its atrial crest. This is shown in Figure 147, in aVR, aVL, and aVF, and in V1 - V3.

Mobitz Type 2 AV Block occurs when, without any warning or any prolongation of the PR interval, beats fail to be conducted. This is therefore a sudden occurrence, which can be disastrous. Mobitz Type 2 block is usually associated with malfunction of cells of the lower AV junction or upper bundle of His, which are not sensitive to vagal tone or acetylcholine and its congeners. Conduction through the His bundle will be good one beat, and may suddenly fail the next. An example is shown in Figure 150, in Leads aVR, aVL, and aVF, and V4 - V6.

Some types of 2/1 or 3/1 block do not permit us to tell whether they are Mobitz Type 1 or Type 2, as they have a stable arrangement and a stable PR interval. An example is shown in Figure 149.

Third Degree or Complete AV Block - Figure 153.

In this situation no impulse passes the AV node. The SA node fires at its own rate, causing normal P waves. The Purkinje fibers fire at their slow

This record shows complete AV block, probable left atrial enlargement, and a ventricular pacemaker functioning in the fixed-rate mode. The first QRS complex in leads V1-V3 is different from the other, has lesser QRS duration, and may in part be conducted down from the P wave, representing a fusion of a conducted and a paced beat.

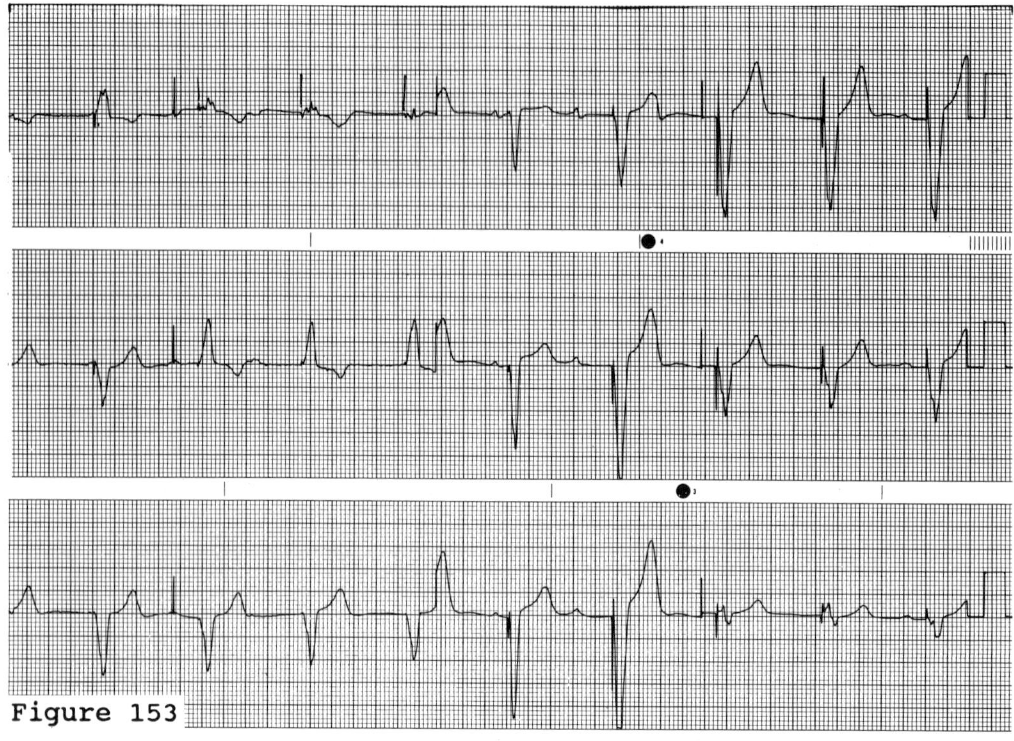

Figure 153

This record shows left atrial enlargement, complete AV block, and a ventricular pacemaker functioning in the fixed rate mode. The QRS axis of the paced beats is -75 degrees in the frontal plane and -90 degrees in the horizontal plane, and is representative of the QRS complexes and axes seen when a catheter pacemaker is placed in the apex of the right ventricle.

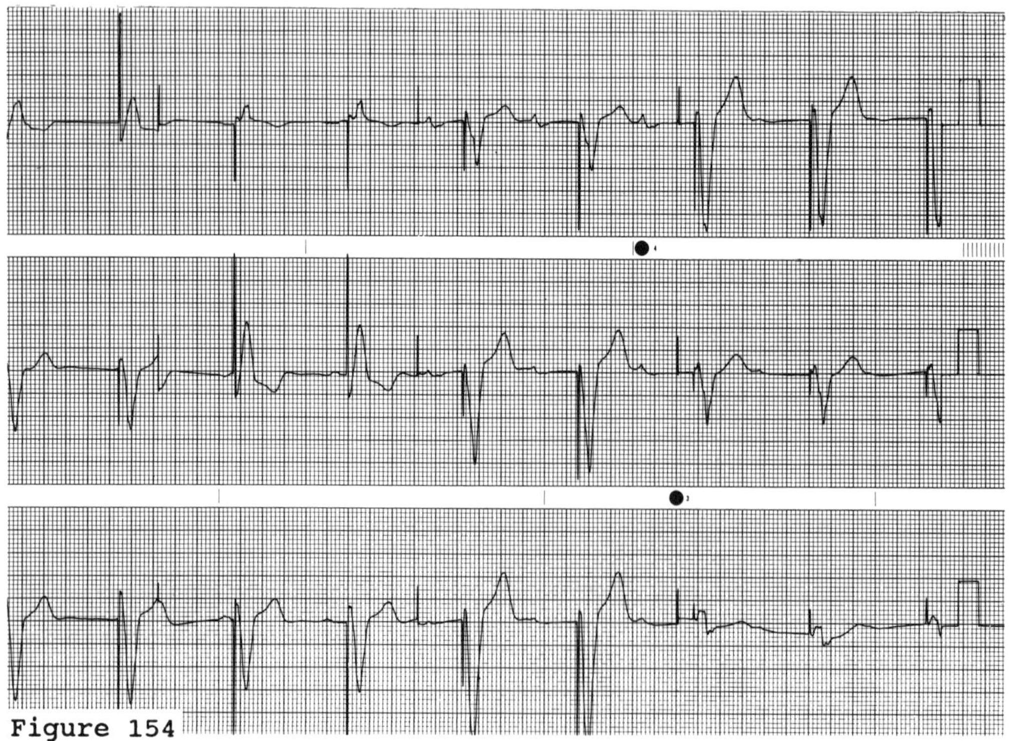

Figure 154

This record shows a slow but quite regular series of narrow QRS complexes at 37/minute. Occasional P waves are present. The rhythm is probably that of complete AV block with the lower focus arising in the bundle of His, below the AV node, but above where the bundle of His divides into its branches. The frontal plane QRS axis is +30, and the T axis is -45 degrees. The horizontal plane QRS axis is -30, and the horizontal T axis is +170 degrees. T changes consistent with inferior, apical, and lateral ischemia are present. Suggest serial records.

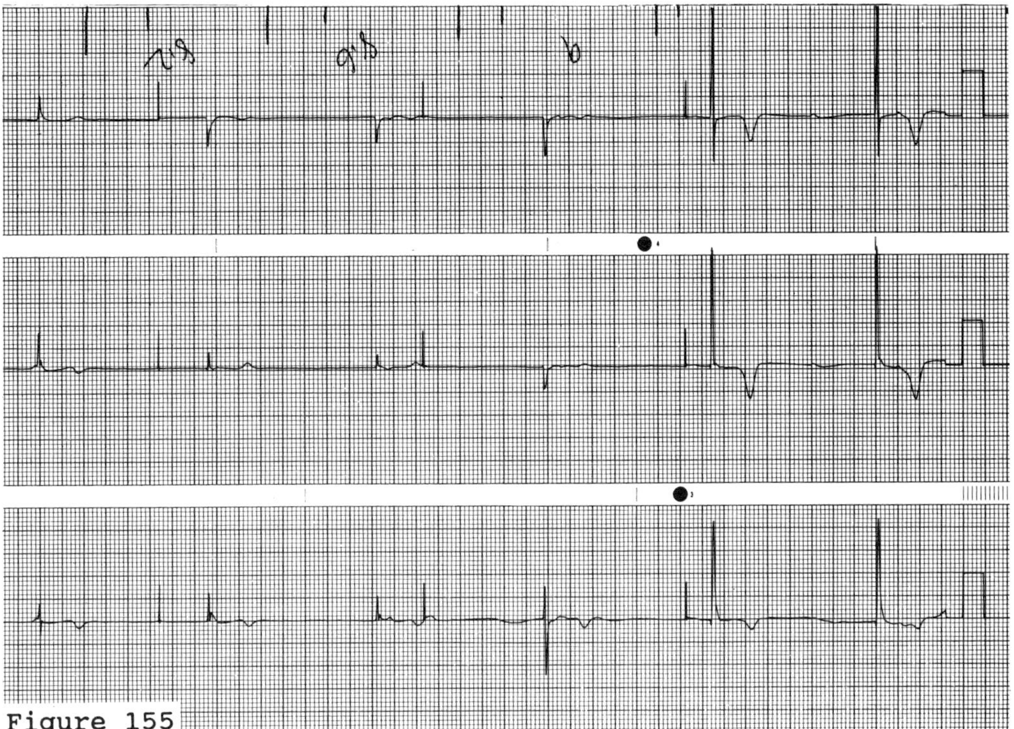

Figure 155

intrinsic rate, causing regular bizarre QRS complexes, (about 30-40/minute), and the two fire regularly, each completely unrelated to each other. Notice that the Purkinje cell focus may be below the division of the Bundle of His, as in Figure 138 earlier, or above it, as in Figure 155.

Stokes-Adams Episodes

When 2nd degree AV block becomes complete, a period of ventricular asystole occurs before an idioventricular focus will arise in the Purkinje system to drive the ventricles. Syncope often results, and the patient is often found awakening with a slow regular pulse of 30-40/minute.

However, ventricular fibrillation may also develop during such a Stokes-Adams episode, probably due to multiple competing spontaneously discharging foci arising in the Purkinje system at about the same time. This then may cause a disorganized depolarization of the ventricles resulting in their fibrillation. If the fibrillation ceases and one Purkinje focus achieves dominance, the patient will probably survive the episode but may have some degree of brain damage. If not, the patient will die of circulatory arrest unless cardiopulmonary resuscitation and defibrillation can be carried out promptly.

8

Pulmonary Disease and Pediatric Tracings

<u>PULMONARY DISEASE.</u> Figures 156 - 157.

Overexpansion of the lungs, with an increased amount of air between the heart and the chest wall, may be associated with generalized low voltage, as shown in Figure 156. Frequently, however, the low voltage is primarily in the limb leads, as shown in Figure 157, while the precordial lead voltage is often quite good, in V2 - V3 of that figure, for example.

How can we have low voltage in the limb leads and not in the chest leads? The answer to this is frequently the same as the answer to the more general question of how the voltage in any single lead can be different from that in some other lead - it is due to the overall QRS axis or vector.

Often with pulmonary disease, as in Figure 157, the overall QRS vector is rotated posteriorly, with the horizontal plane vector being rightward and posterior, at about minus 80-120 degrees. There is relatively little projection of this vector into the frontal plane. Because of this, the voltage in the limb leads is quite low. The low voltage frontal plane QRS vector is at about plus 150 degrees. Therefore the overall QRS axis or vector is going primarily posterior, and slightly rightward and inferior. In addition, the P axis is often vertical, at least plus 60 degrees. Right atrial enlargement may sometimes be seen as well.

<u>Pediatric Tracings.</u> Figures 158 - 159.

You can usually recognize a baby's record when you see the very narrow QRS complex (usually 0.03 - 0.04 seconds), with a rightward and anterior QRS axis or vector resembling that of right ventricular hypertrophy. Remember that in the fetal circulation this is the normal thing, as the pulmonary circuit is a high-pressure one until the lungs expand with air and the

    This record shows sinus tachycardia, generalized low voltage, and nonspecific T wave changes.
The frontal plane QRS axis is +60, the T axis +60, the P axis +70 degrees. The horizontal plane QRS
axis is -60, the T axis is 0, the P axis is 0 degrees. The record is consistent with pulmonary
disease, and nonspecific T changes are also present. Pericardial effusion cannot be excluded.
Suggest repeat record and clinical correlation.

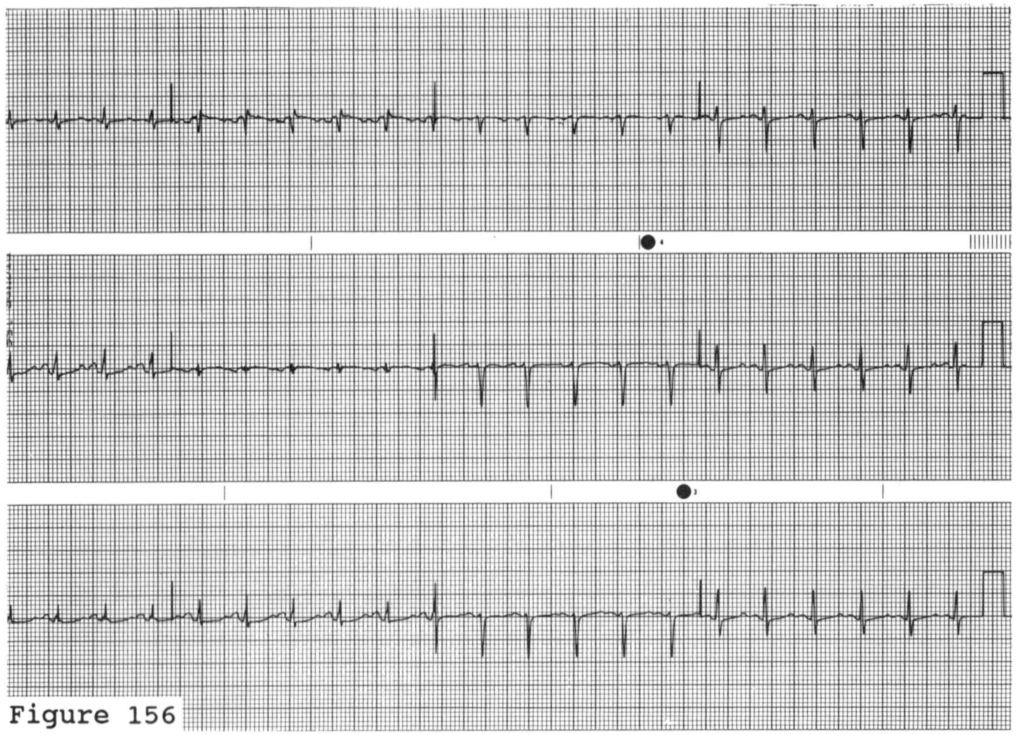

Figure 156

    This record shows sinus rhythm, low frontal plane voltage, Q waves and T inversions in 2, 3,
and aVF, and a marginal precordial R progession in V2 through V5. The frontal plane QRS axis is 180
degrees. The T axis is difficult to plot. The horizontal plane QRS axis is -120, and the T axis is
+90 degrees. The record is consistent with pulmonary disease and inferior infarction. T changes
are consistent with inferior and possible lateral ischemia. An anteroapical infarction cannot be
completely excluded, although it is not clearly seen. Suggest repeat or serial records and clinical
correlation.

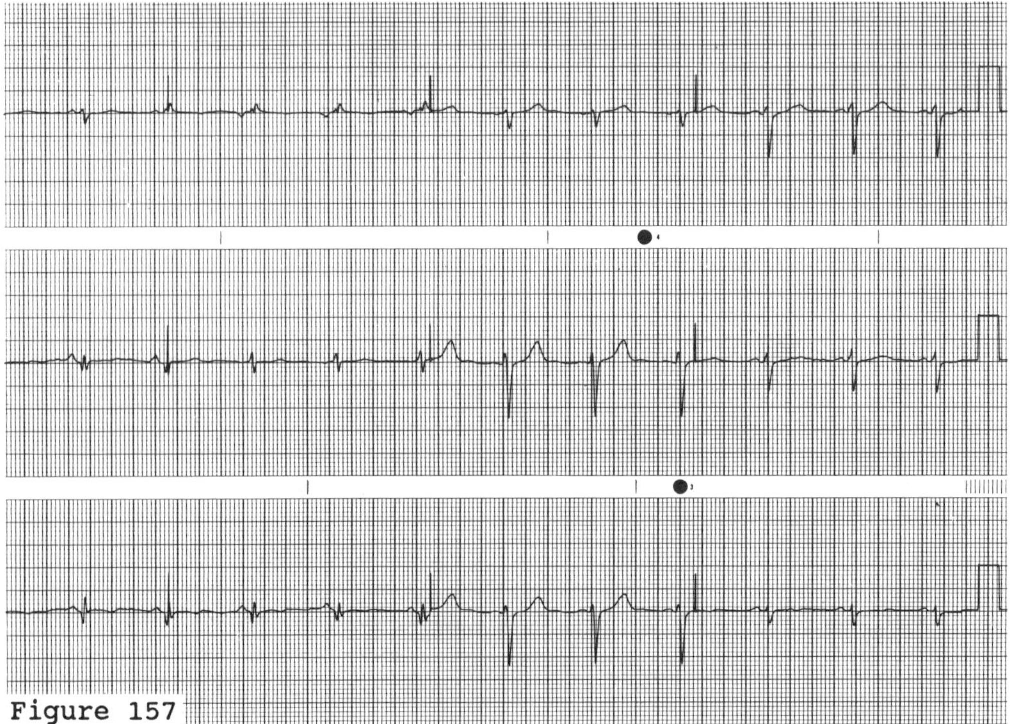

Figure 157

This record shows sinus tachycardia, narrow QRS complexes (.04sec), and evidence of technical misalignment so that the QRS complexes, especially in the middle channel, are not vertical. The frontal plane QRS axis is probably about -115 degrees. Except for the superiority of the frontal plane QRS axis, the record may well be with normal limits for age. The precordial leads show evidence of possible lead misplacement. Lead V1 may be V2, V2 may be V3, and V3 may be V1. This gives the most coherent progression of the P and T wave vectors as well as the QRS vectors. If so, then the horizontal plane QRS axis is +155, the T axis 0, and the P axis +10 degrees. The very narrow QRS complexes and the sinus tachycardia, combined with the evidence of possible right ventricular enlargement (for an adult), suggest that this record probably comes from a normal infant.

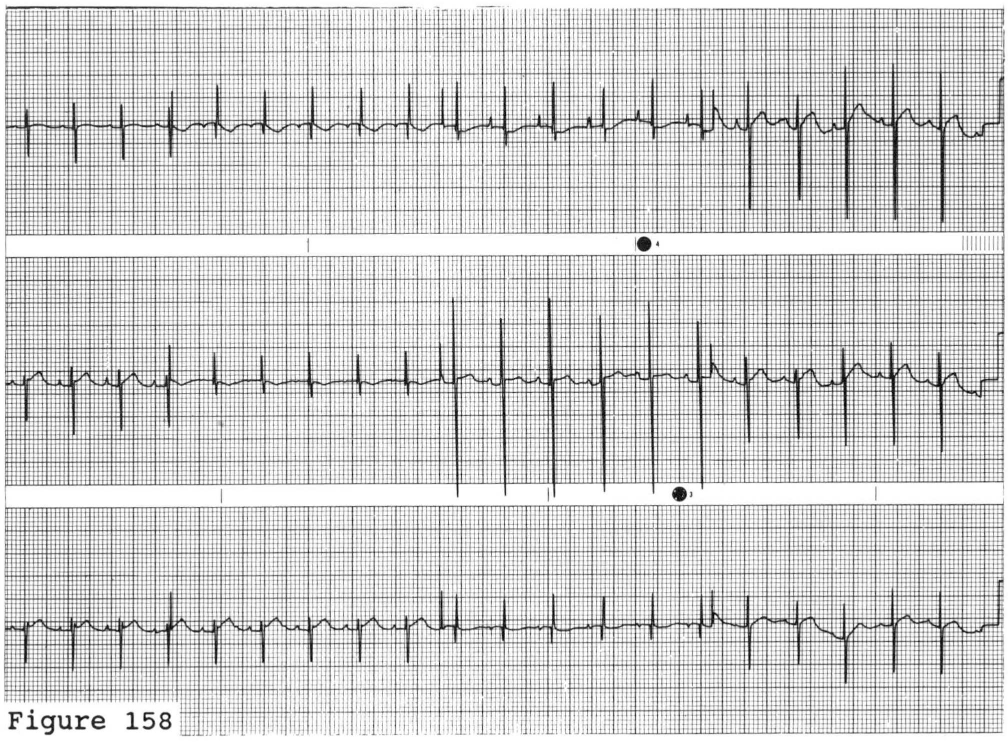

Figure 158

This record shows a sinus tachycardia and might suggest right ventricular enlargement, but again the rapid rate and the very narrow QRS complexes suggest that this is from a baby. The frontal QRS axis is +115, the T axis is 0, and the P axis is +55 degrees. The horizontal plane QRS axis has a double transition on either side of V2, but as shown in V1, excess anterior forces are present for an adult. Nonspecific ST-T changes are noted, especially in leads V4 through V6, but the record otherwise is within normal limits for an infant. Suggest repeat record.

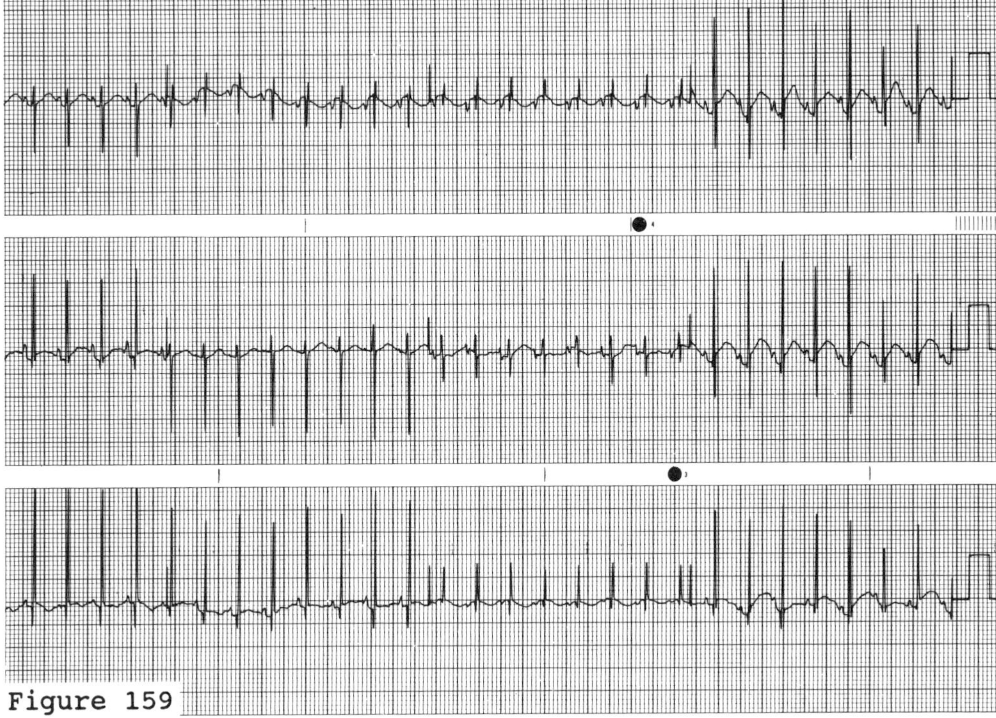

Figure 159

pulmonary vascular resistance drops. After birth, "disuse atrophy" of the
right ventricle sets in rapidly, and the EKG gradually comes to resemble
that of an adult, usually by two years of age. Some typical tracings are
shown in Figures 158 and 159.

9

Drugs, Electrolytes, Pacemakers, and Technical Errors

<u>DIGITALIS</u>

Digitalis compounds have three basic effects on the myocardium. The common theme underlying both desired (therapeutic) and unwanted (toxic) effects of digitalis is the increased availability of calcium within most (probably all) body cells.

1. Increased myocardial contractility and shortening of systole. More myocardial work can be done, in less time, at the same sarcomere length. Thus cardiac power is literally augmented by these compounds. Associated with these events are:

A. Shorter Q-T interval on EKG

B. Shorter individual cell action potentials.

This results in less time spent on the plateau phase of the action potentials, and consequently the ST segment and T wave of the EKG are altered. The depressed ST junction and concave upward ST segment, with flatter or even inverted T waves constitute "digitalis effect" on the EKG, as shown in Figure 135. This may be seen with about one-half of a therapeutic dose of the drug but is very poorly correlated with dose and cannot be used as a guide to dosage at all, unless you know a particular patient extremely well, and have done dose-ranging studies on him or her. Furthermore, it is frequently impossible to tell very marked digitalis effect from ischemia or left ventricular strain.

2. Conduction velocity through myocardial cells is reduced, especially through the AV node. This usually occurs in higher therapeutic doses and serum levels. It is responsible for the increased AV conduction time when digitalis is given to slow and control the ventricular rate in

atrial fibrillation, and for the unwanted (toxic) first and second degree AV blocks in patients with sinus rhythm. It is due to:

    A. CNS effects resulting in increased vagal tone

    B. Direct effects on myocardial cells

    3. Ectopic firing of atrial, junctional, and/or Purkinje fibers, resulting in atrial, nodal, or ventricular extrasystoles or tachycardias.

Because digitalis compounds can produce both AV blocks and ectopic activity, literally _any_ arrhythmia may be a manifestation of digitalis toxicity, as these (along with re-entry) are the two basic mechanisms by which arrhythmias are produced. However, the most common arrhythmias are ventricular extrasystoles, bigeminy, AV blocks, atrial tachycardias, especially with AV block, and ventricular tachycardias. Hypokalemia due to diuretics enhances the likelihood of ectopic beats in patients on digitalis, as the low K leads to increased binding of digitalis to the Na-K ATPase. Poor oxygenation and ischemic heart disease also help to cause arrthymias in patients on digitalis preparations.

When the toxic arrhythmia is predominantly a conduction disturbance, potassium is usually not used, unless hypokalemia is present (see below). When the toxic arrhythmia is predominantly due to spontaneous ectopic activity, that is the usual place to use potassium. This is because the main effects of potassium are:

    A. Slowing of conduction velocity, thus enhancing an AV block.

    B. Abolishing spontaneous firing.

    C. Displacement of digitalis compounds from the Na-K ATPase. This is slow, and requires 1-2 days to be complete. Serum glycoside levels will rise as the patient improves, as the drug is displaced from the receptors.

Management of Severe Digitalis Toxicity

For severe digitalis toxicity, it is most useful to measure RBC Na and K to evaluate the severity of digitalis toxicity. RBC K depletion appears to reflect K depletion in other tissues as well, and is an index of tissue K depletion. In severe digitalis toxicity, a high-normal K (6.0 mEq/L) or even higher (sometimes actually over 7!) may be useful, if tolerated, to help prevent further binding of digitalis to the Na-K ATPase. In severe digitalis toxicity the Na-K ATPase is severely inhibited in all body cells, even the relatively inert RBC's. Tissue K is low. Serum K is high. Usually, though, the EKG shows <u>no</u> evidence of the high K, only severe digitalis effect. The patient will usually rapidly excrete his elevated serum K, causing further attachment of digitalis to the Na-K ATPpase and <u>worsening</u> the toxicity even as his serum digitalis levels <u>fall</u>, due to increased tissue binding. Careful K therapy, to a goal of about 6.0 mEq/L, is helpful in preventing such attachment, getting the digitalis off the membranes and out into the serum again. Serum glycoside levels usually rise and the patient's digitalis toxicity gets better (8). The FAB antibody fragments are also very helpful, and are probably definitive, if needed.

In general, for most digitalis toxicity, one can

1)   Stop the drug. This must be done. Later on, adjust the dose.

2)   Use a temporary pacemaker if needed to control slow rates.

3)   Use K (40-60mEq in 1 L), under careful EKG monitoring, to keep K not only normal, but high normal, and up to 6.0mEq/L for severe

toxicity, or even more, depending on the patient. This is discussed more fully elsewhere (8).

4)   Consider FAB antibody therapy if life-threatening.

<u>PACEMAKERS.</u> Figures 160 - 168.

The earliest type of internal cardiac pacemaker, developed in the early 1960's, was a fixed-rate pacer. You set the rate, put the catheter tip usually in the apex of the right ventricle, and implant the circuitry usually in a subcutaneous site in the chest or axilla.

Pacemakers have been unipolar (only 1 electrode on the catheter tip, the other on the case for the circuitry) or bipolar (both electrodes close together on the catheter tip). Unipolar pacers make a large pacing spike on the EKG, as the voltage difference is present over a wide area of the chest. Bipolar pacers (like the ones shown here in Figures 160 - 168, make a much smaller spike on the EKG, as the voltage is less, and it induces a much smaller field between the 2 electrodes on the catheter tip.

Random variations in height and direction of the pacemaker spike are seen on many EKG's, including the ones shown here. This is because many computerized EKG systems digitize the signal (convert its amplitude to a number) every so often, commonly every 4 msec. Most pacer pulses are much shorter than this, usually about 1 msec. Because of the short pacer pulse, it will play a different role in generating the number digitized by the EKG depending on how much of that particular 4 msec was occupied by that particular pacer pulse. Sometimes such a computerized EKG may even occasionally miss a pacer spike altogether.

180

<u>Fixed-Rate</u> <u>Pacemakers.</u> Figure 160.

Here the pacer simply fires at a regular fixed rate. It does not sense any of the other events taking place. Because of this, one problem with fixed-rate pacers arises when some patients recover from their heart block to a greater or lesser degree, having varying numbers of conducted ventricular beats, and even sinus rhythm once again.

The <u>R-on-T</u> <u>Phenomenon</u> Figure 161.

Such patients who recovered their sinus rhythm, for example, and who still had a fixed-rate pacemaker going, frequently had their pacer fire during the upstroke of their T wave, a very vulnerable period. This <u>vulnerable</u> <u>period</u> (R on T) exists because at that time, some of the myocardial and Purkinje cells have recovered and can conduct a propagated impulse, while others cannot. A stimulus at this time may therefore cause ventricular fibrillation. An example of the R on T phenomenon is shown in Figure 161. Indeed, the mortality of patients who had both sinus rhythm and a fixed-rate pacemaker was found to be about 30% per year because of the R on T problem.   This information led to a development of "smarter" pacemakers.

<u>Demand</u> <u>(QRS-inhibited)</u> <u>Pacemakers.</u> Figures 162 - 163.

One such development (out of many) has been the demand, or QRS-inhibited, pacemaker. Here the pacing electrode also serves a sensing function. It looks for a QRS complex every so often (every second, for example). If one doesn't come along, the pacer fires, doesn't sense for about 0.3 seconds, and then starts looking again to see if another QRS complex is coming along. If it does, the pacer doesn't fire, but simply resets its clock and waits again. This pacer thus not only prevents the R-on-T problem, but also saves power consumption and prolongs battery life. An example

This record shows probable atrial fibrillation, complete AV block, and a ventricular pacemaker functioning in the fixed rate mode.

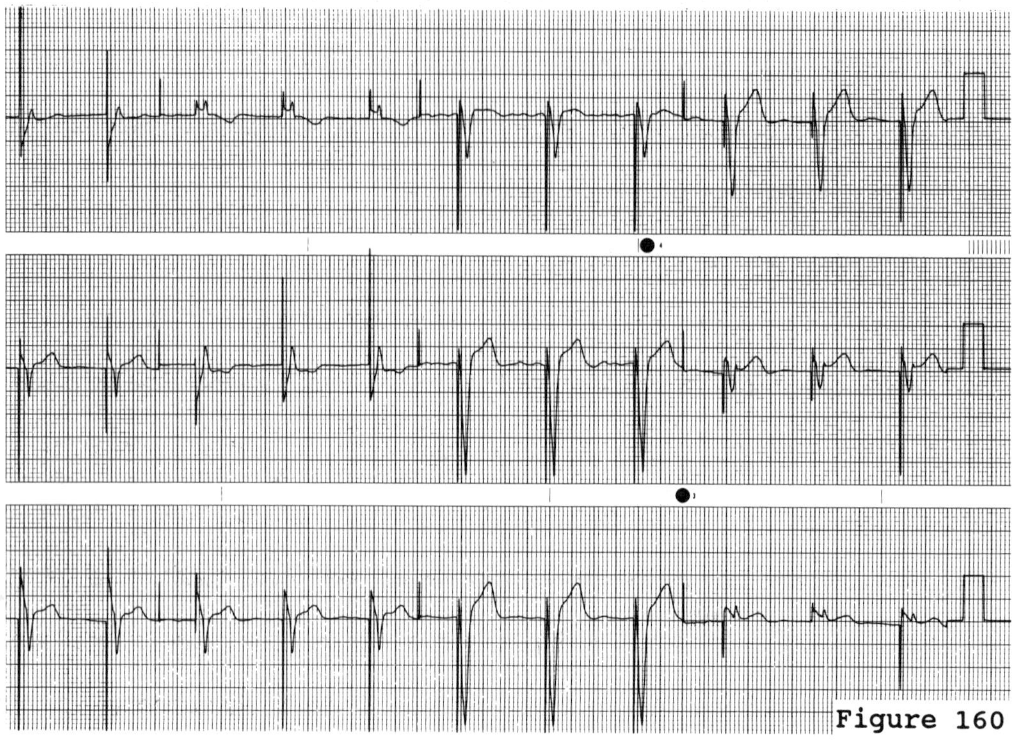

Figure 160

This record shows a combination of regular sinus rhythum and what is probably a QRS—inhibited demand pacemaker which has impaired sensing. As a result, frequent pacemaker spikes are seen, some resulting in a paced beat, others not. Frequent examples of the R on T phenomenon are seen. The record also shows abnormal left axis deviation, possible left anterior superior hemiblock, prominent anterior forces, and T inversions consistent with anterior and lateral ischemia and/or left ventricular strain. Suggest repeat or serial records, clinical correlation, and possible pacemaker removal.

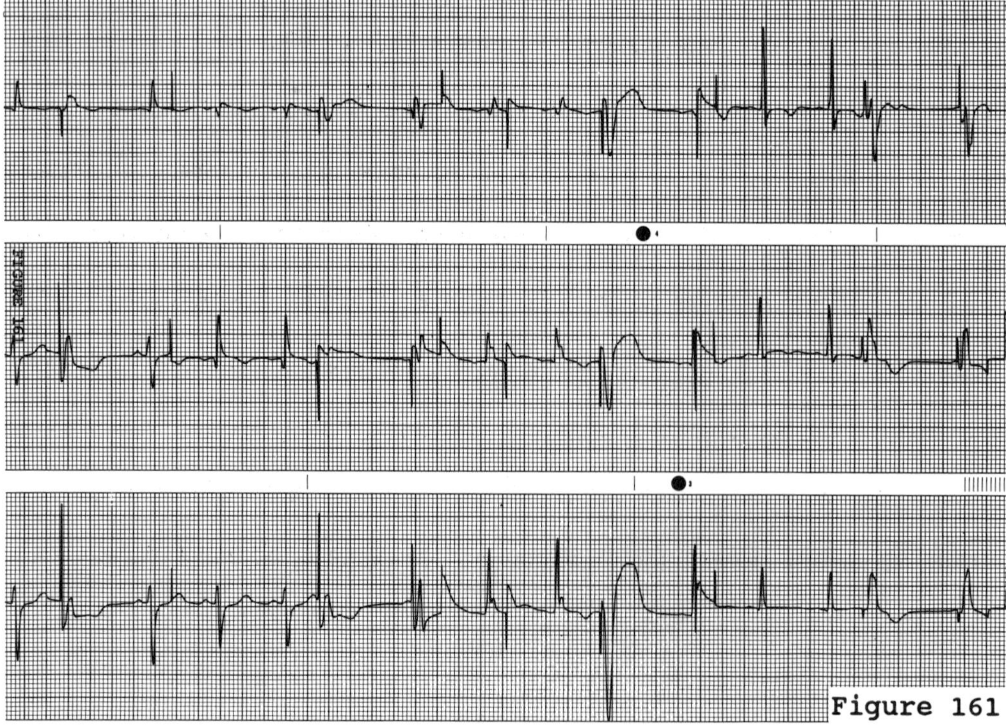

Figure 161

This record shows a ventricular pacemaker functioning in the demand or QRS inhibited mode.
Occasional normally conducted beats are noted. Left atrial enlargement may possibly be present, as
well as anterior ischemia, as judged from the T inversions in the conducted beat in leads V1 through
V3. Suggest serial records and clinical correlation.

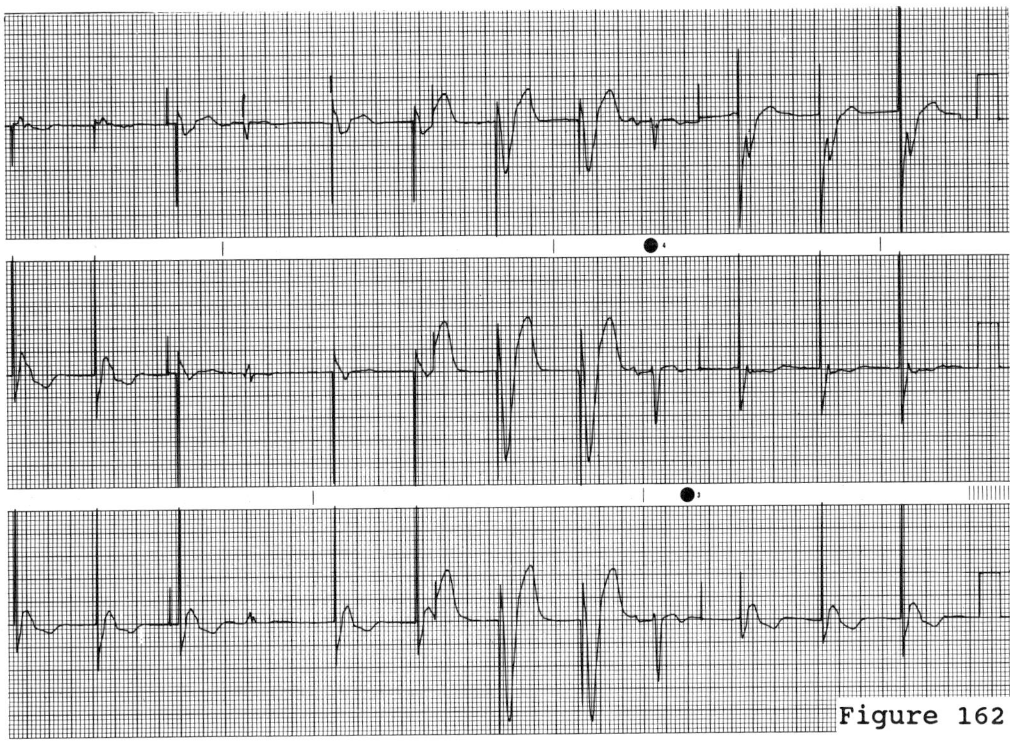

Figure 162

This record shows frequent sinus rhythm and evidence of a ventricular pacemaker functioning in
the QRS inhibited or demand mode. Frequent ventricular extrasystoles are seen following the paced
beats. In the normally conducted beats, inverted T waves are present in leads 2, 3, and V4-V6. In
the very last QRS complex in lead aVF a Q is present. Inferior and lateral ischemia are probably
present. Inferior infarction cannot be excluded. Suggest serial records and clinical correlation.

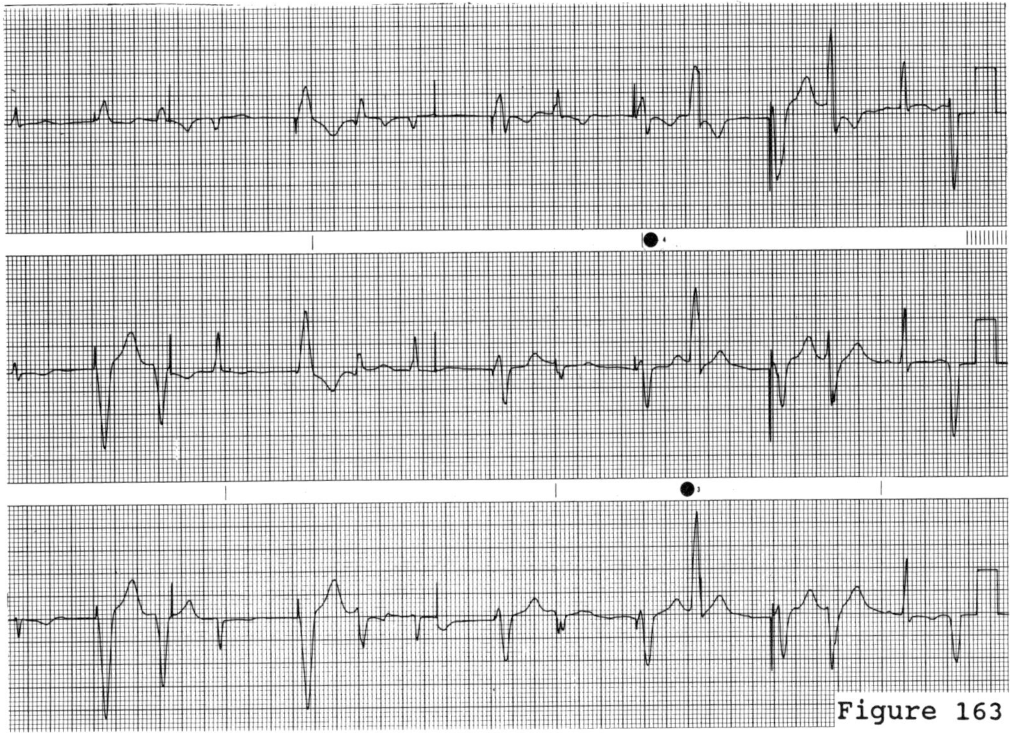

Figure 163

is shown in Figures 162 and 163, where an occasional conducted beat shuts it off and resets its clock. Notice that if these beats had not occurred, we would not be able to distinguish such a demand pacemaker, operating in its "fixed-rate" mode, with nothing to sense, from a true fixed rate pacemaker. The clues to help you tell whether a pacer is the fixed-rate or demand type are whether or not other events are occurring in the EKG which the pacer should be sensing. If not, then you cannot tell them apart. If other events do occur, then you may develop evidence for impaired sensing on the part of the pacer that may lead you to conclude that it is either a true fixed-rate pacer or a demand pacer with defective sensing.

The problem of correctly sensing the QRS complexes was a major hurdle for pacemaker manufacturers to overcome. Microwave ovens, diathermy machines, and automobile ignition systems, for example, will flood the pacemaker with signals that it must distinguish from QRS complexes. Usually when they are so rapid the problem is simple. Nevertheless, most demand pacemakers have fairly sophisticated criteria now to help them distinguish (not always correctly) between a patient's normal QRS complex and other electrical events in the environment.

<u>Dual-Chamber</u> <u>Pacemakers.</u> Figures 164 - 168.

Here, as shown in Figures 164 - 168, there is one electrode placed in or on the atrium, and another in or on the ventricles. With the advent of modern microprocessor technology, each electrode may now serve both a sensing and/or pacing function. In the example shown here, the pacer first senses the P wave with the atrial electrode. It then follows, at the proper PR interval, with a stimulus to the ventricular electrode. It is usually known as an AV synchronous pacemaker. As shown in Figure 164, the pacemaker

At first glance this record appears to show a ventricular pacemaker functioning in the fixed
rate mode. However, every paced complex has a P wave in front of it, with a normal P-R interval.
This record represents an AV synchronous pacemaker which senses the P wave and paces the ventricle
after a proper P-R interval. This particular record shows normally narrow QRS complexes. Because of
this, the pacing may take place not in the ventricle but in the bundle of His. If this is so, the T
inversions in V4 through V6 suggest that lateral ischemia and/or left ventricular strain may be
present. Suggest repeat or serial records and clinical correlation.

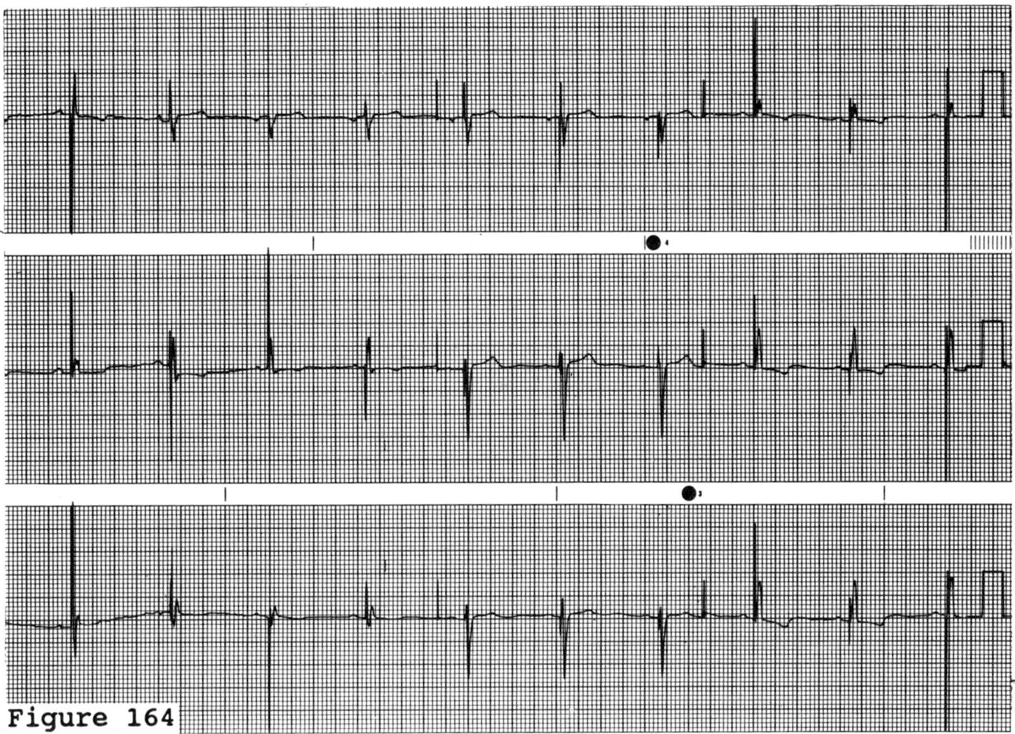

Figure 164

This record shows regular paced ventricular beats each of which follows a somewhat prolonged PR
interval. This record probably represents an AV synchronous pacemaker sensing the P waves and
firing the ventricles. The pacemaker's P-R interval, however, is prolonged.

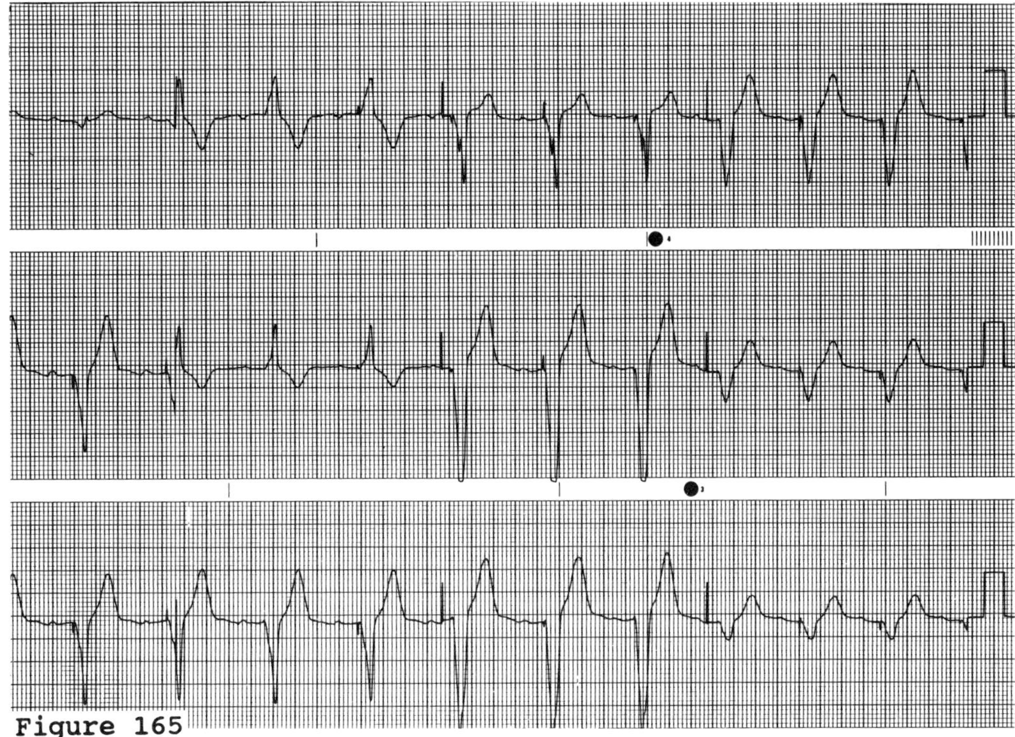

Figure 165

This record shows the dual spikes in each cardiac cycle, consistent with an AV sequential pacemaker firing first the atria and then the ventricles in the proper sequence. The P-R interval of the pacemaker is about .15 seconds.

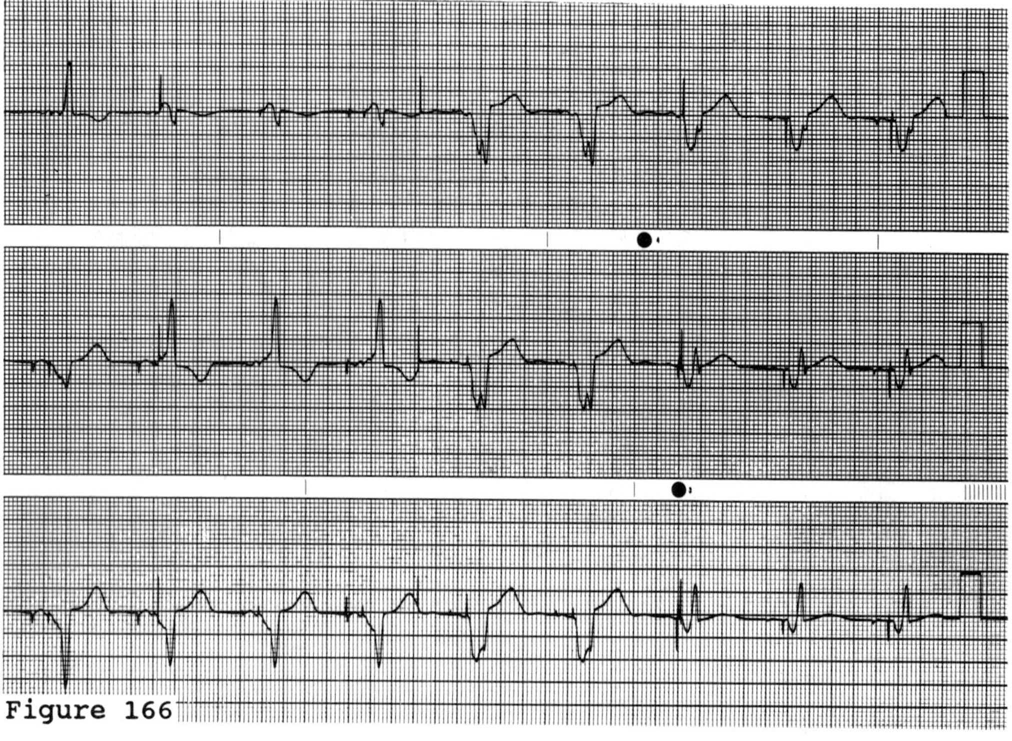

Figure 166

At first glance this record appears to show only atrial pacing. However, in the V leads the spikes associated with ventricular pacing are also seen. The record is that of an AV sequential pacemaker. The P-R interval between atrial and ventricular pacing is prolonged to .23 seconds.

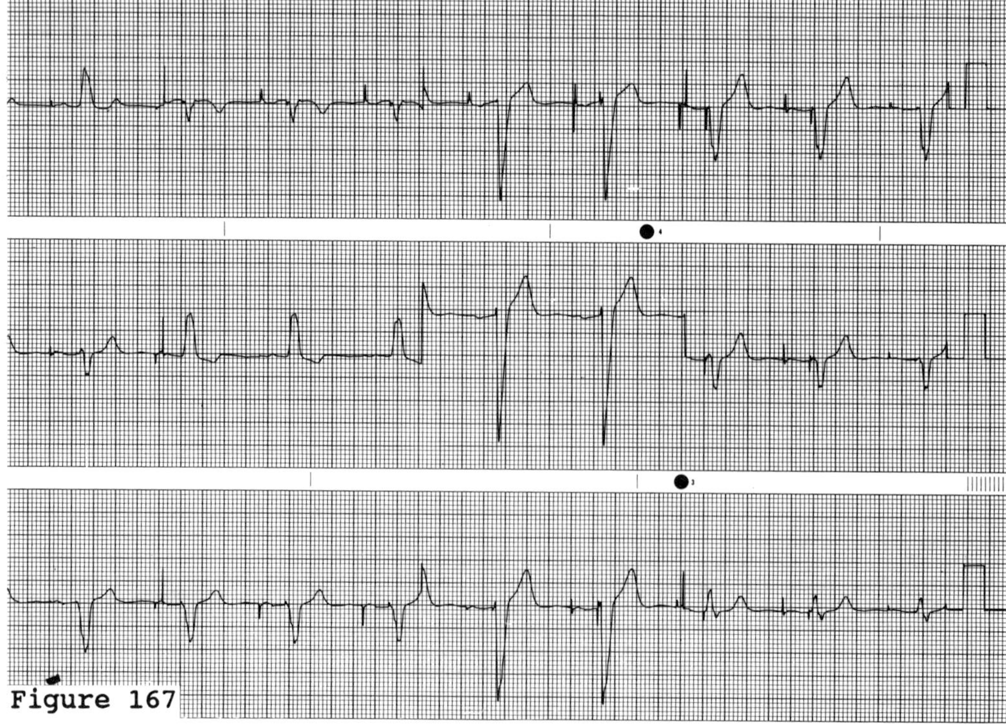

Figure 167

This record shows a probable AV sequential pacemaker functioning at a rate of 92 per minute. The apparent atrial pacing spikes are very large.

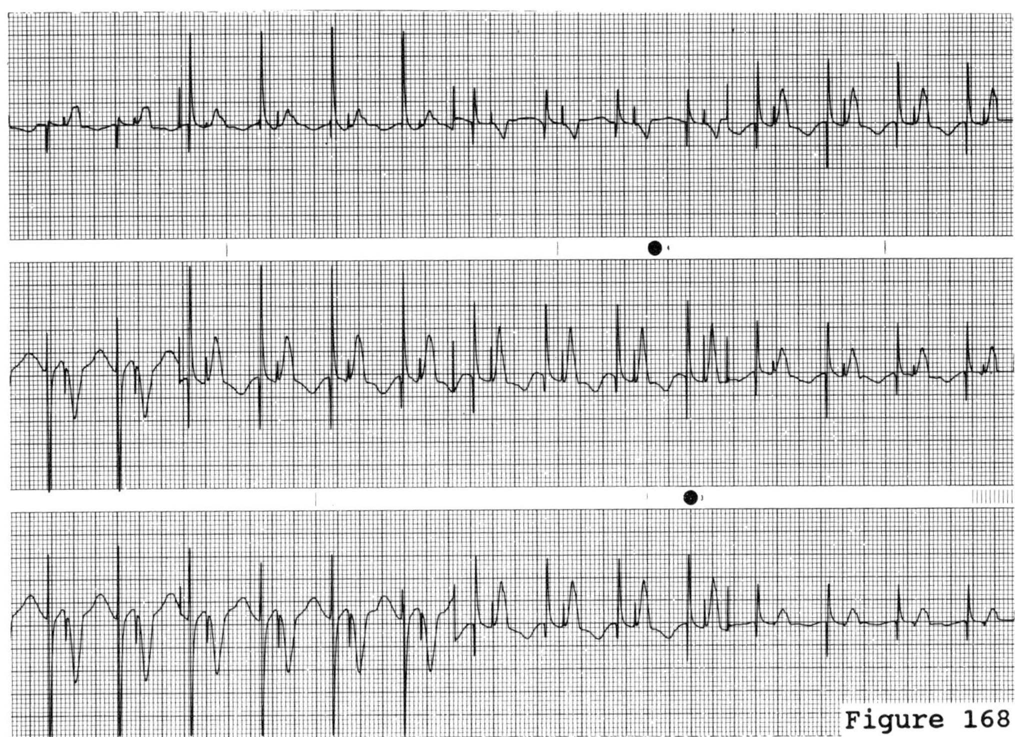

Figure 168

may occasionally appear to fire the Bundle of His rather than the right ventricular apex, the usual location, as shown in Figure 165. Note that Figure 165 also has a slightly prolonged "PR" interval between atrial sensing and ventricular pacing.

In Figures 166 - 168, on the other hand, the AV sequential pacemaker first fires the atrial electrode, followed, at the proper PR interval, by a stimulus to the ventricular electrode. As in Figure 165, Figure 167 also shows a prolonged "PR" interval between the atrial and the ventricular pacing.

<u>TECHNICAL</u> <u>ERRORS.</u> Figures 169 - 179.

<u>Arm</u> <u>Lead</u> <u>Reversal</u>. Figures 169 - 171.

One of the most common technical errors is reversal of the right and left arm leads. As a result of this, Lead 1 will now be written upside down, usually with a downward P,QRS, and T. If the horizontal plane axis is normal, these inversions suggest arm lead reversal, as the discrepancy between frontal and horizontal plane axes is much too obvious to be explained by the 30 degree tilt in the usual horizontal plane.

Further things follow from this. Lead 2 becomes Lead 3, and Lead 3 becomes Lead 2. Even more striking, aVR now becomes aVL, usually with an upward QRS helping to give the clue to the error. AVL also becomes aVR. Only aVF remains essentially unchanged by this error.

<u>Reversed</u> <u>Foot</u> <u>and</u> <u>Right</u> <u>Arm</u> <u>Leads.</u> Figures 172 - 174.

In the tracings in Figures 173 and 174, aVF resembles aVR. If the leads really were correctly placed, the frontal QRS axis would be so superior (about minus 60 degrees), that we should expect to see deep S waves in V5 and V6, due to the 30 degree tilt of the horizontal plane downward and to the left. Since we do not see such S waves, and since the frontal P and T axes would also seem to be very superior if the leads were correctly placed, something must be wrong, and it is likely that the foot lead was placed on the right arm.

We now have two possibilities, as shown in Figures 172a and 172b. In both, the foot lead is on the right arm. In Figure 172a, only the foot and the right arm leads are reversed. This is a more common error than in Figure 172b, where all three leads are misplaced.

This record shows normal sinus rhythm and reversal of the right and left arm electrodes.
As a result, Lead 1 is turned upside down, Lead 2 becomes Lead 3, Lead 3 becomes Lead 2, aVR
becomes aVL, aVL becomes aVR, and only aVF remains unchanged. The record is within normal
limits.

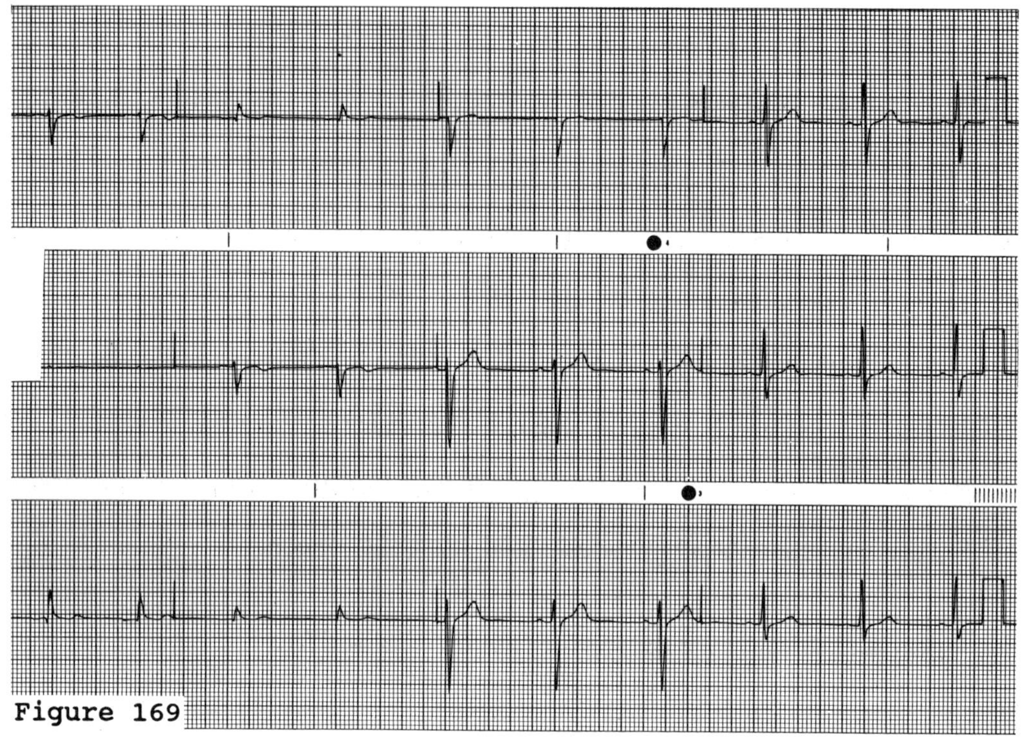

Figure 169

This record shows regular sinus rhythm, evidence of reversal of the right and   left arm leads,
and is probably within normal limits. See text for discussion.

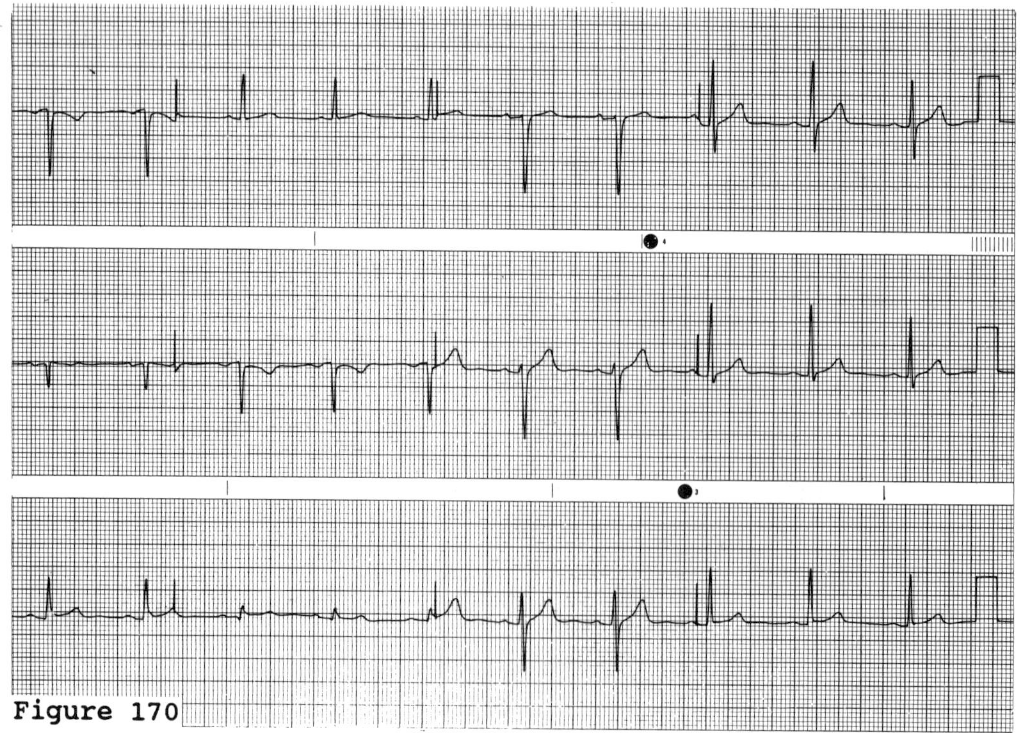

Figure 170

This record shows regular sinus rhythm, evidence of reversal of the right and left arm leads, and is probably within normal limits. See text for discussion.

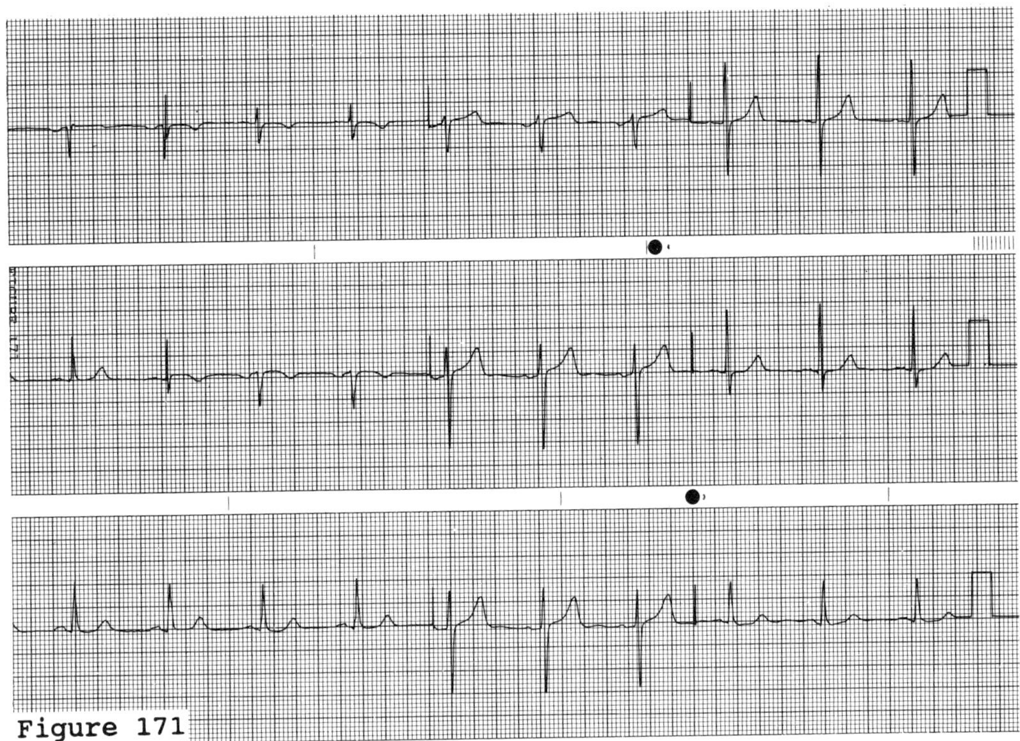

Figure 171

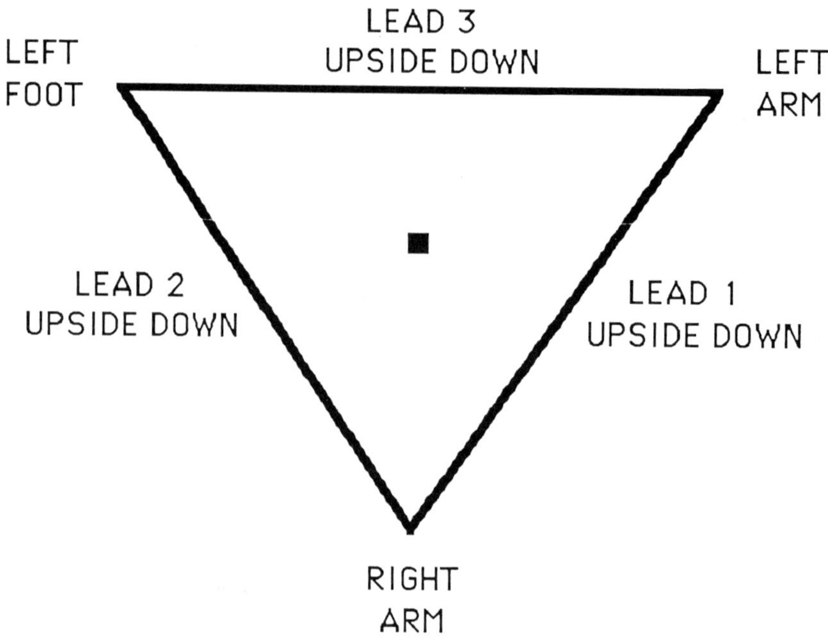

Figure <u>172a</u>

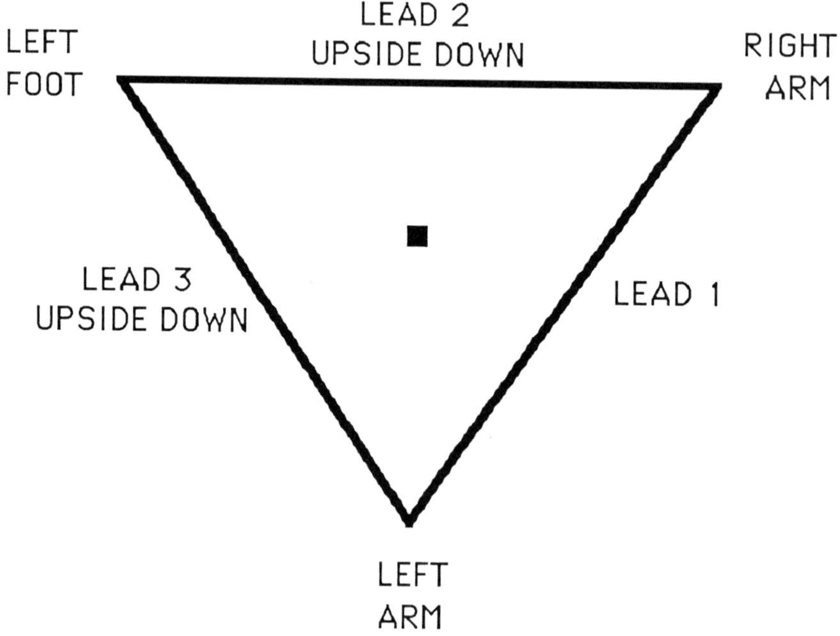

Figure <u>172b</u>

This record shows regular sinus rhythm and evidence of probable reversal of the foot and the right arm leads. It is probably within normal limits. See text for discussion.

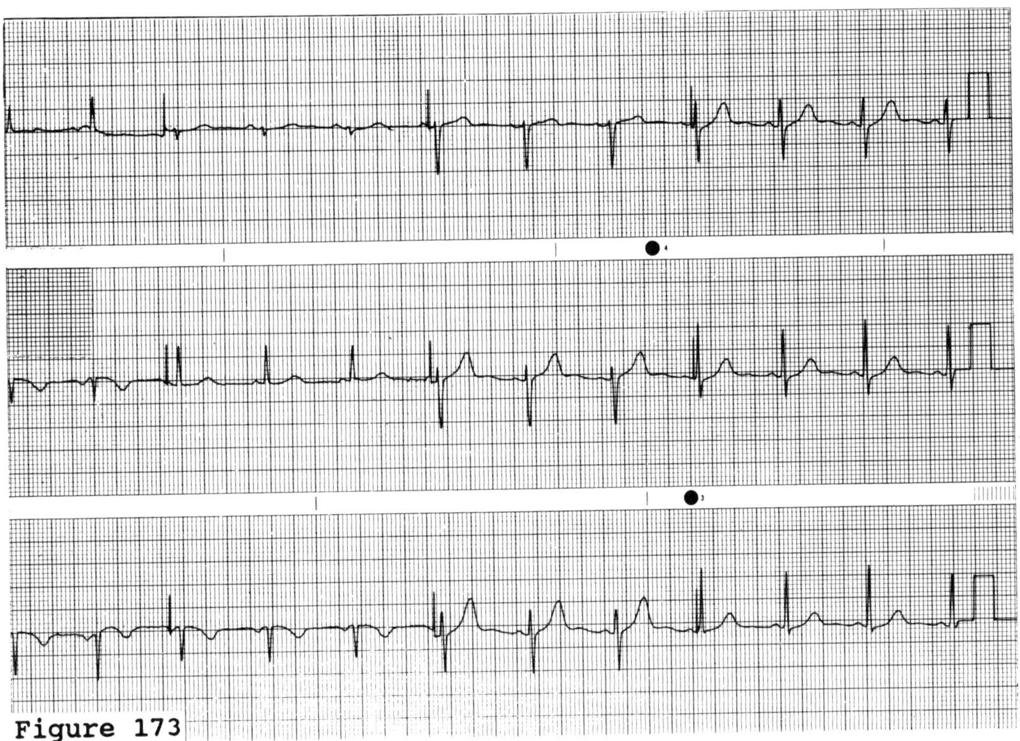

Figure 173

In Figure 172a, Lead 1 becomes Lead 3 upside down, Lead 2 becomes Lead 2 upside down, and Lead 3 becomes Lead 1 upside down. In addition, aVR becomes aVF, aVL remains aVL, and aVF becomes aVR. If this is the case, then for Figure 173 the frontal QRS axis is about 0 degrees, the frontal T axis is plus 30 degrees, and the frontal P axis is about plus 45 degrees. All this is consistent with the precordial leads, and leads to the interpretation of a normal EKG.

On the other hand, if the leads were placed as in Figure 172b, then Lead 1 becomes Lead 2 upside down, Lead 2 becomes Lead 3 upside down, and Lead 3 becomes Lead 1. In addition, aVR becomes aVL, aVL becomes aVF, and aVF becomes aVR. First, let us plot the frontal QRS axis of Figure 173 from Leads 1, 2, and 3. Since the QRS is up in Lead 1, it must really be down in Lead 2 (mostly superior and between minus 30 and plus 150 degrees). Since it is down in Lead 2, it must really be up in Lead 3 (mostly inferior and between plus 30 and minus 150 degrees). Then, since it is down in Lead 3, it must really be down in Lead 1 (rightward). This data suggests that the frontal QRS axis must be very rightward, between plus 150 and minus 150 degrees.

Proceeding to the unipolar leads, aVR (really aVF) suggests the frontal QRS is slightly superior, aVL (really avR) suggests it is rightward, between minus 60 and plus 120 degrees, and aVF (really aVL) suggests it is rightward between plus 60 and minus 120 degrees. All this put together suggests that the frontal QRS axis should be very rightward and slightly superior, between minus 150 and 180 degrees. Such as axis is highly inconsistent with the precordial leads, which then should have deep S waves and downward complexes, especially in V5 and V6.

This record shows regular sinus rhythm. The PR interval is at upper normal limits. Reversed
foot and right arm leads may well be present. The record may well be within normal limits. See
text for discussion.

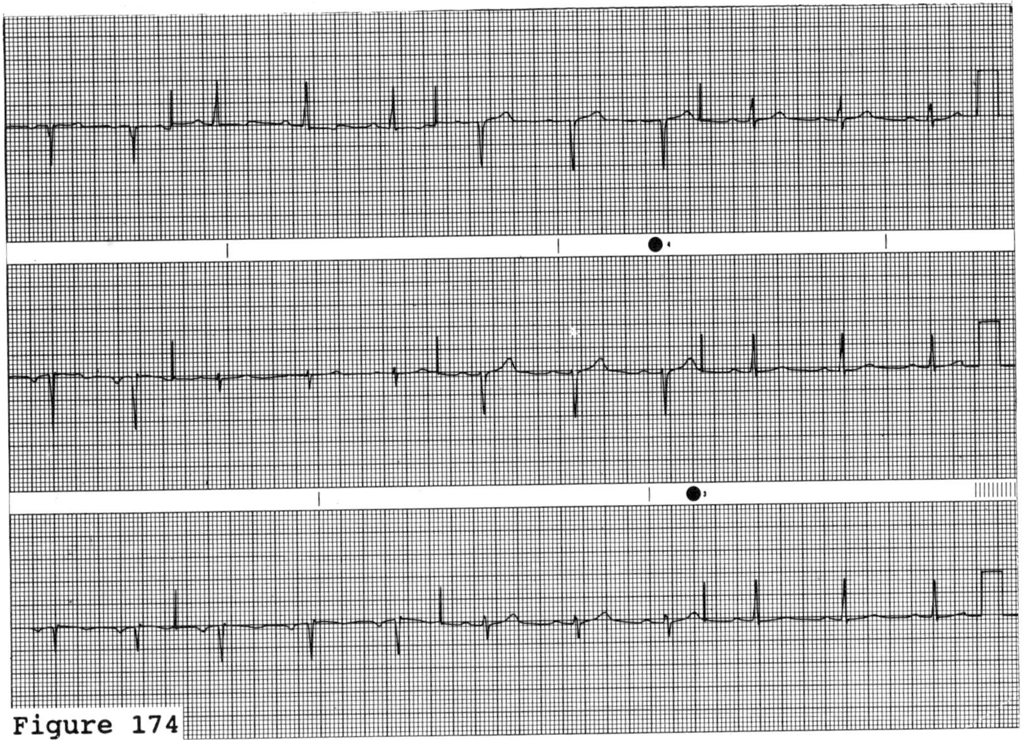

Figure 174

Because of this, it appears much more likely that only the right arm and the foot leads were reversed for the EKG in Figure 173.

If we use the same approach for the EKG in Figure 174, once again only the foot and the right arm leads appear to have been switched. This switch yields a consistent interpretation that the frontal axis is between plus 60 and plus 90 degrees, and is consistent with the precordial leads. If all three leads were misplaced as in Figure 172b, then leads 1, 2, and 3 suggest a frontal axis between plus 90 and plus 150 degrees, while the unipolar leads suggest an inferior axis between plus 90 and plus 120 degrees. Putting this together gives a frontal QRS axis between plus 90 and plus 120 degrees.

This analysis does not solve the problem. Either interpretation is possible. Let us now plot the frontal T axis the same way. If only the foot and right arm leads were switched, then the frontal T axis is about minus 30 degrees. If all three leads were misplaced, then the frontal T axis is about minus 150 to 180 degrees, and this is inconsistent with the precordial leads, which all have upright T waves.

Because of this, it is likely that in Figure 174 the foot and the right arm leads were also switched, as this interpretation seems most consistent throughout.

<u>Reversed Foot and Left Arm Leads</u>. Figures 175 - 176.

Let us use the same approach with Figure 176. Here aVR appears to be correctly placed. Either the foot and left arm leads are switched, or all the leads are correctly placed. These arrangements are shown in Figure 175a and 175b.

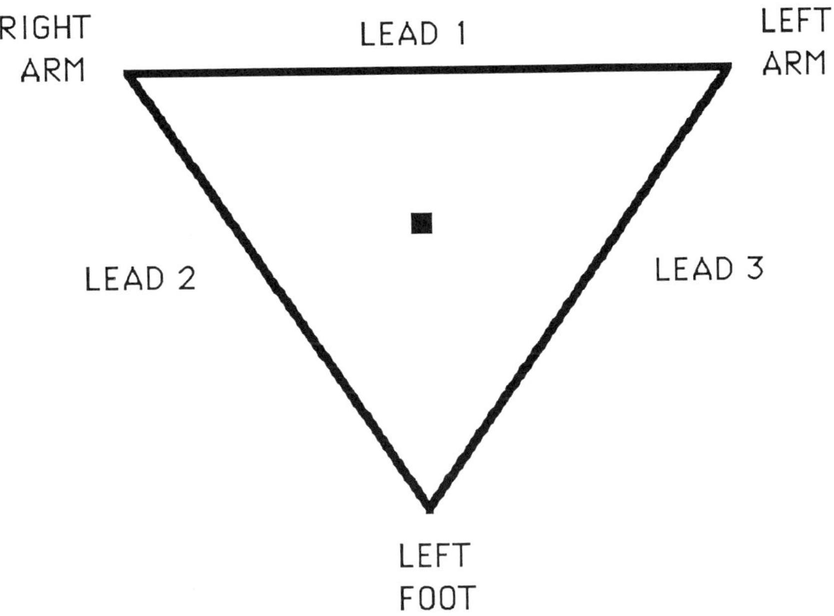

Figure _175a_

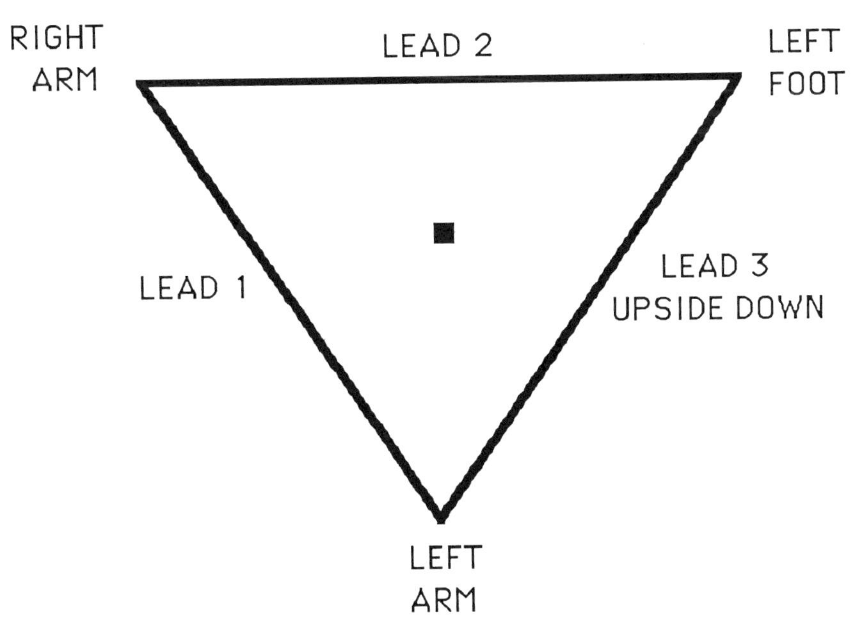

Figure _175b_

This record shows regular sinus rhythm. The foot and left arm leads appear reversed. Right ventricular enlargement, left atrial enlargement, and T changes consistent with right ventricular strain and/or posterior ischemia, and with left ventricular strain and/or lateral ischemia may be present. Suggest repeat or serial records and clinical correlation. See text for discussion.

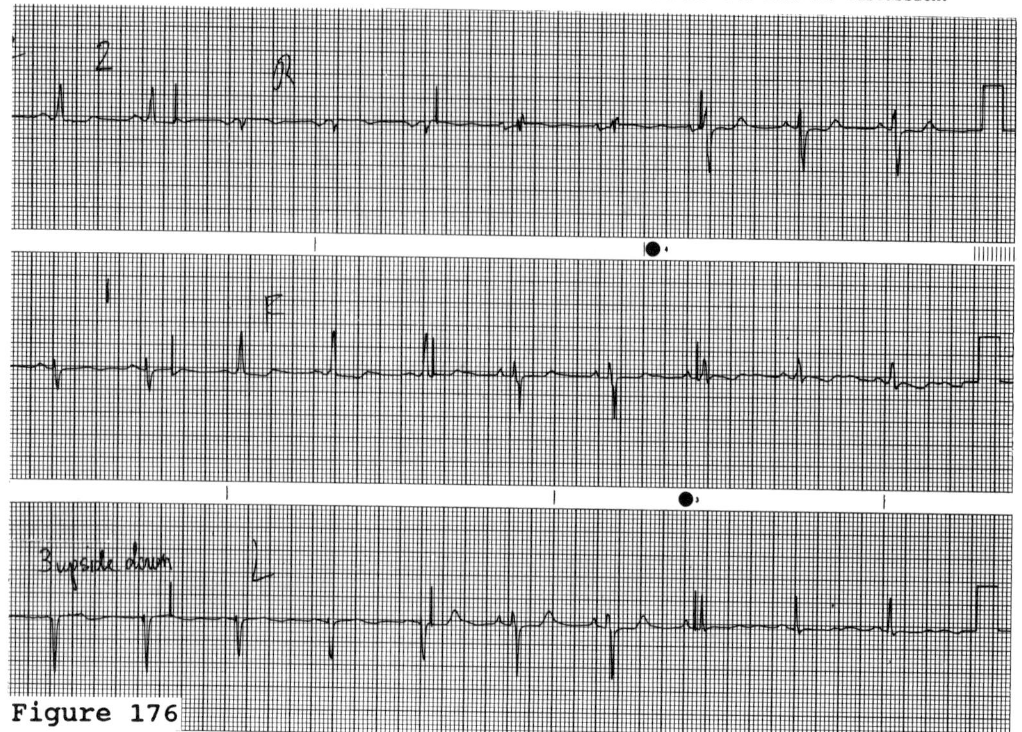

Figure 176

If the arrangement in Figure 175a is correct, then Leads 1, 2, and 3 are correctly placed and give a frontal QRS axis between minus 30 and minus 90 degrees, while the unipolar leads give an axis between 0 and minus 60 degrees. Therefore the frontal axis should be between minus 30 and minus 60 degrees, superior and leftward. However, this is inconsistent with the precordial leads, as there are only minimal S waves in V5 and V6.

If the arrangement in Figure 175b is correct, then leads 1, 2, and 3 give a frontal QRS axis between plus 90 and plus 150 degrees, while the unipolar leads give an axis between plus 60 and plus 120 degrees. Therefore the frontal axis should be between plus 90 and plus 120 degrees, rightward and inferior, and also much more consistent with the precordial leads. Therefore it is quite likely that the EKG in Figure 176 has had the foot and the left arm leads switched.

<u>Misplaced</u> <u>Precordial</u> <u>Leads</u>. Figures 177 - 179.

Here you must check not only the usual precordial R progression, but also the precordial P and T progression. Does everything proceed in the expected fashion as you go around the chest from V1 to V6, or not?

Figure 177 shows an example in which V1 and V2 were reversed. Notice the "abnormal" R progression and also the "abnormal" T progression. The fact that <u>everything</u> is out of the correct progression (especially the T wave) helps us recognize this problem.

Figures 178 and 179 show further examples in which V1, V2, and V3 were simply put on in reverse order as V3, V2, V1. Notice how all the progression makes sense when you put it together in your mind this other way.

This EKG shows a normal sinus rhythm. Leads V1 and V2 are probably reversed.
The record is therefore probably within normal limits. The frontal plane QRS vector
is + 80 degrees. The frontal plane T vector + 50 degrees. The horizontal plane QRS
vector has a transition at V3 and is therefore about minus 35 degrees. The horizontal plane T vector has a probable transition between V1 and V2 (assuming the lead
reversal) and is therefore about + 5 degrees. Once again, V1 and V2 are probably
reversed. The record is otherwise within normal limits.

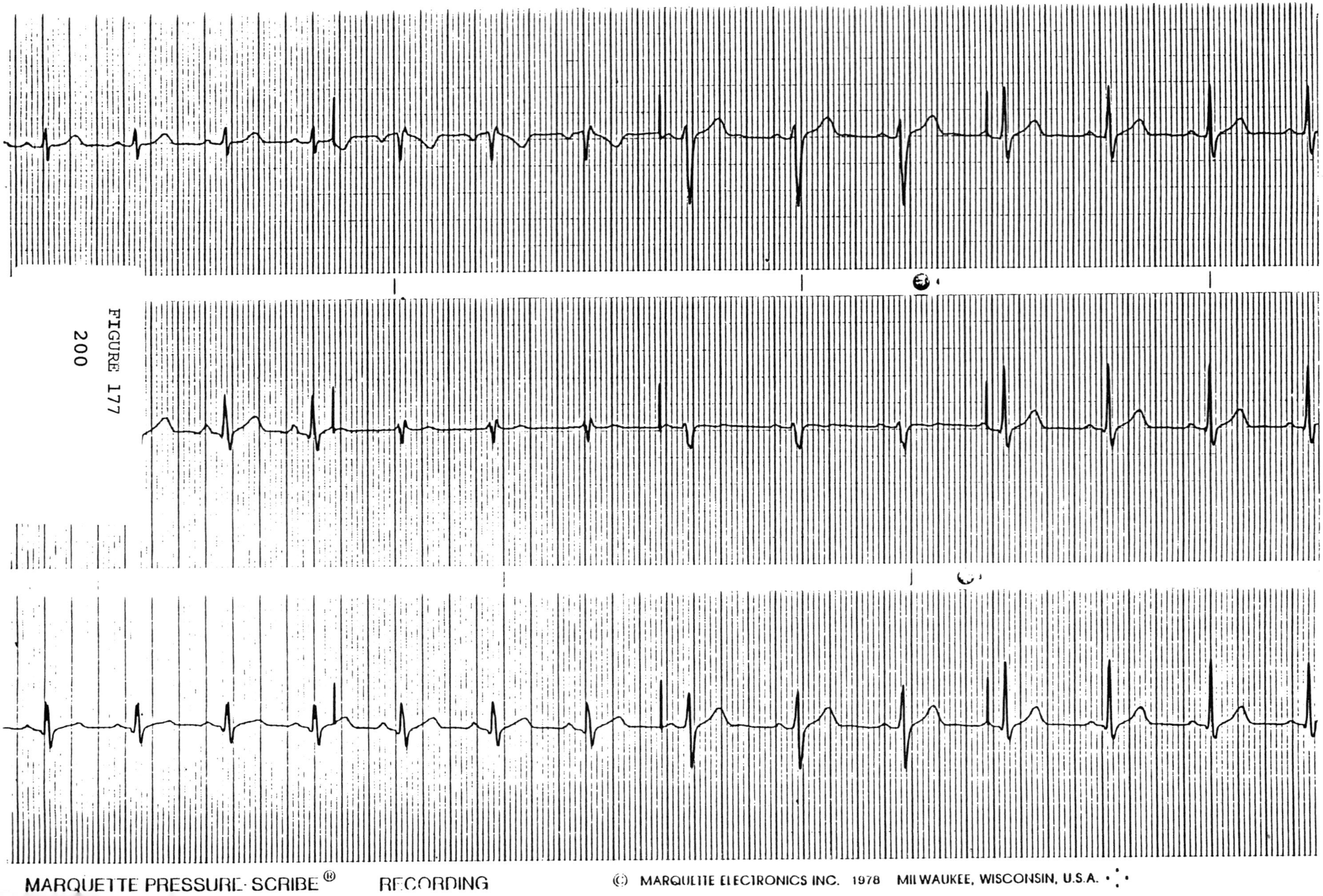

FIGURE 177

200

This record shows normal sinus rhythm and reversal of leads V1 through V3. The frontal plane
QRS axis is +70, the T axis +20, the P axis +30 degrees. Considering that lead V1 is really V3, V2
is V2, and V3 is V1, the horizontal plane QRS axis is -35, the T axis is +5, and the P axis is +20
degrees. Although the T is biphasic in V2, the fact that the T axis is at least 5 - 10 degrees
anterior to the QRS axis probably means that this record is within normal limits. Suggest repeat
record with proper lead placement.

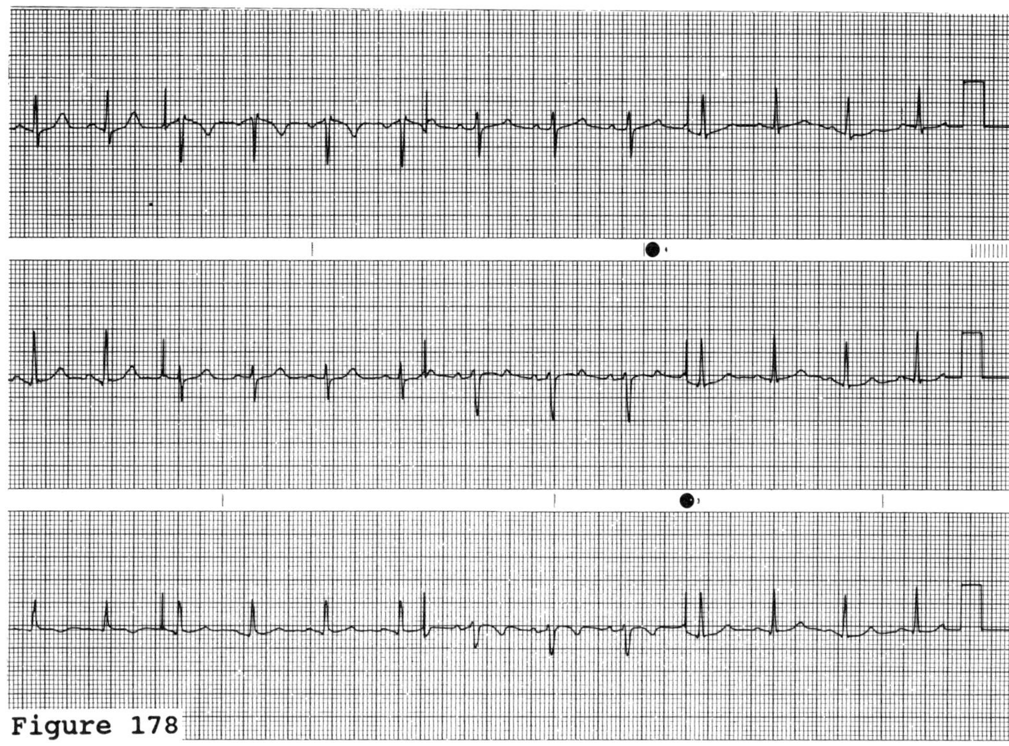

Figure 178

This record shows sinus rhythm and reversal of precordial leads V1, V2, and V3. Lead V1 is
actually V3, V2 is V2, and V3 is actually V1. The frontal plane QRS axis is +15, the T axis +20,
the P axis is 0 degrees. Considering the reversal of V1-V3, the horizontal plane QRS axis is -40,
the T axis +5, and the P axis is +10 degrees. Mild nonspecific ST-T changes are noted. Suggest
repeat record with proper lead placement.

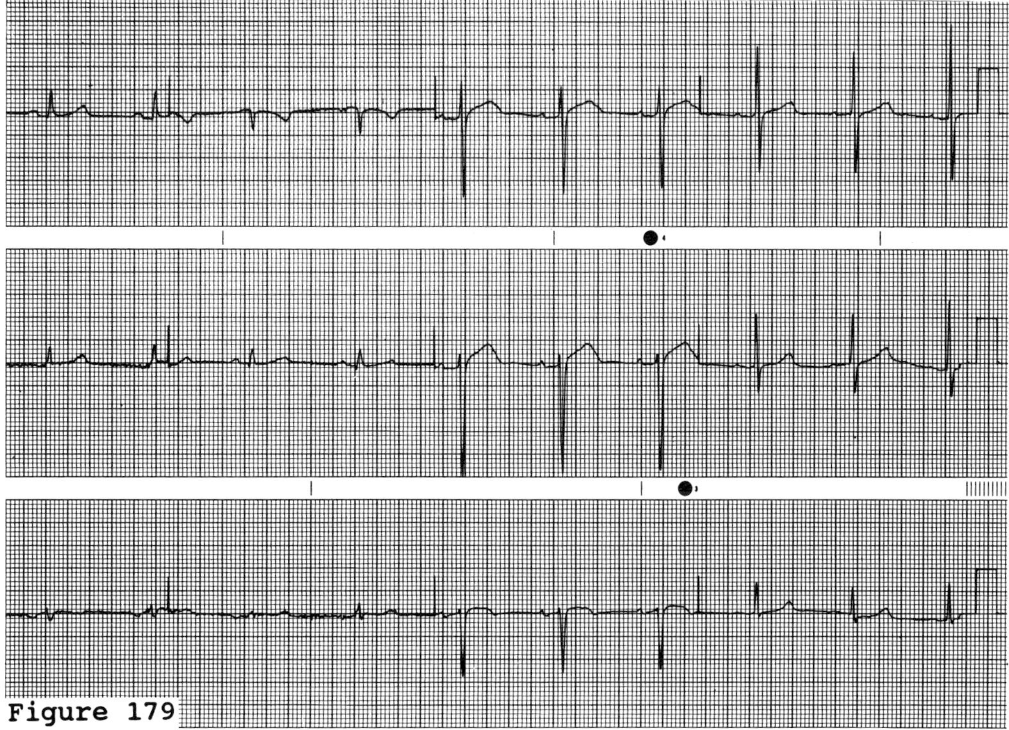

Figure 179

<u>All</u> such lead placement errors need to be <u>proven</u> as such by taking repeat records with careful attention to proper lead placement. Only then can the problem be truly resolved.

<u>Primary, Secondary and Nonspecific T Wave Changes</u>. Figures 179 - 183.

Primary T wave changes are those associated with local ischemia and/or strain. They are the T changes we discussed earlier, in Chapters 2 and 4, which have definite changes in the direction of the T axis or vector.

<u>Secondary T wave Changes</u>. Figures 179 - 180.

Secondary T wave changes take place when there is no local pathology, but when the pathway of ventricular depolarization is altered, thus changing the sequence in which the various ventricular and Purkinje cells regain their resting potentials once again. Secondary T changes are therefore seen with various intraventricular conduction defects (RBBB, LBBB, etc.), and with PVC's and other aberrantly conducted beats. Many earlier figures have examples of such secondary T changes. Examples are also shown in Figures 179 and 180.

<u>Nonspecific T Wave Changes</u>. Figures 181 - 183.

Nonspecific T changes are those which reflect <u>no specific local patho-</u><u>logy</u>, such as ischemia, strain, or pericarditis. Instead, they are due to general metabolic and electrolyte changes that affect all cells together. Because of this, the shape of the T wave is altered, often flattened or rounded in various ways, but the frontal and horizontal T axes or vectors are not shifted from their normal relationships to the QRS axis. Figures 181 - 183 show examples of this. One of the most useful things about plotting both the QRS and T axes in both the frontal and horizontal planes is that doing so lets one recognize many <u>primary</u> T changes as due to local pathology (ischemia, strain, etc.), even when they are of low amplitude, because the T

This record shows an undetermined supraventricular rhythm which may be sinus tachycardia with marked first degree AV block. Probable P waves can be seen on the back of the T waves in lead 1. An episode of probable second degree AV block appears in leads V1 through V3. Right bundle branch block is present. Suggest repeat record.

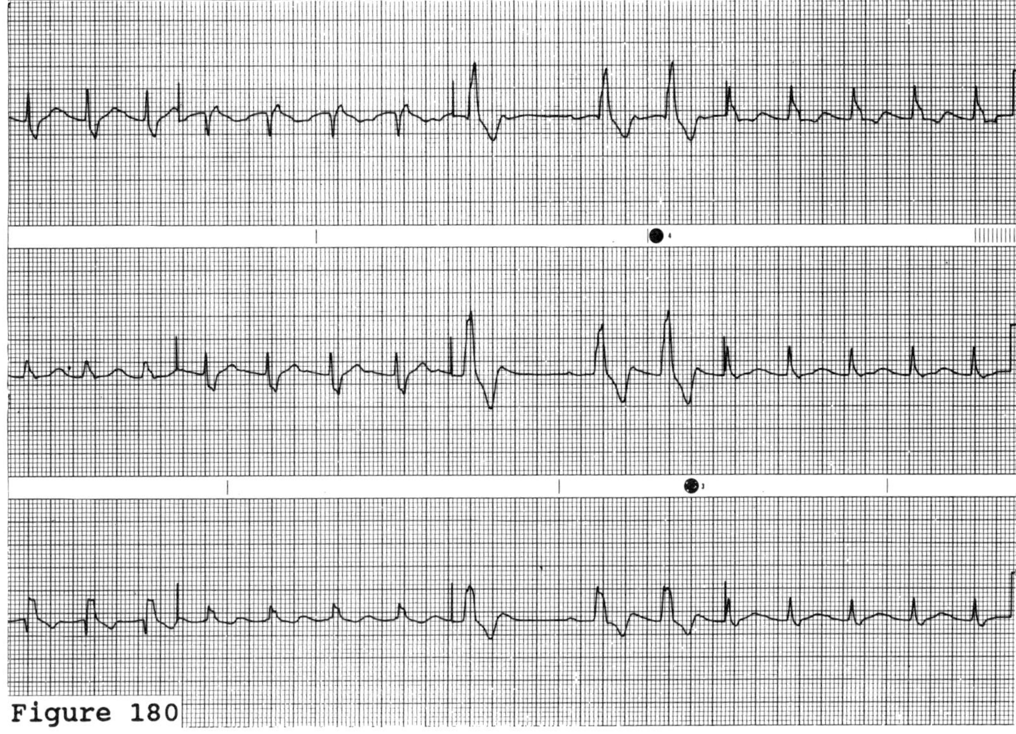

Figure 180

This record shows an undetermined rhythm, possibly atrial fibrillation, with frequent multi-focal PVC's. The QRS duration is .12 seconds. This may represent left bundle branch block, but may also represent severe left ventricular enlargement. ST-T changes are present, consistent with either secondary T changes associated with left bundle branch block, or with left ventricular strain and/or lateral ischemia. A Q is present in lead 1 and an abnormal R progression may be present between leads V4 and V5 (note the early part of the QRS complex in V5), suggesting possible lateral infarction. Suggest serial records and clinical correlation.

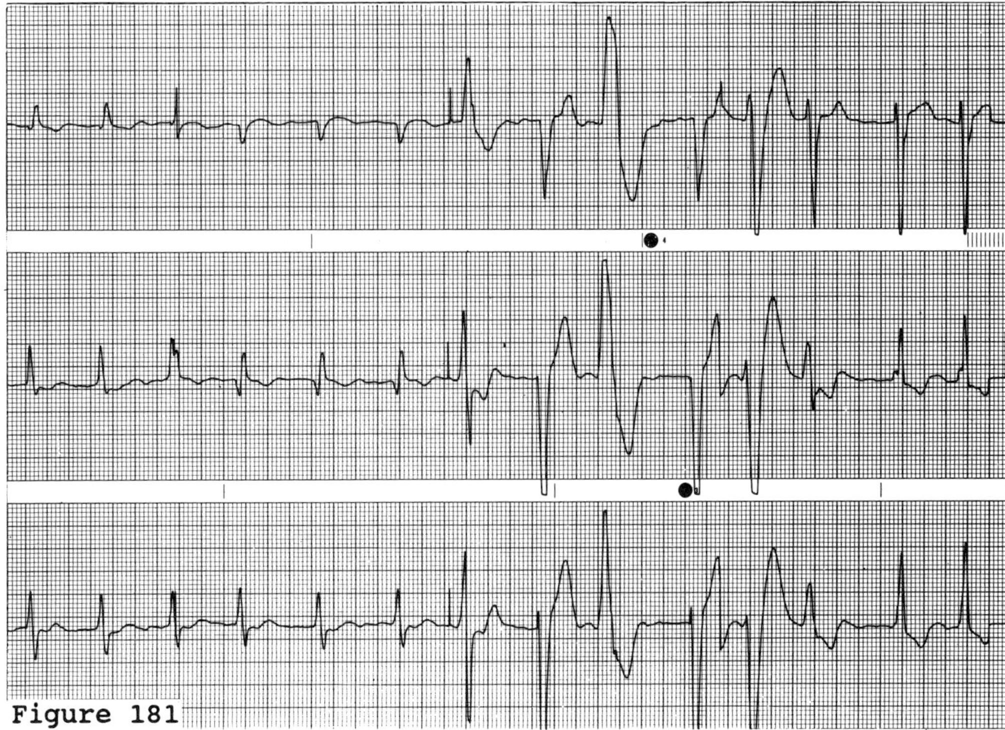

Figure 181

This record shows a probable ectopic atrial rhythm. The frontal P axis is about −90 degrees. Nonspecific T wave changes are also present.

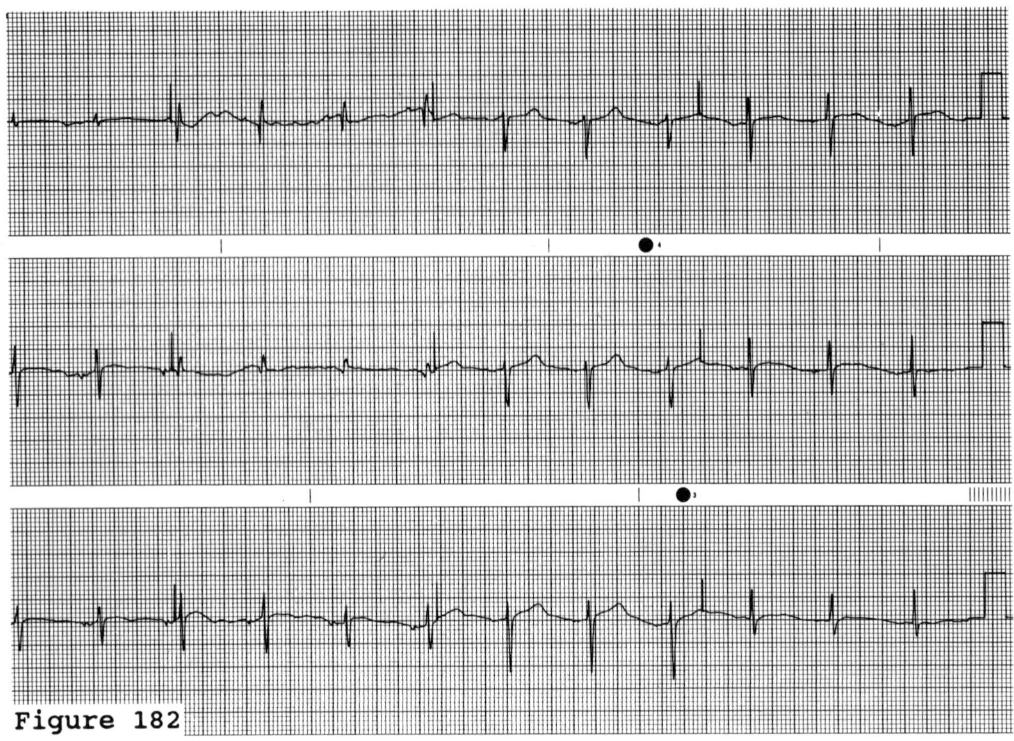

Figure 182

This record shows sinus tachycardia and generalized low voltage throughout, and nonspecific T changes. The record is consistent with pulmonary disease and/or pericardial effusion. Suggest repeat or serial records and clinical correlation.

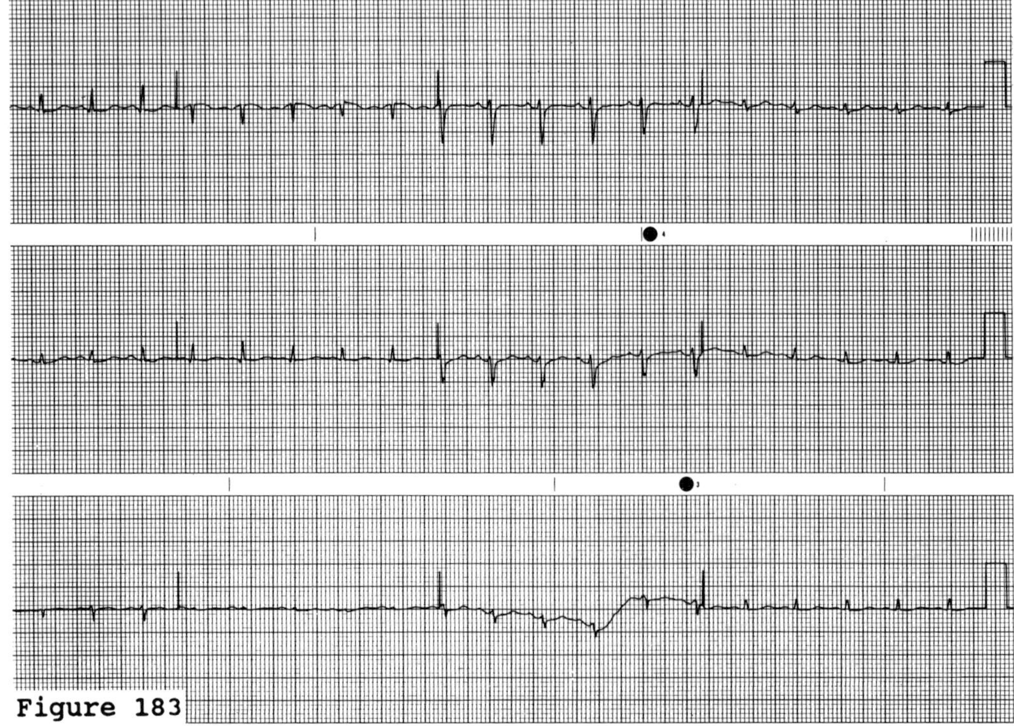

Figure 183

This record shows sinus rhythm, a slightly wide QRS complex, and nonspecific ST-T changes. Suggest repeat record.

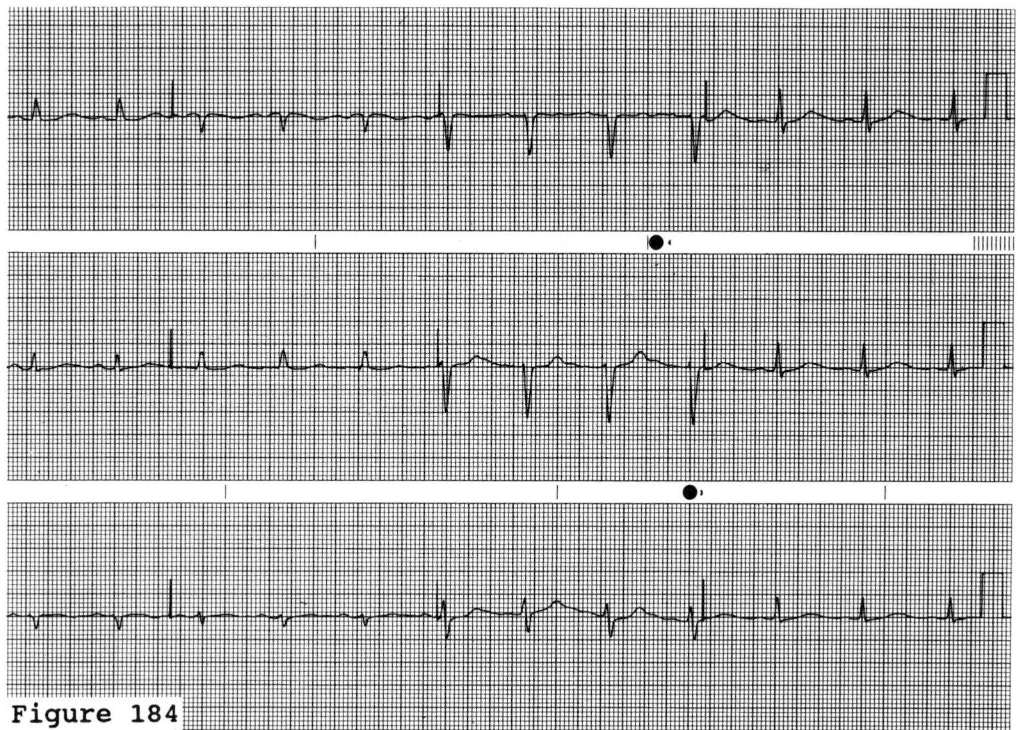

Figure 184

axis is not in its usual relationship to the QRS axis. In contrast, non-specific T changes usually resemble those in Fihures 181 - 183, and their relationship to the QRS vector is within normal limits as discussed earlier in Chapters 2 and 4.

T Wave Changes due to Digitalis. Figure 185, and 135-136.

Digitalis causes a loss of intracellular potassium and an increase in intracellular sodium and calcium. The Q - T interval usually shortens (as with hypercalcemia) and the ST segment scoops downward with an upward concavity. The ST-T changes in Figure 184 are typical except that the Q-T interval is not visibly short. Similar changes are shown in Figures 135-136.

The degree of digitalis effect cannot usually be used as a guide to the degree to which a patient is digitalized, as there is a great deal of variation from one patient to another. However, if one knows a particular patient extremely well, as in a clinical study on a metabolic ward, then one can see that in an individual patient, well studied, the digitalis effect is greater on higher doses and with higher serum levels, other things being equal. Usually, though, we are not this fortunate, and the variability between patients makes it impossible to use the EKG changes as any kind of guide to the degree to which a patient is digitalized. Much better guides are found by noting the various doses and serum levels found, and fitting a 2-compartment pharmacokinetic model to that data, carefully comparing the patient's clinical response with the response of the fitted model (8). Seeing a plot of such a fitted model is quite revealing, while the data of the serum levels alone are often not of much help.

This record shows atrial fibrillation and ST-T changes consistent with digitalis effect. While the QT interval is not noticeably short, the changes are otherwise typical of mild to moderate digitalis effect.

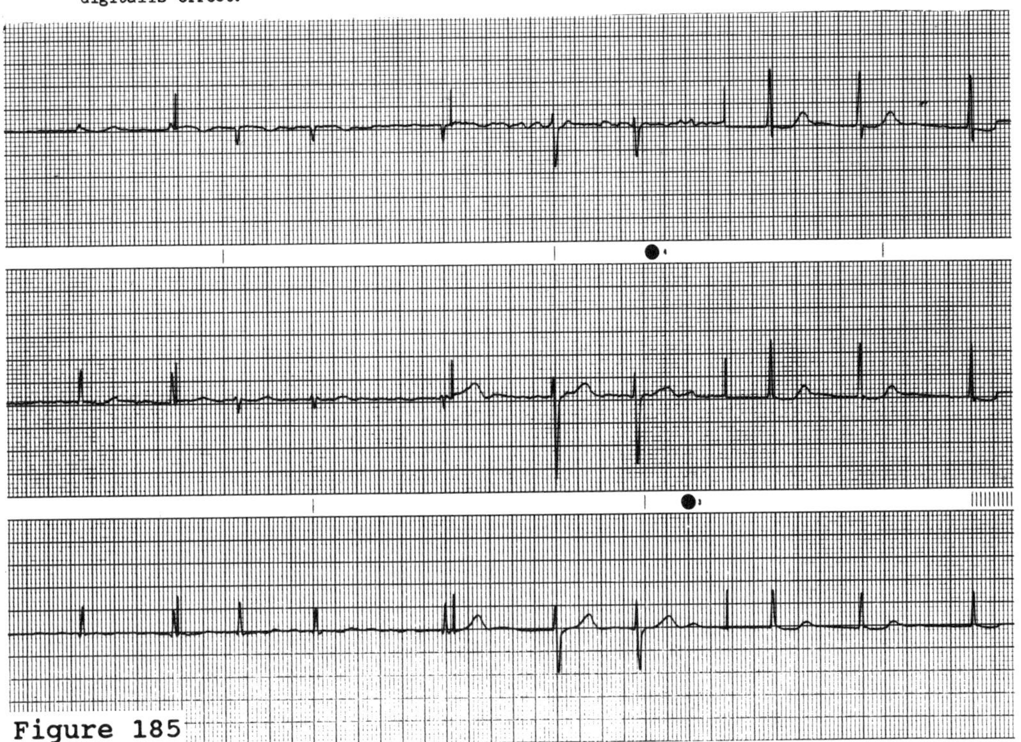

Figure 185

<u>ELECTROLYTE CHANGES</u>. Figures 186 – 191.

<u>A.</u> <u>Hypopotassemia (Hypokalemia)</u> Figure 186.

Repolarization changes in the electrocardiogram reflect the serum potassium in a rather crude quantitative fashion, as myocardial potassium is usually in close equilibrium with serum potassium. As the serum potassium falls below 3.5 mEq/L, U waves may appear following the T waves, and are best seen over the precordial leads. The T wave diminishes in amplitude and sagging of the ST segment occurs. Because of the prominent, broad U waves, the QT interval is said to be lengthened. It is more accurately identified as a prolonged QU interval. In addition, conduction velocity is increased and the QRS may be narrower than usual.

<u>B.</u> <u>Hyperpotassemia (Hyperkalemia)</u> Figures 187 – 190.

When the serum potassium reaches a level of about 6.0 to 7.0 mEq/L, as shown in Figure 187, peaked T waves with narrow bases characteristically appear over the precordium. The QRS may become widened in a progressive fashion at serum potassium levels of about 8 mEq/L. At about that level atrial "arrest" may occur. In any case, sinus rhythm may continue but the atrial waves may not generate any visible P waves, and P waves may no longer be seen. A slow ventricular rhythm with a markedly widened and distorted QRS may be noted at levels 8 to 10 mEq/L.

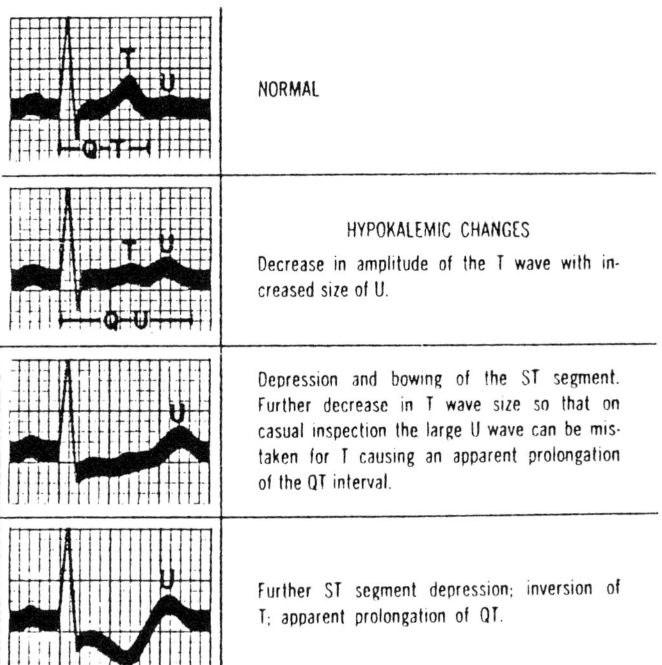

ELECTROCARDIOGRAPHIC CHANGES IN HYPOKALEMIA

FIGURE 186

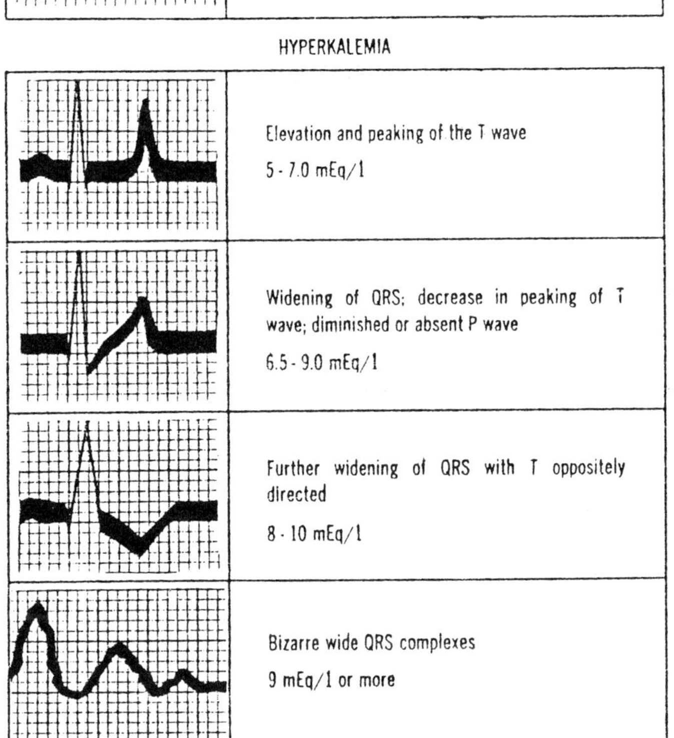

FIGURE 187

NOTE: The levels of serum K associated with the above changes are only approximations; considerable variations may be encountered in individual cases.

This record shows sinus rhythm, possible left atrial enlargement, first degree AV block, and peaked T waves consistent with hyperkalemia. Serum potassium 2 minutes earlier was 6.9 meq/L. The frontal plane QRS axis is +75, the T axis is +45, and the P axis is +60 degrees. The horizontal plane QRS axis is -35, the T axis is +5, and the P axis is +10 degrees. Suggest repeat record and clinical correlation.

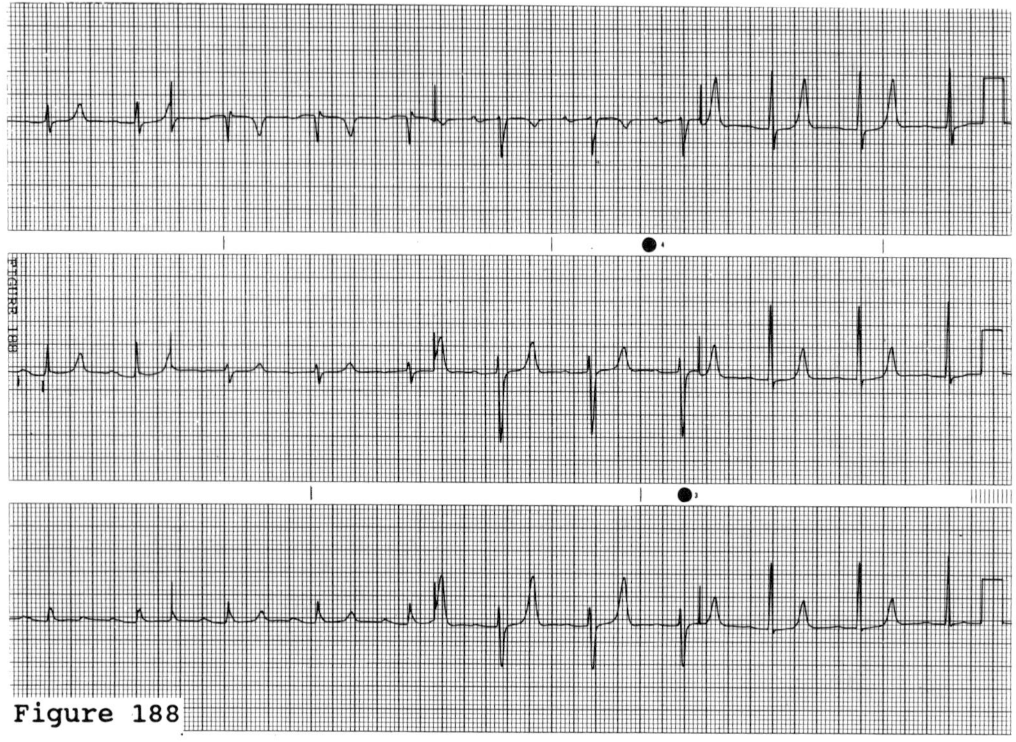

Figure 188

This record shows an undetermined rhythm. No definite P waves can be seen. The QRS duration is .16 seconds. The T waves are peaked, especially in V4 through V6. While this record might suggest an accelerated idioventricular rhythm, it is also known to occur with sinus rhythm (without any visible P waves) in moderately severe hyperkalemia. The serum potassium taken 8 minutes after this record was 7.7 meq/L.

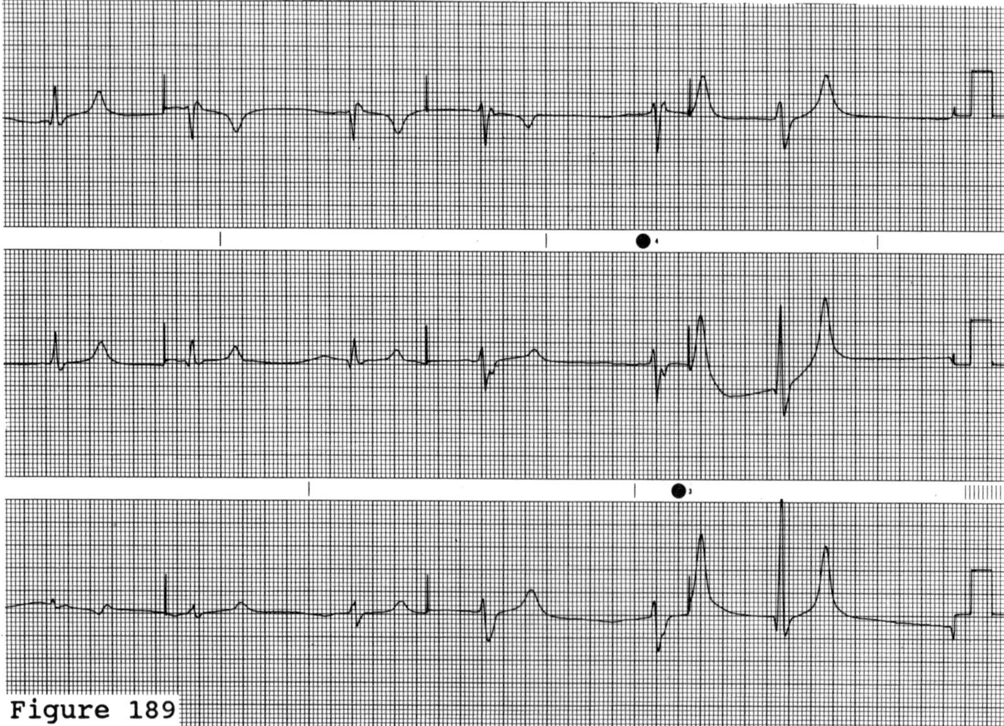

Figure 189

    This record shows an undetermined rhythm, possibly a ventricular tachycardia, but the QRS
complex is so wide (.24 seconds), no P waves are seen, and the T waves are remarkably peaked in many
leads. It is also consistent with severe hyperkalemia. The serum potassium was 7.9 meq/L 37
minutes after this record was obtained.

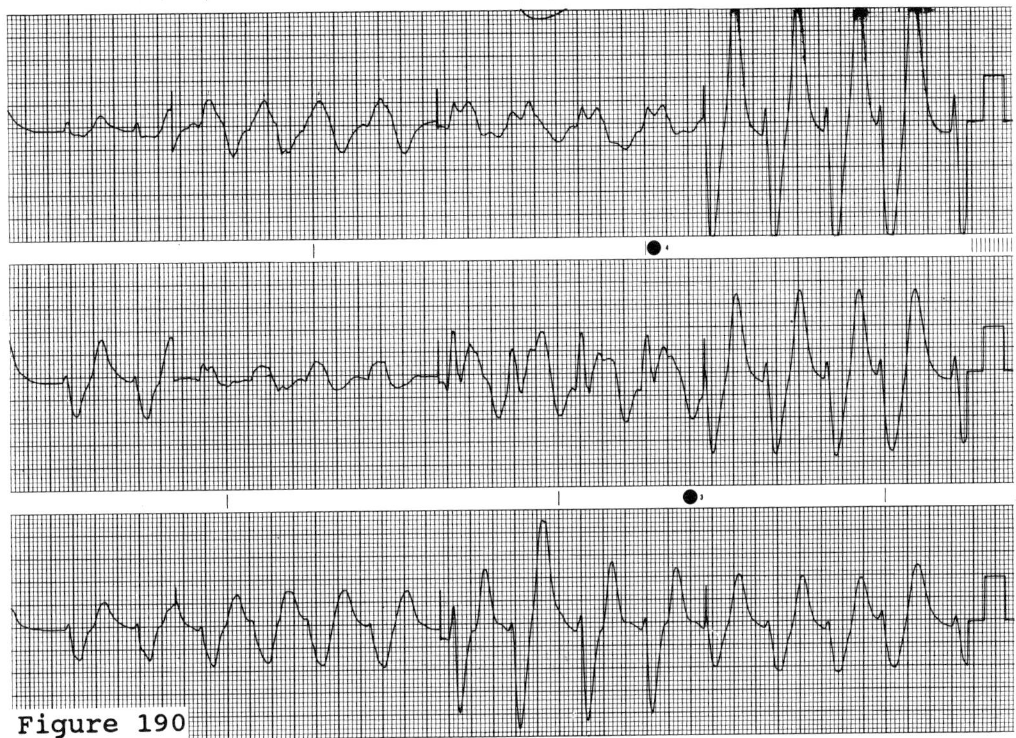

Figure 190

<u>C. Hypocalcemia</u>. Figure 191.

QT prolongation consisting almost entirely of a long, isoelectric ST segment and a normal upright T wave characterizes this disorder. U waves are usually not seen. T wave inversion suggests some other associated disorder, such as uremia with pericarditis and its associated low serum calcium).

<u>D. Hypercalcemia</u>. Figure 191.

The features of this electrolyte disturbance are the reciprocal of hypocalcemia - a shortened QT interval with initial absence of the ST segment, with a normal upright T wave.

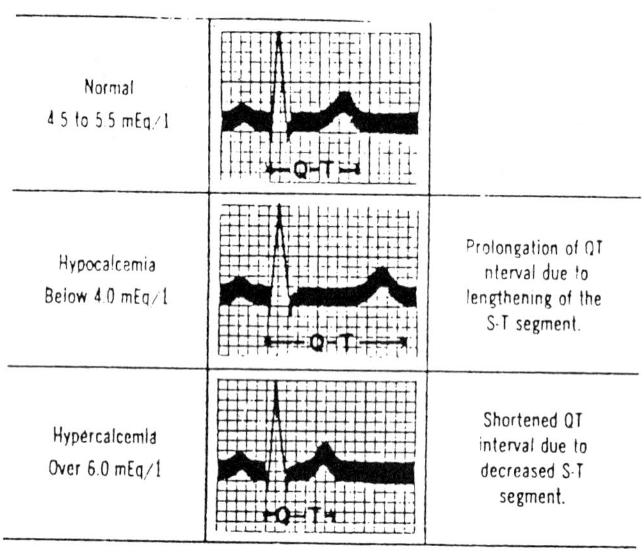

ELECTROCARDIOGRAPHIC CHANGES IN VARIOUS CONCENTRATIONS
OF SERUM CALCIUM

<u>FIGURE 191</u>

Changes in the EKG produced by electrolyte shifts must be carefully interpreted on an individual basis from patient to patient. A low serum magnesium can also give marked nonspecific ST-T changes, and must be considered.

We have had a brief introduction to the pleasures of looking at patients' EKG's and trying to decipher their meaning. There is a wealth of books to go further with. One which I have liked especially well, however, and which is a blend of good science as well as good history (how interesting it is to see how things really <u>were</u> created!) is the excellent HISTORY OF ELECTROCARDIOGRAPHY by Drs. George Burch and Nicholas DePasquale (9). Read it and enjoy!

REFERENCES

1. Sperelakis N: personal communication, 1956.

2. Noble D: The Initiation of the Heartbeat, 2nd ed., Clarendon Press, Oxford, 1979, pp 146-147.

3. Allenstein BJ and Mori H: Evaluation of Electrocardiographic Diagnosis of Ventricular Hypertrophy Based on Autopsy Comparison. Circulation, 21: 401, 1960.

4. Romhilt DW and Estes EH: A Point-Score System for the ECG Diagnosis of Left Ventricular Hypertrophy. Am. Heart. J.,75:752-758, 1968.

5. Boineau JP and Cox JL: Slow Ventricular Activation in Acute Myocardial Infarction. A Source of Re-entrant Premature Ventricular Contractions. Circulation, Volume XLVIII, pp 702-713, October 1973.

6. Rodman JH, Jelliffe RW, Kolb E, Tuey DB, de Guzman MF, Wagers PW, and Haywood LJ: Clinical Studies with Computer-Assisted Initial Lidocaine Therapy. Arch Int Med., 144:703-709, 1984.

7. D'Argenio DZ: Optimal Sampling Times for Pharmacokinetic Experiments. J of Pharmacokinetics and Biopharmaceutics, 9(6):739-756, 1981.

8. Jelliffe, RW: Clinical Applications of Pharmacokinetics and Control Theory: Planning, Monitoring, and Adjusting Dosage Regimens of Aminoglycosides, Lidocaine, Digitoxin, and Digoxin, in Topics in Clinical Pharmacology and Therapeutics, ed. by Maronde, RF. Springer-Verlag, New York, 1986, pp. 26-82.

9. Burch, GE and DePasquale, NP: A History of Electrocardiography. Year Book Medical Publishers, Inc., Chicago, 1964.